fourth edition

Ethical Dilemmas and Nursing Practice

fourth edition

Ethical Dilemmas and Nursing Practice

Anne J. Davis, RN, PhD, FAAN
Professor Emerita
School of Nursing
University of California,
   San Francisco
San Francisco, California

Professor
Nagano College of Nursing
Komagano, Nagano, Japan

Joan Liaschenko, RN, PhD
Assistant Professor
University of Wisconsin, Milwaukee
Milwaukee, Wisconsin

Mila A. Aroskar, RN, EdD, FAAN
Associate Professor
School of Public Health
University of Minnesota
Minneapolis, Minnesota

Theresa S. Drought, RN, PhD
   (candidate)
School of Nursing
University of California,
   San Francisco
San Francisco, California

APPLETON & LANGE
Stamford, Connecticut

97 98 99 00 01 / 10 9 8 7 6 5 4 3 2 1

Prentice Hall International (UK) Limited, *London*
Prentice Hall of Australia Pty. Limited, *Sydney*
Prentice Hall Canada, Inc., *Toronto*
Prentice Hall Hispanoamericana, S.A., *Mexico*
Prentice Hall of India Private Limited, *New Delhi*
Prentice Hall of Japan, Inc., *Tokyo*
Simon & Schuster Asia Pte. Ltd., *Singapore*
Editora Prentice Hall do Brasil Ltda., *Rio de Janeiro*
Prentice Hall, *Upper Saddle River, New Jersey*

Library of Congress Cataloging-in-Publication Data

Ethical dilemmas and nursing practice / Anne J. Davis . . . [et al.]. —
  4th ed.
    p.   cm.
  Includes bibliographical references and index.
  ISBN 0-8385-2283-1 (pbk : alk. paper)
  1. Nursing ethics. 2. Medical ethics. I. Davis, Anne J., 1931–
  II. Davis, Anne J., 1931– Ethical dilemmas and nursing
practice.
  [DNLM: 1. Ethics, Nursing. WY 85 E836 1997]
  RT85.D33 1997
  174'.2—dc20
  DNLM/DLC
  for Library of Congress
                    96-41638

ISBN 0-8385-2283-1

90000

9 780838 522837

Acquisitions Editor: David P. Carroll
Production Editor: Lisa M. Guidone
Designer: Libby Schmitz

PRINTED IN THE UNITED STATES OF AMERICA

Contributor

Marsha Fowler, RN, MS, PhD, MDIV, FAAN
Professor
School of Nursing
Graduate School of Theology
Azusa Pacific University
Azusa, California

Chapter 2: Nursing's Ethics

Contents

Preface

We wrote the first edition of this book in 1978 while we were Kennedy postdoctoral fellows at Harvard University. Since that first edition, a number of important developments have occurred. Ethics has become more central in teaching nursing students and in clinical nursing practice. Nonetheless, there is still room for improvement. Certainly more nursing ethics books are available, which makes the selection of materials more diverse and much richer. More research focused on nursing's ethical issues has been conducted.

In addition to these developments, ethical issues in health care have received more attention in the mass media. At times this attention has come from reports or legal decisions, as in the case of abortion and the right-to-die question. Clinical settings, with new acute care technology or long-term care issues, influenced by the increase in the elderly population and cost containment efforts, constitute a major arena for ethical dilemmas.

Since the first edition, the AIDS epidemic has raised crucial ethical questions, some of which society and health professionals continue to debate. Populations such as the homeless and others without health care insurance reinforce the ethical issues in health policies that stem from a system undergoing change, and hold up to all of us fundamental questions about our shared humanity and the common good.

On the international scene, some areas of the world have experienced profound changes that have the potential to create a brighter future. Other areas have experienced economic and social tragedy. All of these events and changes have an impact on people's health and the health care system. Embedded in change of all types, we find questions of values, rights, and obligations. Concepts of individual rights and the common good present themselves for examination, debate, and solution. Within this international ferment, activities in nursing ethics have continued to increase.

We have been most pleased with the response to this book. It is this response that has led us to prepare the fourth edition. We want to thank all those who assisted with this edition. Two additional authors, Joan Liaschenko and Theresa Drought, are involved in this edition. Both with specialized education and clinical experience in health care ethics, they have agreed to assume responsibility for the next edition. The book is in good hands. Marsha Fowler, whose expertise on ethical codes is well known, has added to the value of this book by writing a chapter on this topic. Hanna Regev typed the manuscript. The people at Appleton & Lange kept us on our toes in the editing process. To all of these colleagues, we acknowledge our thanks. We continue to appreciate the importance of ethical dilemmas confronting nurses and applaud the courage that nurses have demonstrated. This fourth edition is dedicated to them.

Anne J. Davis, RN, PhD, FAAN
Mila A. Aroskar, RN, EdD, FAAN

1

Health Care Ethics and Ethical Dilemmas

Traditionally, philosophy as a body of knowledge has asked and attempted to answer, in a formal and disciplined manner, the great questions of life that any of us might raise with ourselves in our more reflective moments. The branch of philosophy called *ethics*, also referred to as *moral philosophy*, helps us to examine and understand the moral life. It deals with important questions of human conduct that have great relevance to us as individuals and as health professionals. Ethics, as a body of knowledge, has evolved in the Western philosophical tradition since the Golden Age of Greece and deals with the concept of morality and with moral problems and judgments.

The word ethics, derived from the Greek term *ethos*, originally meant customs, habitual usages, conduct, and character, and the word morals, derived from the Latin *mores*, means customs or habit. Today, in the widest sense these two words refer to conduct, character, and motives involved in moral acts and include the notion of approval or disapproval of a given conduct, character, or motive that we describe by such words as good, desirable, right, and worthy, or conversely by such words as bad, undesirable, wrong, evil, and unworthy. Often when we speak of the ethics or morals of an individual or group, we refer to a set of rules or body of principles. Each society, religion, and professional group has its principles or standards of conduct, and as persons concerned with being reasonable in our conduct, we rely on these standards for guidance.

In discussions, the word ethics often becomes synonymous with morality. Morality has been defined as a *social* enterprise and not just an invention or discovery of individuals for their own guidance. This social nature of morality is not limited to its being a system governing the relations of one person to others or one's code of action with respect to others. Obviously, morality is social in this sense, but also, as importantly, morality is social in its origins, sanctions, and functions, since we are born into a society that has developed and continues to maintain mores, laws, and ethical codes. As a societal system of regulations, morality shares some similarities with both the law and social convention or etiquette. Convention, as we usually define it, has to do with considerations of taste, appearance, and convenience, and does not deal with matters of crucial social importance. Convention and morality share similarities in that neither is created or changed by a deliberate judicial, legislative, or executive act; therefore physical force or the threat of it does not serve as a sanction. Verbal signs of approval or disapproval, praise or blame, become social sanctions in these instances. In its focus on crucial matters of social importance, such as individual and groups rights and obligations, morality shares similarities with the law.

There are several approaches to ethics that include normative ethics, practical ethics, descriptive ethics, virtue ethics, ethics of care, and metaethics. Each of these will be briefly defined.

Normative ethics raises the question of what is right or what ought to be done in a situation that calls for a moral decision. It examines individual rights and obligations as well as the common good.

Practical ethics is the use of ethical theory and analysis to examine moral problems. Nursing ethics and bioethics or health care ethics are examples here.

Descriptive ethics describes people's actual moral beliefs and actions. Research in descriptive ethics has been conducted by both nurses and social scientists.

Virtue ethics or character ethics places emphasis on the agents or people who make choices and take actions. A moral virtue is a character trait that is morally valued. Nursing's long interest in and concern about ethics has until recently been an ethics of virtue.

Ethics of care focuses on those traits valued in intimate personal relationships and would include such traits as compassion, love, sympathy, and trust among others. Since the early 1980s, the ethics of care has been written about and found predominantly in feminist and nursing sources.

Metaethics studies the language, concepts, and methods used in ethics. It raises questions about the meaning of the ethical terms that we use in ethical theory and in our discussions of ethical problems.

In a somewhat simplistic way, we can say that normative ethics using ethical principles helps us with the question of what ought I do when confronted with an ethical problem or dilemma. Virtue ethics asks what sort of person ought I be, and ethics of care helps us to determine what the nature of a given relationship ought to be. In nursing, we need all three of these approaches.

While all of these approaches to ethics are important and useful, this book in general discusses normative ethics or principle-based ethics more than the other approaches. While normative ethics is not without limitations, it is, however, this ethics that is widely used in clinical situations, clinical ethics committees, and in policy development. Further reading can enhance one's understanding of normative, virtue, and care ethics.[1-9]

Nurses confront many ethical dilemmas in their practice. Such dilemmas include whether to care for a so-called noncompliant patient, decisions to discontinue intensive therapy, keeping confidences, patient advocacy, or refusing to care for a patient with acquired immunodeficiency syndrome (AIDS). We may be ethical to the extent that our behavior elicits approval and respect from others; however, we still confront moral perplexity and moral doubt. For example, in a situation in which our ethical code guides us to tell the truth, we decide to withhold truthful information because we believe such knowledge will cause psychological harm to the individual hearing it. Such a situation confronts health professionals, particularly in caring for the terminally ill patient. This example shows that in honoring one moral principle we can violate another: If we tell the truth we may risk doing harm to the hearer. On the other hand, if we do not tell the truth, we violate the individual's right to knowledge that affects his or her self-determination. The degree of confidence a community can have in its health professionals remains one critical consideration in the issue of truth telling, or veracity, in the health sciences. Although a set of rules is vital to human conduct, it cannot be wholly depended upon for guidance, since it can never be complete enough to anticipate all possible occasions involving moral decisions.

Socrates, the patron saint of moral philosophy, in the Crito dialogue argued that we must let reason determine our ethical decisions rather than emotion. To accomplish this we must have factual information about the situation and keep our minds clear as we deliberate the issue. We need to be aware of our values and how they influence our definition of an ethical situation. In addition, values held in common by all nurses must be taken into account. It is not enough to appeal to what people generally think, since they may be wrong, but we must, by informed reasoning, find an answer that we regard as correct. And importantly, according to Socrates, we ought never to do what is morally wrong. The proposal of what we should do in a situation must be viewed as to its rightness or wrongness as concluded after informed reasoning and not as to what will happen to us as a consequence, or what others will think of us, or how we feel about the situation. In his arguments, Socrates appealed to a general moral rule or principle that, after reflection, he accepted as valid and applicable to particular situations. But in addition, Socrates, aware of the fact that sometimes two or more moral rules apply to the same case but do not lead to the same conclusion, resolved this conflict by determining which rules take precedence over others. Here he went beyond simply appealing to rules, since they conflict with one another, and established what he called basic rules and derivative rules, which rest on the more basic ones. A reasoning process that establishes basic ethical rules leads to the inevitable question of how ethical principles and judgments are to be justified. A full-fledged discussion develops in moral philosophy when we pass beyond the stage in which we are directed only by traditional rules of conduct, which have limited application to complex ethical situations, and move to a stage where we think critically about an ethical dilemma in ways that allow us to use traditional rules as general principles coupled with ethical reasoning going beyond these traditional rules.

As has been indicated, not all ethical dilemmas can be resolved by an appeal to our common moral rules, and this fact lies at the center of moral philosophy as a field of inquiry. Let it be stressed, however, that the traditional interest in ethics as a subject matter must not be confused with the practical interest of moral beings. To avoid the mistake of supposing that a knowledge of moral theory is sufficient for the improvement of our moral practice, we must realize that the theoretical interest is concerned with knowing and the practical interest with doing. A moralist engages in reflection and discussion about what is morally right or wrong, good or evil. A moral philosopher thinks and writes about the ways in which moral terms like *right* or *good* are used by moralists when they deliver their moral judgments. If our object is to discover unambiguous answers to ethical dilemmas quickly and effortlessly, most likely we will be bewildered by the complexity of these dilemmas. Furthermore, we will most surely experience disappointment if we expect instant truth, for one does not mine ethical dilemmas as easily as one mines for diamonds, but a concern for ethical principles may prove to be the more valuable of the two endeavors.

HEALTH CARE ETHICS

Building on accumulated knowledge, especially from the 17th through the 19th centuries, advances in medical science and technology have progressed triumphantly during the 20th century. In the wake of this progress, two sets of major problems related to optimal health care have arisen. The first set of problems concerns the adequate distribution and availability of health care and the second set concerns the danger of becoming so infatuated with the technological dimensions of health care that we cease to question their limitations. Specifically, we can unintentionally lose sight of the axiomatic foundation of health care, which is that human beings cannot be understood in mechanistic terms only. To do so, though, shows a limited view, a view that could violate that very foundation.

The health sciences make many demands upon the abilities, special training, and character of their practitioners. One of the most basic of these demands requires that we be guided by moral considerations. Health care ethics, also called medical ethics, biomedical ethics, and bioethics, is normative, practical ethics specific to the health sciences—it raises the question of what is right or what ought to be done in a health science situation when a moral decision is called for. Such situations range from moral decisions in the clinical setting focused on one patient and his or her family to those concerned with policy decisions as to distribution of resources. Specifically, health care ethics addresses four interrelated areas: (1) clinical, (2) allocation of scarce resources, (3) human experimentation, and (4) health policy. It has been argued that moral considerations in the health sciences do not differ from normal, everyday moral considerations in that both work with the same moral principles and rules and use ethical reasoning. In health care ethics, the difference occurs only in the special situations and issues confronting the practitioner. The task of health care ethics therefore is neither to discover some new moral principles on which to build a theoretical ethical system nor to evolve new approaches to ethical reasoning, but to prepare the ground for the application of the established general moral principles and rules. In short, health care ethics is practical ethics. As with general ethics, we cannot expect an automatic deductive procedure in health care ethics for arriving at "the" ethical answer, nor can we legitimately expect ethics as a discipline to motivate those of us in the health sciences to be moral or to reprimand us when we are not. Health care ethics does not promote a particular moral life style nor does it campaign for particular life values. Its role has been defined as functioning (1) to sensitize or raise the consciousness of health professionals (and the lay public) concerning ethical issues found in health care settings and policies, and (2) to structure the issues so that ethically relevant threads of complex situations can be drawn out. Health care ethics can illuminate the variety of conflicting ethical principles involved in a particular situation and can isolate pivotal concepts needing definition, clarification, or defense. Principles and theories taken from ethics and applied in the health care arena give us ways to systematically reason through an ethical dilemma.

HEALTH CARE ETHICS AND THE LAW

Law and ethics in a given society are similar in that they have developed in the same historical, social, cultural, and philosophical soil, but they also differ in some important ways. It is possible to view the relationship between ethics and law as a four-way grid. Actions can be (1) ethical and legal, (2) unethical and illegal, (3) ethical and illegal, and (4) unethical and legal. The latter two possibilities confront health professionals and present the most difficult situations to work through to some satisfactory solution.[10]

Because we use the term *right* in a very broad and indiscriminate way, the law can be helpful in giving us clues toward limiting this term to a workable definition and therefore to a more appropriate meaning. Legal rights are grounded in the law whereas ethical rights are grounded in ethical principles and rules. Positive rights mean that one has a right to something and negative rights mean that one has a right to be left alone. Free speech is a positive right, whereas refusing an injection is a negative right.

We have the right to speak and also the right to refuse receiving the injection.

ETHICAL DILEMMAS

As indicated earlier, one of the major difficulties in ethical discourses is that no definite, clear-cut answer exists for all ethical dilemmas. For that reason, critical reflection becomes necessary in any attempt to deal with an ethical dilemma. A dilemma can be defined as (1) a difficult problem seemingly incapable of a satisfactory solution, or (2) a situation involving choice between equally unsatisfactory alternatives. Not all dilemmas in life are ethical in nature, but an ethical dilemma does arise when moral claims conflict with one another. For example, we ought to prolong life and we ought to relieve suffering. Ethical dilemmas are situations involving conflicting moral claims, and give rise to such questions as: What ought I to do? What harm and benefit result from this decision or action? For example, in a situation where moral claims conflict, what one considers good may not necessarily be right. This reveals a conflict between two moral claims, virtue and duty. Assisted suicide may be considered good (a virtue) by some in a particular situation, but it may not be considered right (a duty). Another less dramatic example, but one that may occur more often, concerns the conflict between the patient's right to autonomy and the health professional's interference with and limitation of that right in the name of health. In this instance, the violation of patient autonomy by a decision to withhold information becomes justified because this is considered to be in the best interest of the patient. What is important to note here is that another is determining the best interest of the patient, rather than the patient himself or herself making a decision after discussing the situation with appropriate health professionals. This behavior on the part of health professionals has been referred to by some as paternalism, where the health professional's behavior reduces the adult patient or the parents of the young patient to something less than decision-making, autonomous individuals.

Another example of conflicting moral claims arose in the case in which a hospital superintendent applied to the court for an order authorizing the administration of a blood transfusion. The court held that the adult patient had a right on religious grounds to refuse a blood transfusion, even if medical opinion was that the patient's decision not to accept blood amounted to the patient's taking his own life. The court determined that the patient had been mentally competent at all times when being presented with the decision that he had to make and was also competent when he made the decision. The court then concluded that the individual patient, the subject of a medical decision, must have the final say and that this must necessarily be so in a system of government that gives the greatest possible protection to the individual in the furtherance of his own desire. The court in this case dealt with a conflict between the patient's right to refuse treatment and the doctor's duty to give treatment based on medical judgment.

The 1996 version of the New York Hospital's patient bill of rights contains one section, "Your Right to Decline Treatment," which also addresses this ethical dilemma. It makes the point that patients do have the right to decline treatment but also says that if the hospital staff believes that a patient's decision to decline treatment is seriously inconsistent with its ability to provide the patient with adequate care, the patient may be requested to make arrangements elsewhere for his or her care.[11] This clearly draws the ethical dilemma as a conflict between the patient's right to refuse treatment and the hospital staff's duty to provide treatment.

Yet another example of an ethical dilemma can be found in the clinical research situation. For the purposes of discussion, let us say that a clinical researcher has developed what appears to be an effective therapeutic technique and wishes to test its efficacy among hospital patients who have the disease this technique is designed to cure. For comparative purposes, the patients are divided into two groups by random assignment so that the experimental group will receive the new technique and the control group will receive the currently accepted therapy. After a period of time elapses, the researcher discovers that one group seems to be recovering more rapidly than the other. Regardless of which group recovers faster, an ethical dilemma has been created by the conflict between, on the one hand, the obligation of the scientist to complete the experiment in order to add to knowledge that can help patients in the future and, on the other hand, the obligation of the clinician to provide the present patients with the most effective treatment available. Other research situations call attention to different ethical dilemmas. Research involving children, clinical research using a sample of elderly patients, and research that uses a placebo are only three examples of such situations.

The preamble to the World Health Organization (WHO) Constitution says that the enjoyment of the highest attainable standard of health is one of the fundamental rights of every human being, without distinction on the basis of race, religion, political belief, or economic or social conditions.[12] In the United States at present, fundamental changes are underway in the delivery of health care. Managed care and health maintenance organizations (HMOs) have become the new arrangements with an emphasis on short hospital stays and home or community care. It is still the case that many people in the United States do not have health insurance. Indeed, the United States is the only industrialized country that has not defined health care as a right for everyone but rather continues to think of it as a commodity and big business.

With present economic problems and policies, health and social programs are in danger. The broader ethical question here is: How does one account for societal callousness and indifference when they appear to coexist with a deep and abiding societal concern for others? Perhaps this conflict arises because in our world view we see society as operating in a consistent, just manner, so that the bad are punished and the good are rewarded. But is the world really this simple? Or perhaps the conflict can be explained by the observation that those who are doing well blame the victims, since to do so seems to relieve them of any felt obligation.

Discussion of any number of ethical dilemmas will occur not only during the development of public policy but will continue even after policy becomes enacted into law. The possibility of legislating ethical dilemmas out of the health care scene seems extremely remote. Regardless of the type of health care system, ethical dilemmas will continue to confront health care providers. A recent topic that has received much attention is that of rationing scarce medical resources. Numerous ethical questions arise, such as: who should get what, when not everyone can get what he or she needs to live? If medical resources are rationed, what criteria should be used to determine their allocation? Would such criteria as age, benefit to patient, contribution to society, and so forth be ethical?

PROFESSIONAL OATHS AND CODES OF ETHICS IN THE HEALTH SCIENCES

Health care ethics, concerned as it is with rights, duties, and obligations, calls for an interdisciplinary quest for the structures of responsibility. To understand the present situation, an examination of professional oaths and codes of ethics of the remote and recent past should prove fruitful. Although all health professional groups have codes, this discussion focuses only on those of nursing and medicine. The history and development of nursing's codes will be explored in depth in Chapter 2.

The International Council of Nurses in Geneva updated its code of ethics in 1973. This document addresses the duties, obligations, and rights that nurses have:

1973 Code for Nurses—International Council of Nurses

Ethical Concepts Applied to Nursing

The fundamental responsibility of the nurse is fourfold: to promote health, to prevent illness, to restore health, and to alleviate suffering.

The need for nursing is universal. Inherent in nursing is respect for life, dignity, and rights of man. It is unrestricted by considerations of nationality, race, creed, color, age, sex, politics, or social status.

Nurses render health services to the individual, the family, and the community and coordinate their services with those of related groups.

Nurses and People

The nurse's primary responsibility is to those people who require nursing care.

The nurse, in providing care, respects the beliefs, values, and customs of the individual.

The nurse holds in confidence personal information and uses judgment in sharing this information.

Nurses and Practice

The nurse carries personal responsibility for nursing practice and for maintaining competence by continual learning.

The nurse maintains the highest standards of nursing care possible within the reality of a specific situation.

The nurse uses judgment in relation to individual competence when accepting and delegating responsibilities.

The nurse when acting in a professional capacity should at all times maintain standards of personal conduct that would reflect credit upon the profession.

Nurses and Society

The nurse shares with other citizens the responsibility for initiating and supporting action to meet the health and social needs of the public.

Nurses and Co-Workers

The nurse sustains a cooperative relationship with co-workers in nursing and other fields.

The nurse takes appropriate action to safeguard the individual when his care is endangered by a co-worker or any other person.

Nurses and the Profession

The nurse plays the major role in determining and implementing desirable standards of nursing practice and nursing education.

The nurse is active in developing a core of professional knowledge.

The nurse, acting through the professional organization, participates in establishing and maintaining equitable social and economic working conditions in nursing.*

In order to provide one means of professional self-regulation, the American Nurses Association (ANA) revised its code of ethics, which had originally been adopted in 1950. The Code for Nurses (1976) indicates the nursing profession's acceptance of the responsibility and trust with which it has been invested by society. The requirements of the Code may often exceed, but are not less than, those of the law. While violation of the law subjects the nurse to criminal or civil liability, the Association may reprimand, censure, suspend, or expel members from the Association for violation of the Code. The Interpretative Statements that accompany the ANA Code outline the ethical principles that underpin each section of the Code.

Code for Nurses

1. The nurse provides services with respect for human dignity and the uniqueness of the client unrestricted by considerations of social or economic status, personal attributes, or the nature of health problems.

2. The nurse safeguards the client's right to privacy by judiciously protecting information of a confidential nature.

3. The nurse acts to safeguard the client and the public when health care and safety are affected by the incompetent, unethical, or illegal practice of any person.

4. The nurse assumes responsibility and accountability for individual nursing judgments and actions.

5. The nurse maintains competence in nursing.

6. The nurse exercises informed judgment and uses individual competence and qualifications as criteria in seeking consultation, accepting responsibilities, and delegating nursing activities to others.

7. The nurse participates in activities that contribute to the ongoing development of the profession's body of knowledge.

---

* Reprinted with permission of the International Council of Nurses.

8. The nurse participates in the profession's efforts to implement and improve standards of nursing.

9. The nurse participates in the profession's efforts to establish and maintain conditions of employment conducive to high-quality nursing care.

10. The nurse participates in the profession's efforts to protect the public from misinformation and misrepresentation and to maintain the integrity of nursing.

11. The nurse collaborates with members of the health professions and other citizens in promoting community and national efforts to meet the health needs of the public.*

The Hippocratic Oath for Physicians

I swear by Apollo Physician and Asclepius and Hygeia and Panakeia and all the gods and goddesses, making them my witnesses, that I will fulfill according to my ability and judgment this oath and this covenant:

To hold him who has taught me this art as equal to my parents and to live my life in partnership with him, and if he is in need of money to give him a share of mine, and to regard his offspring as equal to my brothers in male lineage and to teach them this art—if they desire to learn it—without fee and covenant; to give a share of precepts and oral instructions and all the other learning to my sons and to the sons of him who has instructed me and to pupils who have signed the covenant and have taken an oath according to the medical law, but to no one else.

I will apply dietetic measures for the benefit of the sick according to my ability and judgment; I will keep them from harm and injustice,

I will neither give a deadly drug to anybody if asked for it, nor will I make a suggestion to this effect. Similarly I will not give to a woman an abortive remedy. In purity and holiness I will guard my life and my art.

I will not use the knife, not even on sufferers from stone, but will withdraw in favor of such men as are engaged in this work.

Whatever houses I may visit, I will come for the benefit of the sick remaining free of all intentional injustice, of all mischief, and in particular of sexual relations with both female and male persons, be they free or slaves.

What I may see or hear in the course of the treatment or even outside of the treatment in regard to the life of men, which on no account one must spread abroad, I will keep to myself holding such things shameful [more accurately: "unspeakable"] to be spoken about.

---

* Reprinted with permission of the American Nurses Association.

If I fulfill this oath and do not violate it, may it be granted to me to enjoy life and art, being honored with fame among all men for all time to come; if I transgress it and swear falsely, may the opposite of all this be true.

Primarily a pronouncement of medical ethics, this oath is not a set of laws enforced upon physicians by an authority but rather a guide which they accept of their own free will. Far from being a legal document, the Hippocratic Oath is a solemn promise given by the conscience of the physician who swears to it. The doctor's oath can be found in a number of variant forms, such as Christian, Islamic and Buddhist, and the Oath of Charaka used in India, and all share some similarities.

The strengths of the Hippocratic tradition, a vital center of responsible medicine today, emphasize the importance of covenant fidelity between physician and student and physician and patient. Medicine functions, as a social contract, on the basis of this covenant. Justice, fairness, righteousness, faithfulness, canons of loyalty, the sanctity of life, agape or charity are some of the names given to the moral quality of attitudes and of action owed by any individual who steps into a covenant with another. The Hippocratic tradition also reveals several weaknesses. Both the ethical and medical conceptions are pretechnological and thus there are limits in using them to probe the problems posed by technology. In addition, the tradition's focus on crisis treatment, as opposed to health promotion and maintenance, and the model of the physician as a receptacle to whom people come, requires reexamination. Nevertheless, the oath has not only survived all these centuries but, because it anchors responsibility in the moral power and ability of the human being, it exerts influence on the practice of medicine today.

In 1971, the Judicial Council of the American Medical Association (AMA) developed ethical principles to serve as standards of conduct for the physician. They address the duties, obligations, and rights of the medical practitioner. In 1980, these principles were revised, and reduced to seven, and now read as follows:

American Medical Association Principles of Medical Ethics

Preamble:

The medical profession has long subscribed to a body of ethical statements developed primarily for the benefit of the patient. As a member of this profession, a physician must recognize responsibility not only to patients, but also to society, to other health professionals, and to self. The following Principles adopted by the American Medical Association are not laws, but standards of conduct which define the essentials of honorable behavior for the physician.

I. A physician shall be dedicated to providing competent medical service with compassion and respect for human dignity.

II. A physician shall deal honestly with patients and colleagues, and strive to expose those physicians deficient in character or competence, or who engage in fraud or deception.

III. A physician shall respect the law and also recognize a responsibility to seek changes in those requirements which are contrary to the best interests of the patient.

IV. A physician shall respect the rights of patients, of colleagues, and of other health professionals, and shall safeguard patient confidences within the constraints of the law.

V. A physician shall continue to study, apply and advance scientific knowledge, make relevant information available to patients, colleagues, and the public, obtain consultation, and use the talents of other health professionals when indicated.

VI. A physician shall, in the provision of appropriate patient care, except in emergencies, be free to choose whom to serve, with whom to associate, and the environment in which to provide medical services.

VII. A physician shall recognize a responsibility to participate in activities contributing to an improved community.*

In 1948, the general assembly of the World Medical Association in Geneva adopted an International Code of Medical Ethics and the Declaration of Geneva. These documents served to reaffirm the traditional professional commitments of the physician.

One tradition that evolved from historical events in this century must be included in any discussion of health care ethics. The ethos of the health sciences, particularly its experimental concepts, has been profoundly influenced by the Nuremberg experience. The Nazi medical experiments conducted during the Second World War had their genesis in a number of historical and social trends. In the 1800s, German medicine and universities participated in the insidious beginnings of 20th century anti-Semitism. A number of changes affected the physician who, no longer an individual entrepreneur, became responsible for expressing the values of the prevailing

---

* Reprinted with permission of the American Medical Association.

social order. By the 1920s, emphasis on public health and preventive medicine focused on the desire to perfect the Nordic "species" by eliminating all impurities and defects.

The horrors of Nazi medical research included such experiments on concentration camp inmates as sterilization, placing inmates in pressure chambers and forcing them to endure high-altitude atmospheres until they died, tests on the effects of weightlessness and rapid fall, and freezing experiments in ice and snow. The K-technology, or the science of killing, led the Nazis to inject inmates with lethal doses of typhus and other pathogens and to experiment on them with gas gangrene wounds, bone grafting, and direct injections of potassium and cyanide into the heart. The physicians dissected inmates alive to observe brain and heart action. And finally, at the height of sadism, the motivation for the macabre experiments was to collect different shapes of skulls and to retrieve human skin in order to make lampshades. The Nazi physicians' immolation of medical ethics on a massive scale proceeded unopposed by the German medical profession. Out of this experience came the Nuremberg Code, which gives us valuable insights and directives to current research involving human subjects. One of this code's contributions is the precision with which it discusses the criterion of informed consent. The single most important ethical legacy of the Nuremberg experience is that it reminds us of the potential evil in human beings and serves to constantly refute the myth of inevitable progress.

Although not an ethical code per se, the American Hospital Association (AHA) in 1971 developed a Statement on a Patient's Bill of Rights, which had implications for health care ethics. This bill, posted in all hospitals to notify patients of their rights, is addressed in further detail in Chapter 6.

Three other documents, which are not discussed here but that speak of the concepts of human rights and that have implications for health care ethics, are the World Medical Association Helsinki Declaration of 1964, the Preamble to the World Health Organization Constitution, and the United Nations International Covenant on Human Rights. Since so many factors influence health and illness, these documents, addressing the larger social, economic, cultural, civil, and political rights, provide a matrix for health care ethics.

THE ROLE OF THE ETHICIST

To the extent that we confront and attempt to deal with ethical dilemmas in health care by ethical reasoning, we are assuming the role of an ethicist. Although these individuals may not be directly involved in the care of the patient, they can help by bringing their particular expertise to the situation. Such a person can help to structure the ethical issues involved in any ethical dilemma and provide another perspective, drawing not so much from a background in the health sciences but from philosophy and theology. Some health care centers now have an ethicist on the staff to assist the physicians, nurses, and others who ultimately must resolve specific ethical dilemmas and act on the decisions made. Many more have ethics committees.

Although we have ethicists and ethics committees in health care settings, the fact remains that each person is a moral agent. To the extent that we develop moral sensitivity and systematic ways of reasoning through an ethical dilemma, we will do a better job at being a moral agent and a patient advocate. As nurses are even more affected by these situations in the future, they will need to recognize ethical dilemmas as such and will need to be able to think through these dilemmas so that they can participate actively in the decisions on and possible resolution of these dilemmas. It is important to be able to take an ethical stance and to be able to articulate and ethically justify it. Righteous indignation may have its place, but a thoughtful ethical stance may have more impact in the decision-making process.

REFERENCES

1. Beauchamp TL, Childress JF: *Principles of Biomedical Ethics.* 4th ed. New York: Oxford University Press; 1994.
2. Bayles M (ed): *Contemporary Utilitarianism.* Garden City, NY: Doubleday and Co.; 1968.
3. Sherman N: *The Fabric of Character: Aristotle's Theory of Virtue.* Oxford: Clarendon Press; 1984.
4. McIntyre A: *After Virtue.* 2nd ed. Notre Dame, IN: University of Notre Dame Press; 1984.
5. Thomson TT: *The Realm of Rights.* Cambridge, MA: Harvard University Press; 1990.
6. Gilligan C: *In A Different Voice.* Cambridge, MA: Harvard University Press; 1982.
7. Sherwin S: *No Longer Patient: Feminist Ethics and Health Care.* Philadelphia: Temple University Press; 1992.
8. Benner P (ed): *Interpretive Phenomenology: Embodiment, Caring, and Ethics in Health & Illness.* Thousand Oaks, CA: Sage Publications; 1994.
9. Du Bose ER, Hamel R, O'Connell LJ: *A Matter of Principles? Ferment in U.S. Bioethics.* Valley Forge, PA: Trinity Press International; 1994.
10. Smith SA, Davis, AJ: Ethical dilemmas: Conflicts among rights, duties, and obligations. *Am J Nurs* 80(8):1462–1466, 1980.
11. The New York Hospital: *Your Bill of Rights.* New York, 1996.
12. World Health Organization: *Preamble to the Constitution of the World Health Organization.* Geneva: WHO; July 1948.

2

Nursing's Ethics

Marsha Fowler

"Science fiction come alive" is an apt description of the development of medical science and technology since the late 1960s. Its astonishing miracles have also brought moral migraines for all who are or would be nurses or would seek the services of a nurse. As a consequence of the moral uncertainty, dilemmas, and distresses that contemporary health care has generated, and also as a response to the sometimes unwarranted and unwanted technologization of the end of life, the bioethical literature began to explode in that same period. Indeed, the bioethical literature, the creation of ethics centers, and the numbers of conferences, workshops and intensive courses offered since the 1970s seem to indicate that bioethics has reached epidemic proportions.

And yet, ethics has never been a fad in nursing; it has been the very foundation of nursing practice since the inception of modern nursing in the United States in the late 1870s. There is an unbroken thread of ethical literature and activity woven throughout the fabric of the entire profession— its literature, professional association, standards of practice (code of ethics), educational requirements, position statements, and practice. Nothing within the profession has remained untouched by the enduring and intentional commitment to ethics. That commitment has included a massive ethical literature, attention to the ethical formation of the nursing student, development of a code of ethics, ongoing work of the American Nurses Association in addressing ethical issues, and the formulation of ethical position statements with regard to health care and the role of the profession. The history of nursing's ethics is enduring, distinguished, honorable, and worthy of both our respect and our pride.

THE NURSING ETHICAL LITERATURE

As nursing education began to move into the academy in the mid 1960s, the subsequent dissolution of the diploma schools' libraries has proven a substantial loss in the accessibility of early nursing ethical textbooks. Nonetheless, the extant literature is breathtaking in its intensity, commitment, insight, and compass. (A chronological listing of over 40 textbooks on ethics in nursing, dating from 1900 to 1964 is interpolated in the reference section. These textbooks remain fertile ground for scholarly (nonempirical) research.)

Many of the textbooks, beginning with Isabel Robb's work, *Nursing Ethics: For Hospital and Private Use,* went through several editions or were multiply reprinted.[53] The works of Robb, Aikens, Parsons, and Talley (all nurse authors) were apparently particularly influential. A number of ethics textbooks were written by Roman Catholic priests, directed toward students in Catholic nursing schools. Occasionally, works were written by a social worker or directed toward nurses and social workers together. Such a combination would not be untoward given nursing's early involvement in tenements and settlement house work. Though somewhat misleading, nursing's ethics literature was sometimes published under the label "professional problems," "professional adjustments," "the art of conduct," or even more obscurely as "friendly talks to nurses." Most of these books touched upon major aspects of the nurse's private and professional life.

The journal literature is equally impressive in volume and scope. *The Trained Nurse,* the first true journal of nursing, (whose submasthead is "Consecrated to those who Minister to the Sick and Suffering") began in 1888. Beginning in May of 1889, the journal published a six-part series of articles on ethics in nursing. The articles divided "the duties of nursing into seven classes," each class being formed by a different relationship, e.g., the nurse to the patient, the nurse to her friends.[37] This relational motif for the discussion of the ethical duties of the nurse persists into the 1950s when the first officially adopted code of ethics at least overtly abandons that principle of organization, though it retains it in part, intrinsically.

The American Journal of Nursing (AJN), which begins in 1900, also devoted considerable space to articles principally on ethics. In the October 1900 issue, Isabel Robb contributes an article that describes a course of study that she recommends for those graduate nurses who would become superintendents of hospitals or schools of nursing. As one of the required subject areas for potential superintendents, Robb includes a section on nursing ethics, wherein she "levels" the content in terms of what should be taught probationers, juniors, seniors, head nurses, and private duty nurses.[54] "Ethics in Nursing," by Isabel McIsaac, is the first *AJN* article actually devoted to ethics.[42] Thereafter, from the first issue in 1900 to the early 1980s, the *AJN* has published over 400 articles principally devoted to ethics or topics in ethics.[17] Recognizing nurses' need for assistance with specific clinical-ethical problems, the *AJN* included a column entitled "Ethical Problems" that runs from 1926 through 1928, stops for 2 years, then runs again from 1931 to 1934.[7] These columns solicit inquiries on ethical issues or problems in clinical practice from readers, to which the American Nurses Association Committee on Ethical Standards prepared and published a response. In addition, each of the Codes for Nurses has been published in the *AJN*, beginning with "A Suggested Code" in 1926.[4]

The year 1935 marks the beginning of ethics research in nursing. In that year, Sr. Rose Helene Vaughn completed a "dissertation" (thesis) for the Master of Arts degree *The Actual Incidence of Moral Problems in Nursing: A Preliminary Study in Empirical Ethics* at Catholic University of America.[62] The purpose of her study was "to obtain empirical evidence regarding the incidence of questions, doubts, and problems which were confronting the modern nurse, in order to learn the outstanding difficulties present in the lives of a large number of nurses." Vaughn asked nurses to keep diaries; 173 agreed to do so; 95 nurses returned 288 diaries. She gleaned 2,265 ethical incidents, which she categorized in 33 categories, from these diaries. The results of the study indicated that the clinical–moral problem most frequently encountered by nurses was that of cooperation between nurses and physicians. It is not surprising that many of the moral problems encountered by nurses in 1935 persist. A case in point is her category "lust" (6th of 33 categories listed by frequency) that includes a number of incidents that today would be called "sexual harassment."

Given the extent of the early nursing ethical literature, ethics in nursing in nowise constitutes a fad, but rather an enduring and intimate concern of the profession. To say this, however, is to give no indication of the nature and focus of ethics in nursing and its development to the present day. To understand nursing's ethics, it is necessary to turn to a closer look at the nursing ethical literature, tracing its evolution over the past 100 years.

THE FIRST HUNDRED YEARS OF ETHICS

Though it has been characterized as more concerned with etiquette than with ethics, this is to misunderstand early nursing ethics. Early nursing ethics focused on the character of the moral agent, refusing to separate personal from professional behavior. Despite being couched in language about "good conduct," it was what the nurse *was* not what the nurse *did* that was important, the presumption being that good character would produce right action, i.e., that virtue accomplished duty. Concerns for etiquette, then, were simply a part of the larger concern for right conduct as it emerged from right character. Thus, early nursing ethics texts contained sections on personal hygiene, physical self-care and recreation of the nurse, and even dating behaviors. The major emphases were, nonetheless, on more substantive concerns such as confidentiality.

So, what kind of a woman was the nurse to be? Robb quotes a letter she received asking for the recommendation of a nurse to fill a head-nurse position in a hospital that concludes ". . . in short, we require an intelligent saint."[53] This does, in fact, capsulize Robb's understanding of the ideal nurse. It also contravenes the cultural norm of women as bearers of the "finer sensibilities" and men (not women) as the possessors of "intelligence." Indeed, higher education of women was culturally viewed as subversive of the species as it was claimed to reduced female fertility, even to inducing withering of the reproductive organs. Nonetheless, Robb argues vigorously for the higher education of women as nurses.[53]

Nursing students, particularly probationers and junior students, were generally seen to be morally unformed. The task of the nursing school was, therefore, in part, the moral formation of the student, equipping the student for patient care, and for assuming a proper role in addressing the ills of society. Robb writes that:

> . . . the training school of a hospital may, therefore be regarded as a place not only for fitting women to properly undertake the care of the sick, but as an educational institution, where properly selected women are given such educational advantages that they can go forth equipped and ready to aid in the practical solution of social problems, which are to be mastered only by the help of intelligent womanly work.[53]

This sort of passage is important in that it indicates several points common to the ethical literature of the period. First, the training school was about the business of shaping students into moral beings so that they could be trusted to deliver care as graduates, in unsupervised contexts. Second, because the school was a place of moral formation, and because the emphasis was upon moral character, virtually the whole of the student's life was subject to moral scrutiny. Third, nursing was seen to be intelligent work, but womanly work as well, a view that ran countercurrent to societal perspectives on women. And last, that nursing's ethics was from the start not simply an ethics at the bedside, but also at one and the same time a social ethics as well. A quick look at nursing history will give ample evidence of nurses' involvement in causes related to child labor laws, public health, battles against poverty, leagues for animal protection, and a wide range of human and civil rights activism. Nursing's ethics is principally a social ethics that encompasses bioethics.

Robb also holds that while nurses (as even students were called) are being formed morally they also exercise a moral influence. It is an uneasy tension that one finds in the ethical literature. The student is not morally formed thus the school has the right to the moral scrutiny of the student's life, personal and professional. However, the student must not be too morally unformed lest it be inappropriate to unleash the student upon the unsuspecting and vulnerable patient. Thus a compromise had to be forged to relieve the tension. Robb writes that "nurses cannot avoid exercising a moral influence. They exercise it by their characters . . . it is what a nurse is in herself, what comes out of herself, out of what she is (almost without knowing it herself), that exercises a moral or religious influence over her patients." [53] Here the nurse is morally formed, but unaware of it because the formation resides in the character. Parsons, too, acknowledges the importance of character matched by intelligence. She writes that "only the character that is built on a foundation of generosity and sweetness (if linked to intelligence, common sense, and humor) is safe in any exigency that may arise. This character foundation is seldom inherited, but must be built up by training and practice." [47] It was the task of the nursing school to undertake this training and practice.

Early nursing ethics regarded nursing as a *profession,* in the sense of what one professes, that is, as a calling. Robb preferred the terms *call* or *calling* even to that of *vocation* or *profession.*[53] The theme of nursing as a calling is reiterated throughout the nursing literature. Goodrich affirms this perspective. She writes "to no field does the call for the finest expression of womanhood come with greater insistence or greater justification than that of nursing—a call that cannot be denied." [27] Goodrich also believed nursing to be an intrinsically moral endeavor. She writes "so much is nursing of the essence of ethics that it is consistent to assert that the terms good and ethical as applied to nursing practice are synonymous. . . . the calling, vocation, profession, what you will, is in itself intrinsically ethical." [27]

In practice, however, how was the nurse to be toward the patient? Many of these ethics textbooks organize their discussion around the virtues seen as essential to the profession. But, overall, ". . . to the patient laid low by disease or injury she appears as a goddess of healing, and her every gentle movement has a comforting and consoling power." [26] (It is not until well after World War II that this sort of flowery, high-Victorian rhetoric shifts toward a style more consistent with contemporary language.) This goddess of healing nonetheless needed to be protected from certain evils; she was, you must remember, not completely formed morally.

Goodall writes ". . . nursing will disclose the human body in conditions and circumstances that are new to your young eyes. There may be occasions when your only shield from the gross embarrassment will be your purity of mind." [26] In 1947, priest-author McAllister writes more directly that:

> Duty sometimes *obliges* a person to think about things ordinarily dangerous to chastity. Medical students and nurses, to have the professional knowledge they need, must give considerable thought to matters of sex and processes of reproduction. . . . they should guard against *morbid curiosity* and be cautious lest their studies become causes of *venereal pleasure.*[40]

The education necessary to care for patients who might have questions or problems with sex or reproduction posed a grievous moral danger to the nurse. Notice that this perspective, found also in the 1955 edition of McAllister's work, occurs relatively late within the context of the social shifts in society regarding sexual matters. Yet, sex and reproductive education are not the only danger confronting the student and from which the student might need protection. In 1943, Goodall writes:

> In dormitory life or in any other way of life, avoid crushes for they will rob you of all healthy, natural desire to mingle with groups of people and within your life they will harbor evils and miseries that jealousy can bring. When carried too far, they will turn your emotions from their natural bent and cause you to have an unnatural and unhappy attitude toward men . . . the best rule in friendship is to be fond of many and familiar with none.[26]

This expression of homophobia reflected a prevailing though covert fear that women living together in close quarters, as nursing students were required to do, would form emotional attachments that might cause them to become lesbian. Students needed to be protected until they could develop the strength of moral character to weather the moral assaults of sex education, living in close quarters with other women, dating, advances made by male patients or patient relatives, and the temptations of extravagance with one's wages. The world of the nurse was rife with evil influences.

The emphasis on the character of the moral agent, otherwise known as "virtue ethics," was not unique to nursing, but rather reflected the prevailing societal perspective on ethics. However, the emphasis on the moral purity of the nurse endures beyond the point at which society ceases to embrace an ethics that allows scrutiny of the personal life, particularly of public figures. That is to say, long after society began to shift toward a duty-based ethics, nursing retained an emphasis on virtue ethics. This may in part be due to the nature of nursing education that took place in essentially cloistered contexts similar to Erving Goffman's "total institution." [25] In an attempt, by Fowler, to collect the virtues considered essential to the character of the nurse, those that made for a "morally good nurse," the virtues and excellences reflected in the ethical literature of the past 100 years, were compiled into the following list[17]:

Virtues and Excellences in Nursing, Culled from the Nursing Ethical Literature, 1875–1975[17]

absolute accuracy, accepts criticism, adaptable, agreeable, alert, appreciative, calm, charitable, cheerful, Christian, clean, comforting, competent, conscientious, considerate, contented, controlled, cooperative, courageous, courteous, cultured, decisive, decorous, dependable, devoted, dignified, disciplined, discreet, discriminating, eager, economical, economizing, efficient, emotionally mature, enduring, enthusiastic, even temperament, ever ready, faithful, fealty, fidelity to duty, finesse, firm, friendly, gentle words, gentle, gentler virtues, good reputation, good breeding, good grammar, good memory, good posture, gracious, healthy, healthful, helpmeet, high thinking, honest, humanitarian, humble, humorous, impartial, industrious, ingenious, inspires confidence, inspiring, intelligent, intuitive, joyful, kind, liberal of thought, likes people, long suffering, loving, loyal, maintains dignity, meek, mentally fit, morally pure, neat, noble, nonmalevolent, obedient, open minded, patient, patriotic, peaceable, perceptive, perfect woman, physically fit, plain living, pleasant personality, poised, praiseworthy, principled, protective, prudent, public spirited, punctual, pure manner, pure speech, pure heart, quickness, quietness, readiness, reassuring, refined, reliable, resourceful, reserved manner, resistant to infection, respectful of authority, responsible, restful, right living, righteous, satisfied, scientific attitude, seeks perfection, self-controlled, self-respect, self-reliant, self-sacrificing, selfless, sense of fittingness, sincere, skilled, smiling, soft hand, spiritual, spontaneous, stable, strong, studious, sweet, sympathetic, systematic, tactful, tasteful dress, teachable spirit, team worker, tender heart, thorough, thoughtful, thrifty, tolerant, truthful, uncomplaining, unobtrusive, unselfish soul, versatile, vigilant, virtuous, warm, watchful, welcomes criticism, wholesome, womanly

Reducing the list to those habits of character that might be actual virtues or excellences (as opposed to cultural expectations of women) the list includes: benevolence, care, compassion, competence, courage, devotion, faithfulness, honesty, integrity, justness, kindness, knowledgeable, loving, loyal, nonmalevolent, prudent, skilled, teachable, temperate, tolerant, trustworthy, wise, understanding, truthful. This rather more abbreviated list, shorn of some of the more amusing and more troublesome expectations is, in fact, a sound reflection of the moral attributes that one would hope to see in nurses today.

In the late 1960s, nursing, following societal changes and heavily influenced by the rise of the field of bioethics, shifted away from a virtue-based ethics to a duty-based ethics. Yet, it is not an "either–or" situation, but rather a "both–and" necessity. Both a virtue and a duty-based approach to ethics is essential if duties are to have any power and if virtues are to have any direction. The problem of a duty-based ethics is that obligations are empty if the person does not possess the character to meet those obligations. The problem of a virtue-based ethics is that it runs the risk of abuse through unwarranted intrusion into the private life of the individual, an intrusion that was amply evident in our early isolated "live-in education." Nursing needs to avoid any return to such abuses. However, it also needs to reclaim the importance of virtue ethics, not for the purposes of the moral examination of the practitioner, but rather for the scrutiny of the environment in which care is rendered. That environment needs to nurture virtues and to allow them to flourish. For example, can the virtues of knowledge, skill, patience, and caring flourish in an environment where the nurse's patient load is so large that competence and safety are the surpassing concerns? Where the practice environment mitigates against the exercise of specific virtues or excellences it is inappropriate to demand or expect them.

ETHICS CURRICULA IN SCHOOLS OF NURSING

The school of nursing, as a moral training ground engaged not only in the examination of the moral character of the nurse throughout her education, but also offered the nursing student substantial pedagogical content in the field of ethics. In 1917, the National League for Nursing Education (NLNE; later the National League for Nursing [NLN]) published its "Standard Curriculum for Schools of Nursing." It required 10 hours of lecture on ethics in the second year (the same number of hours allotted other major topics). The basic ethics lectures were to include major sections on:

- Introduction—Customary Morality
- Personal or Reflective Morality
- Ethical Ideals and Standards
- Moral Judgement; Conduct and Character
- Place of "Self" in the Moral Life
- Social Virtues
- Ethical Principles as Applied to Community Life
- Principles of Ethics Applied to One's Work or Profession
- Principles of Ethics Applied to One's Personal Life[45]

It is important to note that the NLNE ethics curriculum does not limit nursing ethics to bedside concerns. Beyond the basic ethics lectures, the nursing students received additional ethics-related lectures on "Social and Professional Subjects" that included "ethical and social principles" in the history of nursing, and "modern social problems." [45] Additional ethics content was included under the subject area of "Psychology and Problems of Professional Life." Ethical considerations were also woven throughout the clinical courses.

The 1916 California State Board of Health, Bureau of Registration of Nurses curriculum requirements for schools of nursing also reflects an emphasis upon ethics in nursing. No other subject matter receives more attention than does ethics, and it is equaled only by what would today be called medical–surgical nursing. A course in ethics is required five out of six half years of the curriculum. Again, the ethics content is not limited to bedside nursing. Requirements included lectures and extensive readings in "Democracy and Social Ethics," "Modern Industry," "Housing Reform," "The Spirit of Youth and the City Streets," and other social-ethical concerns.[8]

Though it is beyond the scope of this work to explore more specifically the contents of nursing's ethics curricula or to comment further on nursing's ethics as social ethics, it is important to note the extent to which nursing felt a moral obligation for the shape and reform of society. Within its ethics, *health* was very broadly conceived. It included care for those individuals with disease, illness or debilitating conditions, it included health promotion and maintenance for individuals and families, and it included an attack upon the social ills that brought disease or assaulted the dignity of persons.

Much of the curriculum content on ethics was pinned to an understanding and interpretation of the Nightingale Pledge and the ANA's Codes for Nurses.

CODES OF ETHICS FOR NURSING

The Nightingale Pledge

Though never formally adopted as a code of ethics for the profession, the Florence Nightingale Pledge was influential for generations of nurses. It was penned by Lystra Gretter of the Farrand School of Nursing in Detroit in 1893. The story of the Pledge and its subsequent revision in 1935 is interesting. The original Pledge is:

> I solemnly pledge myself before God and in the presence of this assembly, to pass my life in purity and to practice my profession faithfully. I will abstain from whatever is deleterious and mischievous, and will not take or knowingly administer any harmful drug. I will do all in my power to maintain and elevate the standard of my profession, and will hold in confidence all personal matters committed to my keeping, and all family affairs coming to my knowledge in the practice of my calling. With loyalty will I endeavor to aid the physician in his work, and devote myself to the welfare of those committed to my care.[29]

The revised Pledge reads as follows:

> I solemnly pledge myself before God and in the presence of this assembly to pass my life in purity and to practice my profession faithfully. I will abstain from whatever is deleterious and mischievous, and will not take or knowingly administer any harmful drug. I will do all in my power to maintain and elevate the standard of my profession, and will hold in confidence all personal matters committed to my keeping, and all family affairs coming to my knowledge in the practice of my calling. With loyalty will I endeavor to aid the physician in his work, and as a "missioner of health" I will dedicate myself to devoted service to human welfare.[30]

An accompanying note, written on Farrand School letterhead in Gretter's own hand reads as follows[31]:

> Commensurate with the broader activities of the Farrand Training School of Nurses The Florence Nightingale Pledge has been revised to include service to the community within its scope. [signed] Lystra E. Gretter

The story of its origin and revision is as detailed in the following note from the Alumnae Association of the Farrand Training School for Nurses.[6]

Origin of the Florence Nightingale Pledge

In 1893, 2 years after Mrs. L.E. Gretter came to the Farrand Training School for Nurses (now the Harper Hospital School of Nursing) as Principal and because Florence Nightingale was her ideal of what a professional nurse should be, that she conceived the idea that young women engaged in nursing needed something similar to the Hippocratic Oath, and she presented her idea to the Board of Trustees of Harper Hospital, which appointed a committee of three, namely:

Mrs. Gretter–Chairman

N.E.H. Haight–Supervisor

Louise Tempest Ford–Supervisor

Dr. W.H. Davis–D.D.

Mrs. Gretter was appointed to draft a tentative pledge, as she had in mind, and when presented to the Board of Trustees for consideration, it was accepted without change.

At the time, Mrs. Gretter had only the graduates of the School in mind and it is administered to the graduates at their graduating exercises every year.

During the World War, through the influence of Mrs. Gretter, and as a war measure, it was decided to by the various schools of nursing in Detroit, to combine the commencement exercises, and at that time Mrs. Gretter was invited to administer the Florence Nightingale Pledge to the group.

This had the effect of making the Pledge generally known, and it was not long before advertising firms, book publishers, and many others using it for profit, until in 1933, while the material was being assembled for the "School"—when several of the graduates considered that it was time to do something to protect the Pledge. Agnes G. Deans made a special trip to the Department of Copyright in Washington, and took up the question of having it copyrighted. When the facts were considered, it was found that the time had expired between the time the Pledge had been formulated, and at that time (1933) but the clerk suggested that if Mrs. Gretter was willing to make a slight revision that I could be copyrighted. Mrs. Gretter did, and this was incorporated in the "History of the Farrand Training School," which was incorporated.

As the sale of the History of the School was rather limited, this information did not get over to the public, and the commercial purposes for which it had been used, continued. Another trip was made to Washington by Miss Deans to determine what could be done, and was assured that the pledge was protected by law. As part of the history, and it was suggested that some wider publicity be given the fact.

An appeal was made to the *American Journal of Nursing,* and the *Pacific Coast Journal of Nursing,* and the *Trained Nurse and Hospital Review* for some publicity, which was given. This helped very much. (See correspondence on file under "Nightingale Pledge.")

The Nightingale Pledge (1893) was well received across the country and continued to be administered at graduation exercises nationwide long after the ANA adopted a formal Code for Nurses in 1950.

THE DEVELOPMENT OF AN OFFICIAL CODE OF ETHICS FOR THE PROFESSION

Three years after the appearance of the Pledge, delegates and representatives of the American Society of Superintendents of Training Schools for Nurses convened to establish a professional association for nurses and to write its articles of incorporation. The Nurses' Associated Alumnae of the United States and Canada (later the ANA and the Canadian Nurses' Associations) was formed at that meeting. In the articles of incorporation they identify their purposes, the first of which is ". . . to establish and maintain a code of ethics . . ." [11] It is then another 53 years before a code of ethics is officially adopted. Before it can address the need for a code, nursing must deal with issues of mandatory uniform registration, the evaluation and accreditation of nursing schools, and a number of issues affecting the economic and general welfare of nurses. So, preparation of a code is delayed.

There is, however, continuing demand for a code of ethics, to the degree that, in 1921, the NLNE appointed an advisory Committee on Ethical Standards. The committee studied the need for a code of ethics for the profession and concluded that ". . . nurses throughout the country are desiring something concrete which they may accept as a basis for professional conduct." The committee formally recommended the preparation of a "statement of the principles of nursing ethics." [51] The NLNE received and approved the recommendations of the report. However, at a meeting of the joint boards of the NLNE and the ANA held in 1923, the ANA president (Adda Eldrege) requested that the committee become a part of the ANA rather than the NLNE. The reason given was that the ANA "had planned to compile a code of ethics as a part of the Association's work." [2] Thus, the actual task of preparing a code of ethics was shifted to the ANA.

The ANA committee met in 1923 and after study and discussion concluded that ". . . inasmuch as nursing ideals had been for so many years so beautifully expressed by members of the profession, it seems to us undesirable at this time to outline the elementary principles of good conduct as the code of ethics endorsed by the American Nurses Association." [2] The committee recommended, instead, "a restatement of these high ideals in form somewhat similar to that of the Fellowship Pledge of the American College of Surgeons." However, in January of 1926, a subcommittee presented a proposed code to the parent committee. Suggestions for emendation were then made by the joint boards of directors of the ANA and NLNE, with the recommendation that the amended version be published in the *AJN* as an "editorial," soliciting opinions and suggestions from the readership. The joint boards accepted and approved the code with the provision that it be identified as a preliminary or tentative code.[3]

"A Suggested Code" was published in the August 1926 issue of the *AJN*.[4] (It was also at this point that the Committee decided to institute the *AJN* column "Ethical Problems.") Written in the rhetorically effusive style of the late 1800s and early 1900s, the 1926 code was never formally adopted. It discusses the moral duties of the nurse, organizing its discussion around the various relationships nurses form; specific principles of ethics were not enumerated. Part of the importance of this code, however, resides in its specification of the central moral motif of nursing: *the ideal of service*. The language is stylistically excessive but essentially accurate: "the most precious possession of this profession is the ideal of service, extending even to the sacrifice of life itself." [4] This ideal of service links all the disparate historical forms of nursing into a contiguous whole and finds its distinctive "local" expression in metaphors of each day. For instance, the ideal of service today is expressed in the metaphor of caring, a metaphor that would not have been an adequate expression in earlier generations, e.g., the nursing knights.

In 1940 "A Tentative Code" was published.[5] It retains the relational format of the 1926 code and demonstrates a more overt concern for the status of nursing as a profession and for the public recognition of nursing. This code lists the attributes of a profession and argues for the status of nursing as a profession; unfortunately, this is subject matter that does not properly belong in a code of ethics. Responses were sought from the *AJN* readers following the publication of the 1926 and the 1940 codes. The responses were partly responsible for the reformulation of the 1940 code in 1949. The reformulated code was presented to ANA members, schools of nursing, and health care institutions. Input was also solicited through a questionnaire mailed to individuals (that resulted in replies representing 4,759 persons). The Code for Professional Nurses was accepted, unanimously, at the 1950

ANA House of delegates. At last, the profession had an official code of ethics.[18]

The 1950 Code differed dramatically in style from its predecessors. It had a brief preamble and enumerated 17 provisions. The provisions are organized around a relational pattern that is not made explicit. Several provisions related to the personal ethics (private life) of the nurse. A formal code of ethics is not a static document; it requires periodic revision (probably every 8 to 10 years) in order to keep abreast of changes in clinical practice and in society. While the principles may not themselves change, new situations arise in which they must be applied. In 1957, a minor change was made to the code in relation to nurse participation in advertising.

Nursing was deeply concerned in this period to establish itself as a legitimate "profession" with all the rights and privileges appertaining thereto. As a consequence, it adopted some norms of other groups that society regarded as professions. A case in point is the adoption of a provision against advertising, a long-held norm maintained by both medicine and law. Historically, however, the reason not to advertise services was to prevent fee wars that would drive down the income of the professional. This was usually sanitized for public consumption by declaring that the prohibition against advertising protected the public from quackery. In the 1950s, television used "nurses" (dramatized) in advertising, initiating a flurry of protest and communications. When inquiry was made about the nursing code's proscription of advertising, the response was that it was for the protection of the public. However, the specific products in question were Mum deodorant and Bromo-Seltzer. It is not always the case that all the provisions of professional codes are well grounded in ethical reasoning; codes must always be evaluated for their degree of legitimate self-interest over against self-protectionism.[17] It must be added that nursing's history, and its codes, are remarkably free of self-interest, sometimes perhaps too much so.

Following the adoption of the Code in 1950, responses were again solicited from *AJN* readers. These responses formed the basis of the 1960 major revision of the Code. The code of 1960 reflects the social context of increasing assertiveness of nursing and nurses, and an increasing sense of co-participation (rather than subordination) of nurses in the care of patients. From the vantage point of the 1990s, this code has a greater sense of professional freedom. Between 1950 and 1960, concern arose regarding the enforcement of the Code. The ANA bylaws were subsequently revised to include the obligations of members to uphold the Code. By 1964, the Committee on Ethics developed *Suggested Guidelines for Handling Violations of the Code for Professional Nurses* and distributed them to each affiliate state and territorial association.

The next major revision of the Code was published in 1968. This revision omits the preamble of the 1960 code and reduces the number of provisions from 17 to 10. For the most part, however, it encompasses all of the concerns of the Code of 1960. As this code provides the basis of the provisions of the 1976 and 1985 revised codes, there has, effectively been no revision of the provisions of the code themselves in the past 28 years, though revisions in the interpretive statements have been made.

One of the more significant changes in the Code of 1968 is its omission, for the first time, of any reference to the private behavior of the nurse. A wedge is driven between private and professional ethics when the 1968 Code drops the expectation that the nurse "would adhere to standards of personal ethics which reflect credit upon the profession." [18] Nursing now officially moves into a duty-based ethics, leaving behind much of its traditional ethical focus.

In the 1970s, changes in nursing, medicine, and society made another revision of the Code necessary. The revised Code was published in 1976, giving greater emphasis to the responsibilities of the patient to participate in her or his care. The *Code for Nurses, 1976* was published with *Interpretive Statements* that interpret the provisions in the light of contemporary nursing and health care and professional concerns. It is in this code that the term *patient* is changed to *client*. This Code makes some modest revision to the 1968 code itself, in accord with an increased social consciousness regarding forms of prejudicial discrimination, an increased technologization of the clinical arena, an increased awareness of medical paternalism, and an increased autonomy (and freedom) of nurses. It also gives increased emphasis to the nurse's responsibility and accountability in the relationship with the patient and, overall, takes a more assertive and activistic posture with regard to the nurse and the nursing profession. The streamlining of the language of this code leads to a parsimony that stands in great contrast to the effusiveness and rhetorical elegance of the earliest codes. Nonetheless, it is a more fulsome and professionally energetic code.

In 1985, again in response to changes within the profession, in medicine and medical technology, and in society, another revision was published. This Code retains, intact, the provisions of the 1976 Code and many of that code's categories, but changes the *Interpretive Statements* to reflect the concerns of the day. The 1985 Code, more than any previous Code, attends to the changes that were occurring in the field of bioethics both in relation to specific issues and in relation to professional behavior in general. It relies heavily, too much so, upon a principled approach to ethical analysis and decision making. It also, appropriately, takes a more ethical approach, purging some of the legal language of previous codes. This Code has a heightened awareness of more subtle forms of unjust societal discrimination, of the unwarranted and unwanted intrusion of medical care and the technologization of the end of life, of poor access to care, of the nurse's ever-expanding role as advocate for health, both for individuals and for society. And yet, even this, our present Code has become dated. In 1996, the ANA, through its center for Ethics and Human Rights, convened a task force to examine the Code and to make a recommendation as to whether the Code or its interpretive statements needed revision, in whole or in part.

The task force recommended that the ANA undertake a revision of both the Code itself, which has not been revised since 1976, and its *Interpretive Statements*.[49] A Code of Ethics Project Task force of ten persons has been appointed to begin work on the code and its interpretive statements in late 1996.

Because of changes both in nursing and in the field of bioethics, the forthcoming code should be a substantially new document, extensively revised. It should reflect studies in women's, feminist, Womanist, and Feminista ethics and gender studies. It should be much more broadly based in the field of ethics, rather than relying almost exclusively upon a principled approach to ethics. Work in virtue and communitarian ethics, in particular, should be taken into account. The contemporary clinical environment is economically tense and tends to assert the priority of business values over those of nursing in general or caring in particular; this had profound ramifications for the way in which health care proceeds ethically. Moreover, the potential for moral harm to the nurse in this kind of environment (by preventing the fulfillment of moral duties or the growth of virtues and excellences) should be of grave concern to all who would seek to create a moral milieu consistent with human flourishing. The new code should also reflect an increasing sense of world-community, not just national identity, that is, it should be more globalizing. It should also be more aggressive regarding the social ills that mitigate against care, that foster disease, illness, or trauma, and that see personal health as separate from urban or social health. It would also be hoped that a new code would narrow the wedge that has been driven between personal and professional ethics; one cannot be a rogue and scoundrel in private life and yet a public person of integrity and moral rectitude. This list could continue but need not in order to indicate that times have changed and a more serviceable document needs to be created for the new millenium.

A code of ethics, if it is to serve the profession in assisting to maintain the standards of the profession, must reflect both constancy and change. It must reflect constancy in its commitment to the central values of the profession, its central moral motif of service, its emphasis upon social as well as "bedside" ethics, and its enduring moral tradition. It must reflect change in its application to ever new clinical and professional concerns, moral insights and awarenesses, changes in professional knowledge and role, and social change. Though the norms themselves are stable, they must be reinterpreted afresh for each generation of nurses in accord with the growth of the profession and changes in society.

Nursing's ethics has a long, distinctive, and distinguished history, demonstrating an enduring and intimate concern for the ethical practice of nurses and for the well-being of society. That concern for ethics has suffused its literature, its education, its practice, its research. The Code for Nurses, rooted in the tradition of the Nightingale Pledge, is almost 100 years old. Along the way, nursing has spoken out in society through moral position statements, through testimony before Congress, though its Code, and through its work, to seek to achieve health for all. The nursing ethical tradition is one of which we can be enormously proud.

REFERENCES

1. Aikens CA: *Studies in Ethics for Nurses*. Philadelphia: W.B. Saunders; 1916.
2. American Nurses Association: Report of the Committee on Ethical Standards. In *Minutes of the Proceedings of the 24th Convention of the American Nurses Association*. New York: American Nurses Association; 1924.
3. American Nurses Association: Report of the Committee on Ethical Standards. In *Minutes of the Proceedings of the 25th Convention of the American Nurses Association*. New York: American Nurses Association; 1926.
4. American Nurses Association: A Suggested Code. *Am J Nurs* 26(8):599–601, 1926.
5. American Nurses Association: A Tentative Code. *Am J Nurs* 40(9):977–980, 1940.
6. Anonymous: From the files of Harper Hospital School of Nursing. Paper typed and hand dated "c. 1938," quoted en toto with spelling and punctuation left uncorrected. Used with permission.
7. Brogan JM: *Ethical Principles for the Character of a Nurse*. Milwaukee: Bruce; 1924.
8. Bureau of Registration of Nurses, California State Board of Health. *Schools of Nursing Requirements and Curriculum*. Sacramento: State Printing Office; 1916.
9. Committee on Ethical Standards, American Nurses Association: Ethical Problems. *Am J Nurs* 26(8):643, 1926.
10. Committee on Ethical Standards, American Nurses Association: A Suggested Code. *Am J Nurs* 26(8):599–601, 1926.
11. Convention of Training School Alumnae Delegates and Representatives from the American Society of Superintendents of Training Schools for Nurses: *Proceedings of the Convention, 2–4 November 1896*. Harrisburg: Harrisburg Publishing; 1896.
12. Densford KJ, Everett MS: *Ethics for Modern Nurses: Professional Adjustments, I*. Philadelphia: W.B. Saunders; 1946.
13. Dietz LD: *Professional Problems in Nursing*. Philadelphia: F.A. Davis; 1935.
14. Dietz LD: *Professional Adjustments, I*. Philadelphia: F.A. Davis; 1940.
15. Edgell B: *Ethical Problems: An Introduction to Ethics for Hospital Nurses and Social Workers*. London: Methuen and Company; 1929.
16. Evarts AB: *Ethics of Nursing*. Minneapolis: Burgess; 1935.
17. Fowler M: *Ethics in Nursing, 1893-1984: The Ideal of Service, the Reality of History*. Los Angeles: University of Southern California; 1984.
18. Fowler M: A Chronicle of the Evolution of the Code for Nurses. In White G. ed: *Ethical Dilemmas in Contemporary Nursing Practice*. Washington, DC: American Nurses Association; 1992, pp 149–154.
19. Gabriel S: *Professional Problems: A Textbook for Nurses*. Philadelphia: W.B. Saunders; 1932.

20. Garesche EF: *A Vade Mecum for Nurses and Social Workers*. Milwaukee: Bruce; 1926.

21. Garesche EF: *Couriers of Mercy: Friendly Talks to Nurses*. Milwaukee: Bruce; 1928.

22. Garesche EF: *Ethics and the Art of Conduct for Nurses*. Philadelphia: W.B. Saunders; 1929. Also 1944.

23. Gladwin ME: *Ethics: Talks to Nurses*. Philadelphia: F.A. Davis; 1930. 2nd ed. 1937, 3rd ed. 1938.

24. Godin E, O'Hanley JPE: *Hospital Ethics: A Commentary on the Code of Catholic Hospitals*. Bathurst, New Brunswick: Hotel Dieu Hospital; 1957.

25. Goffmann E: *Asylums*. New York: Anchor; 1961.

26. Goodall PA: *Ethics: The Inner Realities*. Philadelphia: F.A. Davis; 1942. Also 1943.

27. Goodrich AW: *The Social and Ethical Significance of Nursing: A Series of Addresses*. New York: Macmillan; 1932.

28. Gounley ME: *Digest of Ethics for Nurses*. Paterson: St. Anthony Guild; 1949.

29. Gretter LE: *The Florence Nightingale Pledge*. Detroit: Farrand Training School for Nurses, Harper Hospital. Taken from a photograph of the original autograph manuscript (original was discovered to have been removed from the archival scrapbook), dated April 30, 1893. Photograph of original manuscript dates from before 1929. *Used with permission.*

30. Gretter LE: *The Florence Nightingale Pledge*. Taken from autograph manuscript, dated January 1, 1936. *Used with permission.*

31. Gretter LE: Autograph note on letterhead of Harper Hospital, Farrand Training School for Nurses, Principal's Office. Dated January 1, 1936. *Used with permission.*

32. Hansen H: *Professional Relationships of the Nurse*. Philadelphia: W.B. Saunders; 1942.

33. Harrison G: *Ethics in Nursing*. St. Louis: C.V. Mosby; 1932.

34. Harrison H: *Professional Adjustments*. No publisher given; 1942.

35. Hayes EJ, Hayes PJ, Kelly DE: *Moral Principles of Nursing*. New York: Macmillan; 1964.

36. Hayes EJ, et al: *Moral Handbook of Nursing: A Compendium of Principles, Spiritual Aids, and Concise Answers Regarding Catholic Personnel, Patients and Problems*. New York: Macmillan; 1956.

37. HCC (Otherwise unidentified superintendent of a Brooklyn school of nursing): "The Ethics of Nursing." *The Trained Nurse*, Vol. II, 5:179. The remaining articles of the series are found in Volume III, No. 1–6.

38. Jamieson EM, Sewell E: *Ethics Notebook for Nurses*. Philadelphia: J.B. Lippincott; 1931. Also 1933, 1935, 1940, 1944.

39. Lounsberry HC: *Making Good on Private Duty: Practical Hints to Graduate Nurses*. Philadelphia: J.B. Lippincott; 1912.

40. McAllister JB: *Ethics with Special Application to the Medical and Nursing Professions*. Philadelphia: W.B. Saunders; 1947. Also 1955.

41. McFadden CJ: *Medical Ethics*. Philadelphia: F.A. Davis; 1946. Also 1949.

42. McIsaac I: Ethics in Nursing. *Am J Nurs* 1(7):488–490, 1900.

43. Moore DTV: *Principles of Ethics*. Philadelphia: J.B. Lippincott; 1935. Also 1937, 1939, 1943.

44. Murphy, R: *The Catholic Nurse: Her Spirit and Her Duties.* Milwaukee: Bruce; 1923.
45. National League for Nursing Education. Standard curriculum for Schools of Nursing. New York: NLNE; 1917.
46. Parsons SE: *Nursing Problems and Obligations.* Boston: Whitcomb and Barrows; 1916. Also, 1919, 1922.
47. Parsons SE: *Nursing Problems and Obligations.* Boston: M. Barrows; 1928.
48. Pearce ED: *The Nurse and the Patient: An Ethical Consideration of Human Relations.* London: Farber and Farber; 1953.
49. Pelley T: *Nursing: Its History, Trends, Philosophy, Ethics and Ethos.* Philadelphia: W.B. Saunders; 1964. The author was a member of the task force and of the subsequent task force for the actual work of revision.
50. Plachata SMM: *Spiritualize Your Nursing.* No publisher given; 1963.
51. Powell L: Report of the Committee on Ethical Standards. In NLNE: *Proceedings of the 28th Annual convention, Seattle Washington, June 26–July 1, 1922.* Baltimore: Williams & Wilkins; 1923, p. 27–28.
52. Price A: *Professional Adjustments, I.* No publisher given. 1946.
53. Robb IAH: *Nursing Ethics: For Hospital and Private Use.* New York: E.C. Koeckert; 1900. Reprinted without revision in 1911, 1916, 1920.
54. Robb IH: Hospital Economics. *Am J Nurs* 1(1):29–36, 1900.
55. Rothweiler E: *Davis' Cumulative Continued Study Units on Ethics.* Philadelphia: F.A. Davis; 1938.
56. Russell FJ: *Ethics in General and Special.* Emmitsburg, MD: Sisters of Charity; 1929.
57. Spaulding EK: *Professional Adjustments in Nursing, Being Professional Adjustments, II.* Philadelphia: J.B. Lippincott; 1939.
58. Spalding HS: *Talks to Nurses: The Ethics of Nursing.* New York: Benziger Brothers; 1920.
59. Stoney EAM, Catlin LC: *Practical Points in Nursing for Nurses in Private Practice.* Philadelphia: W.B. Saunders; 1917.
60. Talley CE: *Lesson Plans in Ethics for Nurses.* New York: G.P. Putnam's; 1927.
61. Talley CE: *Ethics: A Textbook for Nurses.* New York: Putnam's; 1925. 2nd ed. 1928.
62. Vaughn SRH: *The Actual Incidence of Moral Problems in Nursing: A Preliminary Study in Empirical Ethics.* Washington, DC: Catholic University Press; 1935.
63. Way H: *Ethics for Nurses.* London: Macmillan; 1962.
64. Weis AS: Our Professional Balance. *Am J Nurs* 28(10):1025–26, 1928.

3

Values Clarification, Moral Development, and Other Considerations in Understanding Health Care Ethics

Few things in life are value free. Values are basic to a given way of life and serve to give direction to life. Our values are often similar to our breathing in that they are taken for granted. We do not go through life aware of the fact that we are breathing and therefore we do not think of our breathing. In the same manner, we do not always realize that we have a given set of values or that a decision is based on these values. We do not always examine our values but simply accept them and act on them. Again, as with breathing, we are more apt to think about our values when something goes wrong, because we then become more aware of them, just as we become more aware of our breathing when we experience difficulty. Much of what goes into actual moral choices are unarticulated but remain as unspoken values. In describing an ethical dilemma, we have already structured the situation that now reflects, by our very describing it, our way of seeing the world and our values.

We take moral values and judgments seriously. One's moral convictions are not diminished by the recognition that others have different moral convictions that they take equally serious.[1]

Value clarification is a process that fosters the identification of significant values.[2] In this process we examine what we believe about the truth, beauty, or worth of any thought, object, or behavior. We make value judgments every day, ranging from trivial choices to those that affect our whole lives. Every individual has some sense of value, and there has never been a society that is devoid of a value system. In more traditional societies, values are embedded in habit, custom, and traditions. In societies in which rapid change occurs, values can become a source of controversy and conflict.

The word *axiology*, which comes from the Greek *axios*, meaning "worthy," has come to be used for the study of the general theory of value. Ethics, the study of values in human conduct, and esthetics, the study of values in art, are subspecialties within the larger specialty of axiology.

One of the major issues in the study of values is whether value judgments express knowledge or feelings. Ordinarily we can distinguish between judgments of fact and judgments of value; however, it is difficult to separate them completely. For example, when we say that a Georgia O'Keeffe painting is beautiful, that honesty is good, and that spouse abuse is wrong, are we making assertions about things that are true or false or are we expressing preferences and making entreaties? The observable characteristics of things enter into our appraisals of values, so that if conditions change, our evaluation often changes too. In short, value judgments can be fact dependent.[3]

Philosophers do not agree on the definition of the term *value*, but in general it is possible to say that value judgments are judgments of appraisal. Beyond the basic definition problem, however, other problems exist. For example, how are people to choose the values by which they are to live? Widespread agreement has been reached in the Western philosophical tradition about the existence of certain groups of values: esthetic, economic, intellectual, moral, religious, scientific, and so on, but agreement has not been reached on the number, nature, interrelationship, or rank in a scale of values, or on the principles to be used in selecting them.

Certain principles are generally accepted in philosophical discussions on the selection of values:

1. Intrinsic values are preferred to extrinsic values. When something is intrinsically valuable, it is good in itself—that is, it is valued for its own sake and not for its capacity to lead to something else. Most things we use in our daily life have extrinsic value—that is, they are means to the attainment of other things. These two categories of values are not necessarily mutually exclusive. For example, knowledge is a good in itself but it is also a means to other good things, such as jobs.
2. Values that are productive and relatively permanent are preferred over those that are less productive and less permanent. Social, intellectual, esthetic, and religious values tend to provide us with more permanent satisfaction than do material values.
3. We ought to select our values on the basis of self-chosen ends or ideals. The values we seek should be our values, consistent with each other and with the demands that life makes on us.
4. Of two positive values, the most positive ought to be selected, and, conversely, when we are in a position where we must choose between two evils, we ought to choose the lesser one.[4]

Values clarification is not a set of rules that interfere with conscientious decision-making but rather fosters making of choices and facilitates decision making.[5] Values clarification is a dynamic process that fosters the individuals' understanding of themselves.

An important part of values clarification is the public affirmation of values that we cherish or praise and the act of standing up and being counted as an espouser of one's values.[6] This does not mean that we have the right to impose our values on others. As a profession, nursing embraces certain values, which are reflected in the Code for Nurses found in Chapter 1.[7] Nursing has social responsibilities to society that have been articulated.[8] However, not everyone thinks that nursing's collective values are voiced sufficiently.[9] Within the profession, although certain basic values tend to cement us as a group, we as individual nurses vary in our ethical stances and action.

The American Association of Colleges of Nursing undertook a national survey on preparing students as moral agents. The survey obtained data about ethical dilemmas that senior nursing students had encountered and their assessment of the adequacy of their ethics education.[10] In all the ethical dilemmas identified, questions of value underlie the dilemma. Values are operationalized during moral reasoning.[11]

One first step in dealing with the ethical dilemmas confronting us in nursing practice is to engage in values clarification. Another is to have some understanding of ethical approaches used in thinking through these dilemmas. In addition, some questions need to be considered. One such question is the following: Are socially and politically significant factors—such as gender, race, and ethnicity—morally relevant in dealing with ethical dilemmas?[12] The question will receive more attention later in this chapter.

MORAL DEVELOPMENT

We have moved into the area called *moral development* when we raise such questions as: How does a person become moral? What do we mean when we say someone is a person of principle? What factors influence the way we behave in a moral situation? Moral development has been examined and studied from a variety of perspectives: cognitive–developmental psychology, psychoanalysis, psychobiology, social learning theory, social psychology, education, clinical psychology, political psychology, and social ecology. It is concerned with a vast range of theoretical and empirical issues in child development, adult behavior, violence, altruism, criminality, cooperation, honesty, child rearing, self-control, situational variations in behavior, modeling, social and political attitudes, personality functioning, and the impact of culture on socialization, to list some major foci in the area of moral development.

During the 1960s and 1970s, Kohlberg, an American psychologist, evolved a cognitive–developmental theory of moral development. His theory has three levels of development: (1) preconventional morality, (2) conventional morality, and (3) postconventional or principled morality. According to this theory, most children under nine years of age and some adolescent and adult criminal offenders have limited moral development and are at the preconventional level. People at the conventional level of development tend to conform to and uphold the rules, expectations, and conventions of society or authority. Most adults and adolescents are at this level, according to Kohlberg. The postconventional level is reached by a minority of adults, usually only after the age of twenty. These people have differentiated themselves from the rules and expectations of others and define their values in terms of self-chosen principles.[12–16]

In Kohlberg's theory, there is a parallel between an individual's logical or cognitive stage and that person's moral stage. While logical development is a necessary condition for moral development, it is not in itself sufficient, since many individuals are at a higher logical stage than the parallel moral stage. In addition, one can reason in terms of ethical principles if one is at the postconventional level and still not live up to them. A variety of factors determines whether a particular person will live up to his or her stage of moral reasoning and development. The individual's sense of justice is what is most distinctively and fundamentally moral. One can act morally and question all rules, and one can act morally and question the greater good, but one cannot act morally and question the need for justice.

Students of human development have faced a difficult problem when examining cultural variations in moral judgment. Values found across time and space are remarkably complex and diverse. The substance of morality—the actual rules of ethical conduct, the values and mores that govern behavior—is deeply embedded in specific cultural patterns. When these scholars probe deeper and examine an abstract principle, such as justice, however, they find a more consistent pattern emerging. The structural function of values, or how a culture thinks about these principles, tends to be more stable than their content, or how the culture puts these principles into operation. Thus, values can be analyzed in terms of their common functional purposes and can be viewed as equivalents despite gross differences in specific content. Work done by Piaget and later by Kohlberg does not lend itself easily to the study of cultural variation, since these authors placed emphasis on, essentially, culturally invariant sequences. Others interested in the field of moral development have attempted to overcome this limitation and have developed a conception of moral development using a nonhierarchical typology.

An important question for us to consider is what factors influence the way we behave in a moral situation. Although it is sometimes difficult for us to come to grips with the notion that we are creatures of our environment, the difficulty increases when we examine the idea that some moral behavior is situationally influenced and perhaps determined. This is due in part to the fact that our conception of human responsibility is largely based on the assumption that the individual is responsible for his or her behavior. Nevertheless, analysis of the literature to determine whether morality is more strongly influenced by personality (beliefs, values, attitudes, etc.) than by situations has led several writers to conclude that the latter are far more powerful influences.[17]

Nowhere are the data supporting the importance of situational determinants of moral behavior more compelling than in the reality of and research in the capacity of people to inflict great harm on others. Milgram's classic experiments on obedience provide an excellent example with which to illustrate this point. Milgram conducted research on obedience and in the name of science had his study sample of students "shock" learners with increasing voltages, including one setting marked "severe shock." [18] The results of these experiments do not fit our expectations. That is, we do not expect so many people to obey the experimenter and deliver such harsh pain. Research in this area generally does not point to a relationship between personality variables and behavioral obedience; rather, it seems that the tendency to be critical minded and the possession of a high cognitive energy is related to the capacity to defy authority and to disobey.

The cumulative impact of these studies suggests that we are not always the captains of our moral ships that we would like to believe ourselves to be. Optimism comes from the fact that this research does suggest that situational factors can be arranged to maximize moral and prosocial behavior. It is conceivable that in a society or institution where situational support for prosocial behavior is strongly and consistently provided, many more people will develop the kind of moral system that no longer requires external supports.

MORAL DEVELOPMENT, WOMEN, AND CARING

In the past several years, there has been a growing body of literature that has posed a challenge to both traditional and contemporary assumptions underlying moral theory. The thesis in this new literature is that women undergo a moral development that is distinct from but parallel to that of men. The first to write on this idea that gender is an important variable in our moral life was Carol Gilligan, who studied with Kohlberg. In her book she distinguishes a morality of rights and formal reasoning, which she calls the justice perspective, from a morality of care and responsibility, or the care perspective. In the justice perspective, an autonomous moral agent discovers and applies a set of fundamental rules through the use of universal and abstract reason. In the care perspective, the central preoccupation is a responsiveness to others that dictates providing care, preventing harm, and maintaining relationships.[20] Gilligan also constructed a model of moral development but one that differs from Kohlberg's model. At the preconventional level, the orientation is toward individual survival. At the conventional level, the focus is on care and conformity and there is a concomitant desire to please others. At the postconventional level, care becomes a self-chosen principle, one that recognizes the interdependence of self and other. The individual has developed an increasing understanding of human relationships. As a self-in-relation, one attempts to maintain one's own integrity and care for one's self without neglecting others.

Within the context of feminist research and writings, Gilligan has reconceptualized women's moral perspective. Other writers have added to this literature.[21–25]

A number of nurses have also written about the importance of caring.[26–32] This is a rich literature that addresses both the gender aspects of ethical reasoning and a core value of nursing. The nursing ethics literature has been examined and classified into three categories: (1) the application of the dominant ethical theories to reason through ethical dilemmas; (2) the use of traditional moral principles and ideals to guide discussion of moral problems; and (3) the philosophical foundations approach, in which ethical issues are dealt with from the perspective of a philosophical conception of the nature of nursing.[33] The caring principle is the bedrock of this third category.

It is important to realize that justice- or principle-based ethics, caring, and virtues ethics are different concepts, but are not completely mutually exclusive categories. Fowler has shown that ethics and virtues are interrelated.[34] Gilligan, while pointing to gender differences in moral development, also makes the point that women use both the justice perspective and the care perspective.

Feminists and some nurses have criticized principle-based ethics. Care-based ethics also has its critics.[35–37] One concern about the ethics of care that requires additional examination relates to the criticism that it is too confined to the private sphere of intimate relationships and may reinforce an uncritical adherence to assigning traditional caretaker roles to women.

MORALLY RELEVANT FACTORS

The ethics of care maintains that gender is a relevant factor in defining and dealing with moral issues and ethical dilemmas. But are there others as well? Recently, the question has been probed as to whether there are other morally relevant factors in health care ethics. Some say that culture, race, and ethnicity are morally relevant factors also.[38–44] An important question for our consideration has been raised regarding cultural differences which is as follows: How can we reconcile in a non-ethnocentric fashion, the enforcement of international universal ethics and human rights standards with the protection of cultural diversity?[45] In dealing with this question, we need to think about whether there are universal ethics. In other words, do all people in all places define the ethical dilemmas, ethical principles, ethics of care, and virtues in the same way? Or do we have a situation of ethical relativism in which each culture has a way of life that is of equal validity to all others and moral claims deriving outside any particular culture have no validity within it? Relativism could mean that anything goes, that is, whatever is the norm within a society is ethical. This has obvious problems. But ethical universalism means that all cultures must value the same things, define good and harm in the same way. This too has problems. We must give much more thought to this issue and be flexible in the conceptualization, interpretation, and application of health care ethics and nursing ethics in the international arena. In addition, we will need to look for ethics and human rights cast in other than the western mold.[46, 47]

VALUE CLARIFICATION AND NURSING

It is important for nurses to examine their values and to clarify them. This can best occur in those situations in which we are honest with ourselves. We all have an idea of our selves, referred to as our self-concept. This includes our idealized selves and the values that we think we have and the ones that we really have. In addition, and importantly, there can be a discrepancy between what we value and what we do when these values are called into action.

In the past, socialization into nursing has often dealt with these questions of value by attempting to inject "proper" values into students. There was little, if any, examination of the complexity of values or of the failure to act on one's higher or idealized values. We believe that moral conflict or ethical dilemmas can provide nurses with moments in which they can grow both as moral individuals and as members of the nursing profession. Recently, many in nursing have recognized the place of values in their practice and in their ethical concerns. Indeed, in recent years we find a great deal more in the nursing literature focused on values.[48–67]

REFERENCES

1. Elliott C: Where ethics comes from and what to do about it. *Hastings Cent Rep* 22(4):28–35, 1992.
2. Steele SM, Harmon VM: *Values Clarification in Nursing.* New York: Appleton-Century-Crofts; 1979.
3. Frisch NC: Value analysis: A method for teaching nursing ethics and promoting the moral development of students. *J Nurs Educ* 26(8):328–332, 1987.

4. Fry ST: Teaching ethics in nursing curricula. *Nurs Clin North Am* 24(2):485–497, 1989.

5. Steele SM, Harmon VM: *op. cit.*, p 7.

6. Simon SB, Clark J: *Beginning Values Clarification*. San Diego: Pennant; 1975.

7. American Nurses Association: *Code for Nurses with Interpretive Statements*. Washington, DC: American Nurses Association; 1985.

8. American Nurses Association: *Nursing: Position Statement on Ethics and Human Rights*. Washington, DC: American Nurses Association; 1994.

9. Flanagin A: The ethical voice of nursing—I can't hear it, can you? *J Obstet Gynecol Neonatal Nurs* 17(3):162–163, 1988.

10. American Association of Colleges of Nursing: *Special Report: RN Baccalaureate Nursing Education* (1986–1989). Washington, DC; The American Association of Colleges of Nursing and ASHE/ERIC (HED21745); 1989.

11. Omery A: Values, moral reasoning and ethics. *Nurs Clin North Am* 24(2):499–508, 1989.

12. Davis AJ, Keonig BA: A question of policy: bioethics in a multicultural society. *Nurs Policy Forum* 2(1):6–11, 1996.

13. Kohlberg L: Stage and sequence: The cognitive–developmental approach to socialization. In Goslin DA (ed): *Handbook of Socialization Theory and Research*. Chicago: Rand McNally; 1969: pp 347–480.

14. Kohlberg L, Kramer RB: Continuities and discontinuities in childhood and adult moral development. *Hum Dev* 12(2):93–120, 1969.

15. Kohlberg L: From is to ought. In Mischel T (ed): *Cognitive Development and Epistemology*. New York: Academic Press; 1971: pp 151–235.

16. Kohlberg L, Gilligan CF: The adolescent as philosopher: The discovery of the self in a postconventional world. *Daedalus* 100:1051–1086, 1971.

17. Kohlberg L: *The Philosophy of Moral Development*. New York: Harper & Row; 1981.

18. Rosenhan DL, Moore BS, Underwood B: The social psychology of moral behavior. In Lickona T (ed): *Moral Development and Behavior*. New York: Holt, Rinehart & Winston, 1976.

19. Milgram S: Behavioral study of obedience. *J Abnorm Soc Psychol* 67:371–378, 1963.

20. Gilligan C: *In a Different Voice*. Cambridge, MA: Harvard University Press; 1982.

21. Sherwin S: *No Longer Patient: Feminist Ethics and Health Care*. Philadelphia: Temple University Press; 1992.

22. Cole EB, Coultrap-McQuin: *Explorations in Feminist Ethics*. Bloomington, IN: Indiana University Press; 1992.

23. Brabeck M (ed): *Who Cares? Theory, Research, and Educational Implications of the Ethics of Care*. New York: Praeger; 1989.

24. Gudorf CE: A feminist critique of biomedical principlism. In Du Bose ER, Hamel R, O'Connell LJ (eds): *A Matter of Principles? Ferment in U.S. Bioethics*. Valley Forge, PA: Trinity Press International; 1994.

25. Noddings N: *Caring: A Feminine Approach to Ethics and Moral Education*. Berkeley: University of California Press; 1984.

26. Benner P, Wrubel J: *The Primacy of Caring*. Menlo Park, CA: Addison-Wesley; 1989.

27. Benner P (ed): *Interpretive Phenomenology: Embodiment, Caring, and Ethics in Health and Illness*. Thousand Oaks, CA: Sage Publications; 1994.

28. Tanner C, Benner P, Chesla C, Gordon D: The phenomenology of knowing a patient. *Image J Nurs Sch* 25(4):273–280, 1993.

29. Bishop A, Scudder J: *The Practical, Moral and Personal Sense of Nursing*. Albany: State University of New York Press; 1990.

30. Watson J, Ray M (eds): *The Ethics of Care and the Ethics of Cure: Synthesis in Chronicity*. New York: National League of Nursing; 1990.

31. Cooper MC: Principle-oriented ethics and the ethics of care: A creative tension. *Adv Nurs Sci* 14(2):22–31, 1991.

32. Millette BE: Using Gilligan's framework to analyze nurses' stories of moral choices. *West J Nurs Res* 16(6):660–674, 1994.

33. Pence T: Approaches to nursing ethics. *Philos Context* 17:7–16, 1987.

34. Fowler MD: Ethics without virtue. *Heart Lung* 15(5):528–530, 1986.

35. Beauchamp TL, Childress JF: *Principles of Medical Ethics*. New York: Oxford University Press; 1994: pp 85–92.

36. Allmark P: Can there be an ethics of care? *J Med Ethics* 21(1):19–24, 1995.

37. Nelson HL: Against caring. *J Clin Ethics* 3(1):8–15, 1992.

38. Flack HE, Pellegrino ED (eds). *African-American Perspectives on Biomedical Ethics*. Washington, DC: Georgetown University Press; 1992.

39. Jecker NS, Carrese JA, Pearlman RA: Caring for patients in cross-cultural settings. *Hastings Cent Rep* 25(1):6–14, 1995.

40. Muller JH, Desmond B: Ethical dilemmas in a cross-cultural context: A Chinese example. *West J Med* 157(3):323–327, 1992.

41. Orona CJ, Koenig B, Davis AJ: Cultural aspects of nondisclosure. *Cambridge Quar Health Care Ethics* 3(3):338–346, 1994.

42. Koenig B: Cultural diversity in decision-making about care at the end of life. In *Dying, Decision-Making and Appropriate Care*. Washington, DC: Institute of Medicine, National Academy of Science; 1994, pp 1–18.

43. Carrese JA, Rhodes LA: Western bioethics on a Navajo reservation: Benefit or harm? *JAMA* 274(10):826–829, 1995.

44. Paul EF, Miller FD, Paul J: *Cultural Pluralism and Moral Knowledge*. New York: Cambridge University Press; 1994.

45. James S: Reconciling international human rights and cultural relativism: The case of female circumcision. *Bioethics* 8:1–26, 1994.

46. Renteln AD: *International Human Rights: Universalism Versus Relativism*. Newbury Park, CA: Sage Publications; 1990.

47. Kearly MC, Rigney D: Moral relativism and moral health. *Second Opinion* 20:73–83, 1995.

48. Sawyer LM: Health and human rights: Can nurses work for one and not the other? *Calif Nurse* 86:8–10, 1990.

49. Davis AJ: Professional obligations and personal values in conflict. *Am Nurse* 22(5):7, 1990.

50. Thompson JE: Values: Directional signals for life choices. *Neonat Netw* 8(4):83–84, 1990.
51. Raya A: Can knowledge be promoted and values ignored? Implications for nursing education. *J Adv Nurs* 15(5):504–509, 1990.
52. Oberle K: Measuring nurses' moral reasoning. *Nurs Ethics* 2(4):303–313, 1995.
53. Aroskar MA: Managed care and nursing values: A reflection. *Trends in Health Care, Law Ethics* 10(1–2):83–86, 1995.
54. Moss MT: Principles, values, and ethics set the stage for managed care nursing. *Nurs Econ* 13(5):276–284, 294, 1995.
55. Wurzbach ME: Long-term care nurses' moral convictions. *J Adv Nurs* 21(6):1059–1064, 1995.
56. Viens DC: The moral reasoning of nurse practitioners. *J Am Acad Nurse Pract* 7(6):277–282, 1995.
57. Rushton CH: When values conflict with obligations: Safeguards for nurses. *Ped Nurs* 21(3):260–261, 1995.
58. Sim J: Moral rights and the ethics of nursing. *Nurs Ethics* 2(1):31–40, 1995.
59. Mohr WK: Values, ideologies, and dilemmas: Professional and occupational contradictions. *J Psychosocial Nurs Mental Health Serv* 33(1):29–34, 1995.
60. Davis AJ, Stark R: Ethics of nursing and midwifery: Responding to change. *World Health Forum* 16(2):127–130, 1995.
61. Camunas C: Organizational tax status, values and nursing. *J Nurs Admin* 24(12):5–6, 1994.
62. van Aswegen E, van Niekerk K: Do we need to clarify our own values to be effective carers? *Nurs Rsa* 9(6):40–44, 1994.
63. Gournic JL: Responses of clinical nurses about what is moral in nursing. *Nurs Connections* 7(4):33–37, 1994.
64. Aroskar MA: A plea for revisiting values in nursing and health care. *J Prof Nurs* 9(5):253, 1993.
65. Seroka AM: Values clarification and ethical decision making. *Semin Nurse Manag* 2(1):8–15, 1994.
66. Gold C, Chambers, J, Dvorak EM: Ethical dilemmas in the lived experience of nursing practice. *Nurs Ethics* 2(2):131–142, 1995.

4

Selected Ethical Approaches: Theories and Concepts

Ethical issues and questions confronted nurses even before the founding of modern nursing by Florence Nightingale. Yet, the late 20th century brings new and daunting challenges. Development of new patient care technologies, cost-containment efforts, downsizing of health care organizations, and the emergence of managed care affect the nature and substance of ethical issues in the interactions of nurses, patients, and physicians as individuals and as members of an increasingly complex pluralistic society. These realities increase the responsibilities of all health professionals to make ethically supportable decisions and choices for action. Additional decision-making burdens fall on consumers of health care as well.

Nurses as both individuals and health care professionals make judgments everyday that involve human lives and have an impact on the welfare of patients, families, and others. Many of these situations involve relationships and decisions in which there are conflicts of values, priorities, and duties related to what is "good" or "right" for individuals, families, communities, and society as well as the nursing profession. Nurses encounter situations in their daily work in which ethical questions and concerns require a different order of judgment from what would commonly be considered a clinical judgment such as encouraging ambulation after surgery. Even this situation has some ethical dimensions in the broadest sense as consent of a patient with decision-making capacity is still required for ambulation. Decision-making at the end of life and the allocation of professional nursing expertise in downsizing hospitals, including intensive care units (ICUs), are additional examples of situations that require attention to ethical aspects of practice. These situations often have no ready-made answers to be found in codes of ethics or law.

A more systematic way of approaching ethical aspects of practice is required in responding to difficult decisions and choices in which ethical principles and values such as respect for persons and avoiding harm often conflict in decisions about nursing duties and obligations. Such situations confront nurses at levels ranging from the individual provider–patient encounter to levels involving organizational and public policy making for delivery of health and nursing care. An ethical approach requires the use of a reasoned process in which explicit attention is paid to the ethical aspects of nursing practice. A reliance on answers or decisions based only on gut-level feelings or past practice is not adequate when the well-being of patients and other persons is at stake.

The content of ethical decisions in nursing and health care is changing as the field of bioethics is evolving from a primary focus on philosophical theories that emphasize principles to a broader array of ethical approaches. This chapter is a brief introduction to selected ethical theories and concepts that can be considered in responding to patient care situations where the right decision is unclear and there are conflicts of nursing duties and obligations. Ethical theories and approaches presented here are virtue ethics with a focus on individual character, utilitarianism, and deontology that focus on principles, and caring as one aspect of feminist ethics with a focus on relationships and responsibilities.

The concerns of ethics have to do with examining the moral basis for our judgments and actions, our duties and obligations. Moral philosophers, beginning with Socrates, Plato, and Aristotle, have for centuries attempted to answer two major questions of ethics: What is the meaning of right and of good? What is the morally right thing to do in this particular situation? The first question is in the area of metaethics; the second is in the area of normative or applied ethics. Nurses and other health professionals are primarily concerned with the second question, concerning normative or applied ethics. Normative ethics attempts to justify one form of behavior over another, and to determine the characteristics of an action that make it right, for purposes of identifying and carrying out one's professional duties and obligations when they are unclear. Nurses often find themselves in ethical dilemmas that require choices between alternative courses of action that seem equally unattractive. Choices must be made that have significant implications for patient well-being and often the well-being of others. A decision-making framework, along with standards of nursing practice and codes of professional ethics, are helpful in reflecting on such situations and making decisions about what action(s) to take. The framework presented here contains elements that are familiar from the nursing process and adds ethical considerations in a more systematic way. These ethical elements will be discussed in more detail later in this chapter as ethical theories and concepts.

ELEMENTS OF A DECISION-MAKING FRAMEWORK

The ability to provide an ethically supportable rationale for decisions and actions is foundational to professional practice and the integrity of practitioners. The reflective decision-making framework presented here can be used in responding to the ethical questions posed by the case studies found at the end of each of the following chapters. The first task is to identify whether a situation presents an ethical dilemma or problem recognizing that the nurse–patient relationship always has ethical dimensions whether problematic or not. Three characteristics of an ethical problem are the existence of a conflict of values, obligations, loyalties, interests, or needs in a patient care situation such as disagreement about treatment between health professionals and patients or health team members and patients' family; ethical principles or values are at stake such as respect for patient autonomy, doing the least harm, or the values of caring and patient advocacy; and the situation involves the feelings and values of all key persons involved in the situation.

Once a situation is identified that constitutes an ethical problem consideration of the following elements assists with the discussion, analysis, and development of ethically supportable decisions. These elements can be adapted for use at the policy development or evaluation level as well as used for ethical problems related to individual patient care decisions. They include:

1. Review of the overall situation to identify what is going on
2. Identification of the significant facts about the patient–client, including medical, social history, decision-making capacity, existence of an advance directive for treatment
3. Identification of the parties or stakeholders involved in the situation or affected by the decision(s) that is made
4. Identification of relevant legal data
5. Identification of specific conflicts of ethical principles or values
6. Identification of possible choices, their intent, and probable consequences to the welfare of the patient(s) as the primary concern
7. Identification of practical constraints, e.g., legal, organizational, political, and economic
8. Make recommendations for action that are determined to be ethically supportable recognizing that the possible choices often have positive and negative aspects
9. Take action if you are the decision-maker and implementer of the decision(s) made
10. Review and evaluate the situation after action is taken in order to determine what was learned that will help in resolution of similar situations in patient care and related policy development

This process indicates that the methods of thinking in science and ethics are not mutually exclusive. One goes through a similar process of discernment in asking questions about the world of nature, on the one hand, and the world of ethics and values, on the other hand. The data base is different as are the variables considered but both are reflective processes that can be learned.

Different ethical theories provide different emphases and ways of reasoning in an ethically substantive way about the data gathered and may lead to the same or different decisions for action that are ethically supportable. For example, nurses frequently make decisions with and for dying patients where choices are made about withholding or withdrawing medical treatments that merely prolong suffering or they make decisions about allocation of the scarce resource of professional nursing expertise when patient care needs conflict with organizational cost-containment goals. Because these situations are often frustrating and painful to deal with, as they involve the values and feelings of all involved, a spirit of compassion and caring is necessary in making the difficult choices involved at the bedside or in policy making when ready-made answers do not exist. The first theoretical approach to be discussed focuses on the character or virtues of the decision makers.

FOCUS ON VIRTUE AND CHARACTER

For the past two decades, the bioethics literature has focused primarily on the process and content of ethical decision making with less attention to character. Now there is a resurgence of concern for the character of decision makers as well as the content and process of decision making, a traditional concern of ethics and moral philosophy. Issues of character are significant to professional practice broadly and more narrowly to development of responses to ethical issues in patient care and policy making. It can be argued that the character and integrity of nurses as individual moral agents determine or, at the very least, influence whether ethical problems are identified and how responses are developed to such problems in patient care and policy arenas. Virtues refer to particular dispositions or character traits such as integrity, trustworthiness, respectfulness, honesty, and kindness. They are evidenced by our behavior and express ethical principles such as truthfulness or respect for individuals as self-determining and as interconnected members of the human community. While the major provisions of the ANA Code for Nurses (1985) allude to virtues such as individual responsibility that are necessary for ethical nursing practice, the code acknowledges that it cannot assure the character of each individual nurse.

Philosopher of clinical ethics, James Drane, describes what he calls a virtue approach to bioethics in which he argues that considerations of character and virtue, often considered to be too subjective, do have a place in today's professional health care ethics in order to enrich a field currently characterized by a focus on right decisions and acts based on consideration of more abstract ethical principles[1]. Descriptions of character and character traits portray a way of *being* instead of a way of acting. Character has both positive and negative affective elements. The nurse who responds to a difficult patient care situation with respect, patience, and an attitude of care is described as a "good" nurse or a "good" person. Whereas the nurse who responds to the same situation with impatience and disrespect for a patient and family would not be viewed in the same way. Character, according to Drane, refers to the structure of one's personality with special attention to its ethical components. From one's way of being flows one's way of conducting the business of one's personal and professional life in ways that are identifiable and dependable over time. These two elements, nurses' ways of being and acting, are integral to the integrity of nursing practice and patient care. One's character is a source as well as the product of one's value commitments and actions. In turn, one's character and behaviors are also influenced by one's social (work) environment. This provides an argument for attention to organizational ethics in health care systems where existing power differentials between nurses, physicians, patients, and payers and differing goals for health care must be considered as part of the milieu of nursing practice and decision making.

FOCUS ON PRINCIPLES

Two ethical theories or approaches that have been emphasized in bioethics over the past few decades are deontology or Kantianism and utilitarianism. These theories are now being critiqued using the language of "principlism," that is, an overreliance on unrelated and often conflicting principles in dealing with moral problems in medicine and health care.[2] Deontology uses several principles in considering what is right while utilitarianism uses a single principle. They provide us with different ethical arguments from which to consider decisions in troubling patient care or policy development situations. They are discussed here in more detail than the other theoretical approaches because they continue to dominate the thinking of clinical ethics and health policy development implicitly or explicitly in our society.

Ethical Theory Based on Multiple Principles

The deontological or Kantian ethical approach, attributed to 18th century moral philosopher Immanuel Kant, focuses on duties and obligations.

Whether an act is right or wrong depends on more than an individual's pleasure or the consequences (utilitarianism) of the proposed action. Rightness or wrongness depends on the nature or form of these actions in terms of their inherent moral significance such as respect for persons or considerations of fairness. A deontological position requires commitment to the principle of universalizability. That is, when one makes a moral judgment in a given situation, one will make the same judgment in any similar situation regardless of time, place, or persons involved. If one judges X to be right or good in this situation, then one must judge that anything like X is right or good in any similar situation.[3] Prior to the work of philosopher W.D. Ross on ways of responding to conflicting principles and rules, Kant had acknowledged this problem of conflicting rules and principles. He stated that one should "act only on that maxim which you can at the same time will to be a universal law," the major form of his categorical imperative.[4] An example of this imperative is a nurse asking another nurse, "What if everyone did what you're doing?" when the first nurse sees the second nurse taking patient medications for her own use. Another form of the categorical imperative says that persons should always be treated as ends and never solely as means. This represents an ethical challenge to nurse researchers who use hospital patients or nursing home residents primarily as means to nursing research goals. Kant said that categorical imperatives are unconditional commands, morally necessary and obligatory under any circumstances.[5] It is one's duty to obey categorical imperatives with no exceptions. One does not focus on the consequences and there is no external authority to tell one what to do.[6] Moral significance is also attached to certain relationships. Relationships of parents and children or nurses and patients are examples of certain types of human relationships that serve as a basis for determining one's duties and obligations as a parent or a nurse in these instances.

Deontologists may focus on acts or rules to justify decisions and actions, that is, obligations in the nurse–patient relationship are based on performing certain actions or adhering to certain rules or principles that determine the "right" behavior. In act-deontology, the moral values of individual nurses are of major significance. For example, in a given patient care situation in a home setting, the moral values of the community health or home care nurse would play an important part in decisions made about kinds of information on birth control methods or cancer chemotherapies provided to a patient. According to act-deontology, one has only rules of thumb to go by. There are no identified criteria, standards, or guiding principles used in decision making as in rule-deontology. One simply gets all the facts and makes a decision. An act is made right simply by choosing it and by the individual's commitment to universalizing it.

Critics of act-deontology claim that it is not helpful in terms of moral guidance, because it is difficult to do without rules. Furthermore, one may not always have the time and energy to carefully judge each situation in and of itself.[7] Think of a busy clinic where nurse practitioners are required to see a certain number of patients per hour based on cost-containment goals rather than more patient-oriented goals.

A rule-deontologist uses established standards for choosing, judging, and reasoning morally before responding to an ethically troubling situation. The standard consists of fairly specific rules such as keeping promises or principles such as avoiding or preventing harm to the degree possible. Identified moral rules and principles provide guidance then for how we should act in a given situation—one role of professional codes. One problem with rule-deontology is that rules or principles sometimes conflict, as previously noted, and one has to decide which takes precedence over the other(s). Another problem is the exception to the rule. In dealing with these problems, Ross distinguished between actual duties and prima facie duties. He said that every rule of actual duty has exceptions, but prima facie duties have no exceptions. They are obligations that one must always try to fulfill—for example, fidelity, gratitude, and justice.[8] But what if even prima facie duties conflict with each other in a given situation? For example, if a nurse is spending most of his time caring for a critically ill patient when the patient should be in intensive care but there is no bed and staffing is inadequate, he cannot give needed nursing care to other patients on the unit. While caring faithfully for one patient, the nurse may not be providing fair and needed treatment to other patients on the unit. In complex nursing care dilemmas or in health policy development and implementation, ethical principles of respect for persons, beneficence, and justice may all be at stake or in conflict. Rule-deontology is not adequate for dealing with conflicts of what Ross identifies as prima facie duties when they conflict in such real-life situations.

Each of the three major ethical principles mentioned in previous paragraphs will now be discussed briefly. They are the principles of respect for persons, beneficence, and justice. The principle of respect for persons is broader than a principle that speaks to respect for individual autonomy and self-determination. In addition to respect for individual autonomy, it also recognizes that individuals are interrelated and interconnected members of the human community. The broader principle recognizes that many of the decisions we make as individuals affect others, directly or indirectly, and rejects an extreme ethic of individualism with its focus on individual rights.

Respect for individuals requires that each individual be treated as unique and as equal to every other individual. Special justification is required for interference with an individual's own purposes, privacy, or behavior.[9] It rules out paternalistic decisions made by health professionals for patients with decision-making capacity and requires that patients' own goals and values be taken into account in decisions about care and treatment if patients are unable to make their own decisions. Respecting persons as individuals and as interconnected community members requires consideration of duties and obligations to others as well as to one's self whether patients or professionals. Commitment to the principle of respect for persons affects whether and how ethically troubling situations are dealt with on a patient care unit and influences all of the relationships on that unit. It can be used as one ethical benchmark for evaluating nurse–patient interactions and organizational policies. In addition to considering the patient as an autonomous individual, nurses would think about patients as members of families and communities when considering their obligations as patient advocates. On this principle, nursing action or nonaction is justified on the moral basis of whether or not it enhances the uniqueness of the individual, taking into consideration the consequences of choices for significant others, rather than just using a legalistic, bureaucratic justification based on "following the doctor's orders," patient wishes, or institutional policy.

Respect for persons as a general guide to decisions and actions has consequences for individual patients, health professionals, and health care organizations. Decision making becomes a more time-consuming process in many instances. There will still be emergency situations in which health professionals will make decisions without immediate patient input based on standards of practice and ethical norms of the profession. This principle places the burden for justifying why patients should not participate in major decisions that affect them on health professionals who often automatically make decisions for patient care and treatment in the paternalistic, bureaucratic, and authoritarian structures that still exist in some health care institutions. Nurses and other health professionals such as administrators can consider respect for persons and other ethical principles in evaluating organizational structures and relationships among health professsionals that impede respectful care.

The principle of beneficence may be viewed on a spectrum extending from noninfliction of harm or nonmaleficence to benefitting others or positive beneficence. The two aspects are sometimes separated into two separate principles of nonmaleficence and beneficence. The duty not to inflict harm takes precedence over providing benefits with other things being equal in situations where the two conflict. According to moral philosopher William Frankena, both are obligations that one must try to fulfill.[10] They are always to be taken into account, even though there are other considerations that may sometimes take precedence when there is conflict about what action to take. One example is infant immunizations. Overall, they inflict some degree of short-term pain but have long-term health benefits. Or one might consider a surgical procedure that inflicts some immediate harm in order to promote a positive outcome such as saving a life, diminishing pain and suffering, or increasing mobility. Frankena points out that these principles apply to everyone and thus are universal. Philosophers Tom Beauchamp and James Childress take the position that nonmaleficence also requires moral agents such as nurses to be reflective about their decisions and actions and to follow professional standards of care as moral obligations.[11]

The beneficence principle requires the provision of benefits and a balancing of harms and benefits as well.[12] Benefits are considered to have positive value that promotes health or welfare, such as the prevention of illness or premature death. Costs, while usually thought of in financial terms, can be anything that detracts from human health and welfare, such as physical or psychological pain. Since costs are frequently not quantifiable, they are often referred to as risks. Risks refer to possible future harms. Consideration of risks and benefits in patient care decision making, human subjects research, or policy development can be considered as part of the thoughtful and careful action required by the principle of nonmaleficence. This dimension of beneficence requires assessment and balancing of trade-offs in situations where decisions are made against a background of uncertainty. Examples include balancing of the trade-offs required in development of organ transplant policies when there is a scarcity of available organs for the people who could potentially benefit or disagreements between nurses and physicians about the use of costly technologies for prolongation of life in an elderly patient when they seem to add to patient suffering with little or no hope of long-term benefit.

In situations of conflict, while the principle of beneficence does tell us to promote good while preventing or minimizing harm, it does not provide guidance as to how we are to distribute burdens and benefits when not all will benefit from the required decisions. Such decisions range from determining the number and kind of nursing home beds in a given geographic area to deciding who should get what levels of nursing care in a hospital that is downsizing or in a home care agency that provides care for people with a variety of health problems. Such decisions require attention to principles of justice.

Ideas about justice are basic to the structure of a society and to structures for delivery of nursing and health care. There are many ways of talking about justice in our pluralistic society. We do not currently have a social consensus as to what exactly constitutes justice, although it is recognized that most people have a sense of justice, and most of us could probably agree on what constitutes injustice, such as lack of access to needed health care for the uninsured.

Distributive justice is one form of justice and has to do with the distribution of goods and evils, of burdens and benefits, in any society in which resources are limited. It is a matter of comparative treatment of individuals. One needs to consider the morally relevant differences between individuals that justify differential treatment. There are several ideas as to what might serve as justification for different distribution of benefits and costs of health care to individuals or groups. These ideas include individual need, individual effort, ability to pay, societal contribution, contract, and equal shares. Age is a suggested and very controversial criterion for the distribution of benefits of health care, specifically high tech care at the end of life. Different bases for distribution are used in different contexts. For example, welfare payments are distributed on the basis of need, while jobs and promotions are usually distributed on the basis of individual achievement or merit.[13]

Individual need is commonly invoked in nursing documents such as the ANA Code for Nurses (1985) to justify the distribution of the benefits of nursing and health care. Health maintenance organizations and other types of managed care organizations use the language of medical necessity to determine plan benefits. One issue in using the concept of need as a basis for just distribution is who defines needs vis-a-vis demands, wants, or fundamental needs. A fundamental need for something such as emergency care for chest pain indicates that a person will be harmed if that thing is not obtained.

The work of philosopher John Rawls on justice as fairness and justice as the foundation of social structures provides another way of looking at a more just distribution of social goods, such as work, income, and self-respect.[14] According to Rawls, the principles of justice have to do with distribution of what he called primary goods: income, wealth, liberty, opportunity, and the bases of self-respect. His theory offers us another perspective from which to view ethical decision making and the basis for moral decisions in health care even though Rawls made no claim that his theory could be applied directly to economic or social issues in contemporary society. His ideas about justice are based on a re-thinking of the social contract theory of obligation in the Kantian tradition. The heart of the theory is the notion of the "original position" in which people come together to negotiate the principles of justice by which all are bound to live. The negotiators are rational, intelligent people who wish to pursue their own life plans in a more just society.[15]

Rawls placed these rational negotiators under the constraints of what he called a "veil of ignorance." They have knowledge and facts about general areas such as sociology, political science, and economics. They do not know any particular facts about themselves or others—for example, health status, race, sex, or socioeconomic class. The purpose of the "veil of ignorance" is to remove from the negotiations any possibility of individuals seeking to satisfy their own interests at the expense of others. This is the situation referred to as the "original position." The negotiators must favor only those principles that advance everyone's best interests. Any of the negotiators might turn out to be one of the least fortunate or less advantaged individuals in a given community.[16] In the end, the negotiators must arrive at what Rawls called "justice as fairness," because they negotiate behind the "veil of ignorance" to form the basic principles of society.

The concept of "justice as fairness" is articulated in two basic principles of justice: (1) each person is to have an equal right to the most extensive system of liberty for all; and (2) social and economic inequalities are to be arranged so that they are to the greatest benefit of the least fortunate and are attached to offices and positions open to everyone under conditions of equality of opportunity.[17] The first principle, maximizing liberty for all, has absolute priority over the second if and when the two principles conflict. Rawls also discussed five criteria for judging the "rightness" of any ethical principles: (1) *universality* (i.e., the same principles must hold for everyone in similar situations), (2) *generality* (i.e., the principles must not refer to specific people or situations, such as my mother or your marriage), (3) *publicity* (i.e., they must be known and recognized by all involved), (4) *ordering* (i.e., they must somehow order conflicting claims without resort to force), and (5) *finality* (i.e., they may override the demands of law and custom).[18] Nurses could use these criteria to examine their own moral principles used in decision making, those proposed by other health professionals, or those assumed in a policy for health care delivery to those who are uninsured.

In Rawls' theory of "justice as fairness," inequalities are allowed only to improve the condition of the least fortunate or most vulnerable—for example, children, the frail elderly, and the poor. The least advantaged then are in the normative position in society. Basic rights and obligations proceed from the notion of fairness for these disadvantaged groups. Justice as fairness to the least advantaged becomes a categorical imperative in the Kantian tradition. Rawls has provided us with a new way to look at moral problems in society generally and more specifically to examine more critically the distribution of finite economic and nursing resources in health care. Meeting health care needs in our society amid changes such as development and use of new health care technologies and rationing of health care for the poor and uninsured require attention to issues of distributive justice and Rawlsian ideas of justice as fairness. Using income inequalities and ability to pay as screening devices for access to health care is ethically unjustifiable under this view of justice.

Briefly returning to Kantian ethical theory, it does not help us with the resolution of conflict between moral principles as Ross attempts to do with the ideas of actual and prima facie duties. When one tries to apply the Kantian theory of obligation, it is difficult to separate the idea of duty and obligations from ends, purposes, wants, and needs in any given situation. For example, if the goal is to return the institutionalized mentally retarded to the community, what happens to the specific needs of a mentally retarded adult who may not be able to live outside an institution and has no family? What is a health provider's obligation or what type of health policy is required to respond to this and similar issues?

In summary, the deontological or Kantian theoretical approach focuses on the moral significance of the values of the moral agent or decision maker and on duties and obligations guided by specific rules and principles without regard to consequences. This position does not help nurses as moral agents resolve situations in which duties and obligations conflict and choices must be made. It does not resolve the dilemma for the nurse who decides to follow the rule that one should always tell the truth and realizes that the truth will undoubtedly hurt a particular patient in a given situation where the rule of telling the truth conflicts with the principle of doing no harm. Kantian ethics, however limited, does provide us with one way to consider what counts from an ethical perspective in a patient care situation where there is disagreement about medical interventions or in health policy development that has consequences for the most vulnerable. From an ethical perspective, we cannot ignore considerations of respect for persons, avoiding harm, beneficence, and justice in healthcare decision making.

Ethical Theory Based on a Single Principle

The theory of utility or utilitarianism is one form of consequentialist theory using the single principle of utility. It focuses on consequences of decisions and actions and defines "good" as happiness or pleasure and "the right" as maximizing the greatest good and least amount of harm for the greatest number of persons. Whatever maximizes utility as happiness or pleasure is to be pursued. This position assumes that one can weigh and measure harms and benefits and arrive at the greatest possible balance of good over evil for most people.

Bentham and Mill have presented the major historical arguments for the position of utility as a standard against which the rightness and wrongness of actions are to be compared. This position, sometimes known as "calculus morality," calculates the effects of all alternative actions on the general welfare of present and future generations in a given situation. Some moral philosophers distinguish between rule- and act-utilitarianism. One seeks to determine acts and rules having the greatest utility in a broad sense of usefulness, pleasure, and happiness. The agent looks at actions and rules in terms of what the consequences would be for the general welfare if everyone acted similarly in a given situation.[19] What if every hospital decided to perform heart transplants and to close its emergency room? What would be the consequences for a population group that uses an emergency room as its only source for primary care?

One is immediately faced with the problem of aggregation in this theory focused on consequences. Does this theory involve aggregation of total happiness for a few or average happiness for all? A crucial question is whether or not what one does in a particular situation contributes to the greatest general good or the least amount of harm for everyone. But how can everyone's welfare really be considered in a large and pluralistic society of millions of people or even in large hospitals or nursing homes? Critics bring up several other problems. They accuse the utilitarian of ignoring the personal nature of good as exemplified for example in truth telling and promise keeping. All actions need not be considered in light of the overall general welfare. Each individual does count as one of the aggregate in this theory but one could end up in a minority group rather than the majority when consequences are identified.

A utilitarian approach is often invoked in making decisions about the funding and delivery of health care. This is in direct conflict with the medical ethic in which everything possible is done for the individual patient. Also, some individuals or groups may accept benefits without making any sacrifices raising the "free rider" issue. Questions of justice and fairness, rights and responsibilities are not adequately addressed by utilitarianism. Utility is not the only criterion in making moral judgments. If one does add the notion of distributing the good as widely as possible through society, one adds the principle of justice to the principle of utility for making ethical judgments. This is no longer pure utilitarianism. From this point of view, utility by itself cannot be the only basic standard or first principle of right and wrong and requires consideration of at least two principles, that count from an ethical perspective, in decision making.[20]

To summarize, deontological and utilitarian traditions offer different perspectives from which moral judgments might be made and ethical problems assessed using a "principled" approach of multiple principles or a single principle. Each position has strengths and limitations when considered in the context of specific ethical dilemmas in nursing and health care delivery where ready-made responses do not exist and moral discernment is required. Kantian theory could be viewed as more sympathetic with virtue or character ethics given its consideration of persons as moral agents. Even in a theory of utility, it is hard to totally ignore the moral character of decision makers who do the aggregating and decide ultimately what counts as morally significant consequences such as in development of institutional or public policy that involves financing and delivery of health care.

FOCUS ON CARING

Today's philosophers and bioethicists offer other theoretical positions from which to look at ethical dilemmas and problems in a richer and more comprehensive way than the use of abstract principles alone, such as theoretical approaches focused on character and caring as points of departure for ethical discussion and decision making. Even in these approaches, one can discern hints of principles although the substantive content of these theories is not couched in the language of abstract principles. These perspectives also have their strengths and limitations and demonstrate that we do not have a single overarching ethical theory to explain how we identify the rightness or wrongness of decisions and actions. An ethic of caring with a focus on relationships and responsibility will be discussed here as one aspect of the broader field of feminist ethics. According to Christine Gudorf, a professor of religious studies, feminist approaches to biomedical ethics in the United States have developed primarily from women's life experiences of alienation within the health care system rather than as a critique of principlism as ethics based on abstract principles.[21]

The idea of an ethic of caring is appealing to nurses who consider the foundations of their practice to be about caring—caring for people, for the environment, for society, for the profession. Contemporary nurse philosopher Sarah Fry proposes caring as a fundamental value for the development of a theory of nursing ethics.[22] Caring, viewed as a value ". . . is of central importance in the nurse–patient relationship . . . ," is considered as ". . . a pre-condition for the care of specific entities, whether things, others, or oneself . . . ," and ". . . is identified with moral and social ideals. . . ."[23] Care for particular others is a core notion in an ethic of care according to philosopher Nel Noddings.[24] This core notion is evident in the ANA Code for Nurses (1985), which emphasizes respectful care of individuals as its major tenet. In an ethic of care, decision making focuses on identifying decisions and actions that promote and maintain relationships as an individual responsibility. Patients are viewed as unique individuals within networks of relationships rather than as isolated bodies or members of a population group— more akin to the ethical principle of respect for persons as interrelated members of the human community rather than an emphasis on individual autonomy. In health care settings, persons significant to the patient would be included in discussions and decision making under this idea of caring.

In her critique of ethical theories based on abstract principles, philosopher Susan Sherwin reminds us that Western philosophical ethics, focused on more abstract principles, was developed primarily by males who considered women to be morally inferior to themselves.[25] Moral thought was considered to need a level of generality of which most women were not capable. Psychologist Carol Gilligan's research in the early 1980s found that women bring a different focus to deliberating about moral questions. The focus is on care and responsibility in relationships rather than on the application of abstract principles such as respect for individual autonomy and justice. Ideally, according to Gilligan, moral agents, including health professionals, are concerned about both relationships and ethical principles as they make decisions and establish practices that are morally sensitive and justifiable.

From a societal and historical perspective, caring has usually been the responsibility of women in the home and workplace. That continues to be the case when one looks at the majority of caregivers for children, the chronically ill, elderly, or people with AIDS. Sherwin makes the point that ". . . most women experience the world as a complex web of interdependent relationships where responsible caring for others is implicit in their moral lives" implying that this reality must be accounted for in theoretical and applied ethics.[26] Caring as a concept or theory for discerning "right" responses in ethically troubling situations is not yet well developed and requires further philosophical, scientific, and historical work.[27] This limitation is significant for nurses and the nursing profession to consider, if caring is to serve as the basis for its professional ethic beyond nursing's current principle-based codes.

Caring focused on individuals and relationships is one aspect of feminist ethics. Another equally compelling dimension of feminist ethics is the analysis of oppression and dominance wherever they occur in relationships and social institutions. Oppression and dominance are found in relationships within health care organizations and in the ways that these organizations are structured to meet their goals. Power differentials between nurses, physicians, patients, administrators, and payers illustrate some of the relationship inequalities that exist in most health care organizations. A concern of Sherwin's is that some women may be so focused on caring for others and meeting their needs that they may even protect those who oppress them. In doing so, they maintain a morally problematic status quo. The ability to care, respect for persons, avoiding harm, and justice as fairness may all be at stake or in conflict in such morally troubling situations. This aspect of feminist ethics, as a critique of caring serving alone as an ethic, is of further import for nursing.

Nursing is still predominately a female profession and should explore both dimensions of feminist ethics in development of decision-making processes and policies in patient care situations and organizational arrangements. Additional features of feminist ethics include incorporation of efforts to develop new nonoppressive relationships and structures for political and social interaction and to incorporate more socially oriented principles such as mutuality, community, empathy, solidarity, and integrity. Gudorf maintains that we do not need to reject principles *per se* but need to connect the use of principles with an examination of the concrete situation of those who are most vulnerable or most at risk.[28] All of these aspects and values are significant to the development of an adequate nursing ethic for the new millenium. An ethical benchmark for relationships in and structures of health care financing and delivery is how they contribute to the humanity of all the participants in our health care systems—systems in which no one is exluded from decisions and deliberations based on personal characteristics such as gender, race, or socioeconomic status. Such an approach links nursing's focus on respectful care of individual clients and Florence Nightingale's focus on nursing's obligation to create healing environments with the foundational values of public health—promotion of the common good and assuring conditions in which people can be healthy. This is a very different model and starting point for considering what is "right" in an ethically problematic situation than a focus on individualism and individual rights—still a dominant value perspective in United States society and in medical care.

ETHICAL THEORIES AND CONCEPTS IN NURSING PRACTICE

This brief discussion of theoretical approaches and concepts is not meant to provide the reader with "formulas" for resolution of ethical dilemmas in practice. They do serve as examples of the ethical elements to be considered in using the decision-making framework presented at the beginning of the chapter. In complex decision-making situations where ethical concerns predominate, ethical theories and concepts may well conflict or be inadequate for the task at hand. Yet, one may find any of these theories, concepts, or a combination of them represented in health care deliberations about ethical problems whether or not they are made explicit. Ethical problems and concerns are found on a spectrum that range from morally troubling individual nurse–patient, nurse–nurse, or nurse–physician relationships to policy making for health plan benefits or for population-based health programs.

Nurses, both as individuals and in collaboration with others, may consider these theories and concepts as they deliberate and develop responses to questions of what is the morally right thing(s) to do in situations of moral conflict. A key objective is that decisions be made in a more thoughtful, reasoned way incorporating explicit attention to ethical considerations. Part of learning skills to initiate and participate in such decision-making processes and organizational structures is to gain familiarity with ethical theories and concepts in the search to determine one's professional obligations when there are no ready-made answers, confidence in developing an ethically supportable rationale for one's decisions, and the capability to understand why and what ethical and value disagreements occur in a given situation.

Nurses might also take a look at recurrent ethical dilemmas in their practice, whether service, education, research, or administration, and take action to modify or prevent them from happening in a spirit of preventive ethics. Some recurring dilemmas could be prevented from occurring at the primary level of prevention through listening, careful assessment, and education in dealing with hard choices about care and treatment in patient, colleague, and family relationships. Such ethical issues as informed consent and decision making, humane care of the terminally ill and dying, and experimentation with human subjects better lend themselves to a preventive approach when considered in non–crisis settings such as in planned ethics rounds, in the work of institutional ethics committees, and in the deliberations of review boards for protection of human subjects in clinical research. Such activities are an expression of the concept of fidelity, that is, faithfulness and commitment to patients as foundational to the nurse–patient relationship and to the integrity of the nursing profession as an essential service in society.

REFERENCES

1. Drane JF: Character and the moral life. In DuBose ER, Hamel R, O'Connell LJ (eds): *A Matter of Principles? Ferment in U.S. Bioethics*. Valley Forge, PA: Trinity Press International; 1994, pp 284–309.
2. Clouser KD, Gert B: A critique of principlism. *J Med Phil* 15(2):219–236, 1990.

3. Frankena WK: *Ethics*. 2nd ed. Englewood Cliffs, NJ: Prentice-Hall; 1973.

4. *Ibid.*, p 30.

5. Kant I: The Metaphysical Elements of Justice. *The Metaphysics of Morals, Part I.* Indianapolis: Bobbs-Merrill; 1965.

6. MacIntyre A: *A Short History of Ethics.* New York: Macmillan; 1966.

7. Frankena WK: *op. cit.*, p 24.

8. Ross D: What makes right acts right? In Sellars W, Hospers J (eds): *Readings in Ethical Theory.* Englewood Cliffs, NJ: Prentice-Hall; 1970, pp 484–485.

9. Jonsen A, Butler L: Public ethics and policy making. *Hastings Cent Rep* 5(4): 19–31, 1975.

10. Frankena WK: *op. cit.*, p 47.

11. Beauchamp TL, Childress JF: *Principles of Biomedical Ethics.* 4th ed. New York: Oxford; 1994.

12. *Ibid.*, pp 292–293.

13. *Ibid.*, p 331.

14. Rawls J: *A Theory of Justice.* Cambridge, MA: Harvard University Press; 1971.

15. *Ibid.*, pp 17–22, 62, 136–147.

16. *Ibid.*, pp 136–142.

17. *Ibid.*, p 302.

18. *Ibid.*, pp 131–135.

19. Frankena WK: *op. cit.*, pp 39–41.

20. *Ibid.*, pp 42–43.

21. Gudorf CE: A feminist critique of biomedical principlism. In Dubose ER, Hamel R, O'Connell LJ (eds): *A Matter of Principles? Ferment in U.S. Bioethics.* Valley Forge, PA: Trinity Press International; 1994, pp 164–181.

22. Fry ST: Toward a theory of nursing ethics. *Adv Nurs Sci* 11(4):9–22, 1989.

23. *Ibid.*, p 15.

24. Noddings N: *Caring: A Feminine Approach to Ethics and Moral Education.* Berkeley: University of California Press; 1984.

25. Sherwin S: *No Longer Patient: Feminist Ethics and Health Care.* Philadelphia: Temple University Press; 1992.

26. *Ibid.*, p 47.

27. Morse JM, Bottorff J, Neander W, Solberg S: Comparative analysis of conceptualizations and theories of caring. *Image J Nurse Sch* 23(2):119–126, 1991.

28. Gudorf CE: *op. cit.*, pp 168, 171.

5

Professional Ethics and Institutional Constraints in Nursing Practice

This chapter focuses on the nature of professional ethics in nursing and some of the institutional and social constraints that can act to inhibit the ethical practice of nursing. The discussion will be generally focused on those nurses who practice in hospitals, for two reasons. First, we have more data on this group, and second, over 50 percent of all employed nurses have worked in hospitals.

The overriding ethical issue for nurses, especially those working in hospitals, can best be described as one of multiple obligations coupled with the question of authority.[1] As professionals, nurses have a code that maintains that their primary ethical obligation is to the patient.[2] This, in general, means that when an ethical dilemma arises, the nurse places the patient at the center of the dilemma and seeks to discover the patient's ethical position based on deeply held values. The main question is: What does the patient think is the right thing for him or her in this situation? In some ethical dilemmas, nurses simply want to replace the physician's ethical stance with their own, without either physician or nurses having full knowledge of the patient's ethical stance.

Nurses have an ethical obligation to the patient, but they also have an ethical obligation to the physician and to the institution in which they work.[3] As professionals, nurses owe their primary ethical obligation to the patient; however, as employees, nurses also have ethical obligations to the institution and the physician. To the extent that these multiple ethical obligations mesh so that no conflict develops among them, the nurse should have a clear idea of the right action. However, when conflicts arise between or among these obligations, the nurse has an ethical dilemma.[4,5] One can argue that nurses are not professionals by certain criteria, but the important fact to remember is that many nurses define themselves as professionals with ethical obligations.

Several examples will help in understanding the concept of multiple obligations better. If the physician makes the decision to withhold information about Mr. Brown's diagnosis and prognosis on the basis of his or her best clinical judgment, but the nurses, in their best clinical judgment, believe that Mr. Brown should be given this information so that he may function as an autonomous person, the ethical dilemma involving multiple obligations has occurred. Should the nurses go along with the physician and support the decision to withhold information or should they attempt to change the situation so that Mr. Brown will know his health status and be able to plan his life accordingly? It will make a difference if there is evidence that Mr. Brown does or does not want to know this information.

Further, what should the nurse, Ms. Hyde, do in a situation where information has been withheld or distorted by the hospital authorities to prevent a legal suit by the patient's family when a mistake was made in surgery? If the family knows this information they may sue and such a legal suit, if won, can hurt the hospital's reputation and financial stability. Should Ms. Hyde go along with the hospital's definition of events that transpired in the operating room because of her obligation to her employer or should she attempt to have the patient's family told what really happened? What is the ethical thing to do regarding this patient? What is the common good?

Ethical decisions are usually made in a social context, and that context often has within it constraints that make taking an ethical stance and acting on it a complex matter. The physician has a special legal and ethical relationship with the patient, as well, but as an employee, the nurse also has obligations to the institution. This social reality of ethics makes being ethical both more difficult in many situations and more complicated. The simple answer to this problem is that the nurse should do what is right and abide by the Code for Nurses. However, an examination of any situation of multiple ethical obligations brings into sharp focus the fact that answers to ethical dilemmas are not usually so easily answered.

In the first example given above, the nurse must make a choice between the physician's decision to withhold information and the patient's right to have this information. Let us assume that the physician's stance is based on the ethical principles of nonmaleficence (do no harm) and beneficence (do good) and that he or she believes that to tell Mr. Brown would do harm, since Mr. Brown does not seem emotionally able to cope with the facts of his case. Suppose that Mr. Brown has indicated to the nurse that he has some questions about his illness and wonders if he has been told the facts. The nurse, then, becomes concerned about the ethical principle of autonomy as well as the meaning of caring in relationship with Mr. Brown and wonders if withholding information from this patient is really unethical. The nurse then takes the stance that the patient should be told. Both the nurse and the physician are acting to meet what they think is their ethical obligation to the patient. Yet, it is the nurse who confronts a situation of multiple ethical obligations, obligations to both the patient and to the physician. This is complicated by the fact that the physician is viewed as having more authority to make this type of decision because of the physician's role and clinical judgment.[6,7]

When nurses confront situations involving multiple ethical obligations, the first question is: What is the right thing to do, and in what ways can I think about this problem that may help me to know what the right action is? Along with this question, another one comes into play, which is: How far does the nurse's ethical obligation extend? If, in this situation the nurse reasons that the right thing to do is to withhold information, there is no problem of multiple ethical obligations. However, if the nurse does not agree with this decision to withhold information, the second question arises: How far and in what directions does the nurse pursue this obligation to the patient? Should the nurse tell Mr. Brown his diagnosis and prognosis? One can argue that this is the ethical and legal obligation of the physician. What if the nurse goes to the physician and explains that Mr. Brown is asking for information about his diagnosis and that she thinks that the physician should talk with Mr. Brown about this? What if the physician continues with the decision to withhold the information even after the nurse has given these additional data? Has the nurse met the ethical obligation to Mr. Brown? Should the nurse go to other sources, and, if so, which ones? Suppose the nurse goes to the head nurse, but the head nurse does nothing about the situation. Has the nurse's ethical obligation been met? All of these and similar questions stem from several questions:

1. What is the nurse's ethical obligation in those situations of multiple ethical obligations?
2. What is the extent of this obligation?
3. What ethically ought the relationship between the nurse and patient be?
4. What does it mean to be a virtuous person in this situation?
5. What is caring in this situation?

NURSING HISTORY AND ETHICS

As far as we can glean from history, the establishment of the first hospital occurred in India before the birth of Christ. Not until the Middle Ages did such institutions develop in Europe. As long as the sick remained at home, their care naturally fell to the women in their families. With the shift from the home to the hospital, the services of some attendants to care for the sick—in addition to the physicians—became a necessity. Early on in this development, two problems regarding these attendants received consideration: (1) how to secure nurses who would provide devoted service, and (2) how to train them to give this service in an efficient manner. The first concern reflects a matter of ethical or religious ideals, while the latter reflects a scientific objective. These considerations, in turn, involve many questions concerning the relationship of nurses to patients and the relationship of nurses to physicians. Both considerations for ethical ideals and scientific objectives, along with the attendant questions regarding the nursing role and how it interacts with the other roles such as the roles of the patient and the physician, remain with us today.

In the early development of these hospital attendants—who would evolve into the nursing professionals we know today—it is unclear whether they were thought of as glorified servants or viewed as professional personnel. In all probability, a mixture of both attitudes coexisted and created a confusion regarding role and function that persisted through many later periods. Women, who constitute the great majority of nurses today in the United States, did not enter nursing at this earlier period. The fact that the first nurses were men has been explained by the generally inferior status of women at that time in those places where hospitals developed. The status of women throughout the world continues to affect nursing in some crucial ways today.

Our knowledge of nursing generally goes back to the growth and spread of Christian influence in Europe. At that time, the Church held nursing in high regard and made this known by bestowing sainthood on the nursing leaders. Later, in the 16th century, secular trends in nursing began to evolve. The paucity of scientific medicine made the situation such that nurses required no training beyond what could be gained by experience as they worked in the hospital. Nursing practice was, more often than not, a matter of difficult and unpleasant routines. In the past, religious devotion had ennobled this toil and made it worthwhile, but now the religious basis for nursing practice was lacking. For more than three centuries after the Reformation, secular nursing carried with it no promise of a respectable career, and the so-called better types of women tended to avoid it. For many years, nursing was best described as a poorly paid, confining discipline of unpleasant routines, and the typical nurse was depicted as Sairey Gamp, the unpleasant, uneducated, uncouth character in Dickens' *Martin Chuzzlewit*, published in 1844.

The history of nursing in England and the United States since the mid-19th century has evolved from the reforms that Florence Nightingale instituted in nursing education and practice. She maintained that a nursing school should teach the mind as well as form the character. The latter imperative resulted in indoctrination and practice in the middle-class values of the period. Many remnants of the Victorian era and some strands from earlier times remain with us today and reflect the checkered history of nursing, which has included the images of both the saint and the immoral prostitute. One important historical study examining early American nursing points to another factor that has greatly affected the profession. This factor, the systematic oppression of the nursing profession, has affected the quality and delivery of health care.[8]

NURSING ETHICS—A BRIEF BACKGROUND

Many books on nursing ethics in the past have in large part restricted their content to professional etiquette. In 1900, the early nursing leader, Robb wrote of a breach of etiquette, but her comments reflect the sociology of the situation, including differences in role, function, and status. She remarked that occasionally we find a nurse who, through ignorance or from an increase of her self-conceit and an exaggerated idea of her importance, may overstep the boundary in her relationship with the doctor and commit some breach of etiquette. The point being driven home here is that not only will the individual nurse be made to suffer most acutely, but also her school and the profession at large come in for a share of criticism and blame.[9] Aikens, in 1937, devoted two chapters to what she called old-fashioned virtues and included in this category such items as truth in nursing reports, discreetness of speech, obedience, being teachable, respect for authority, discipline, and loyalty.[10]

Perhaps one of the most interesting books on nursing ethics, published as a fourth edition in 1943, has a chapter entitled "Master and Servant: Physicians and Nurse." The author says that if the hospital employs the nurse, she is a servant of the hospital and as such the hospital becomes responsible for her acts. With this status, any disobedience to the physician's orders is not only a matter of professional etiquette but a violation of the employee contract. In those situations in which the nurse knows that the physician is mishandling the patient's treatment, she must either continue to carry out his orders or give up the case. This latter choice seems to reflect the fact that many nurses at the time this book was written worked as private duty nurses. The author continues by pointing out that the nurse has no duty to enlighten the public on the relative merits of physicians and the value of their treatment. In short, the nurse ought to remember that she has "a duty of charity as a faithful servant to a master to protect the good name and reputation of the physician under whom she works." [11]

Some years later, another author quoted a remark made by a physician to a nursing school graduating class; he said that to be a successful nurse, one must also be a successful liar. This quote led the book's author into a discussion of loyalty as the nurse's first duty. By virtue of her profession as well as of her implied contract, the nurse owes the physician not only efficient care of patients but also such evidence of loyalty as will strengthen the patient's confidence in him.[12]

All of the above references on nursing ethics were written in this century, and some practicing nurses today read these books or ones similar to them when they were students. Among other things, such input reflects the nature of the socialization process into nursing, the role of women and nurses, and the hierarchical organization in the health care system. Many of these early ethics books delved into the private life and morality of nurses, reflecting the status of nursing students in an apprenticeship system and the stereotype of the intellectually and morally weak woman. Such concerns focused on the individual's morality, and the nurse's duties, obligations, and loyalties referred to a situation in which nurses were, on the one hand, expected to exhibit a dedication of almost a religious nature while, on the other hand, their morality was open to suspicion.[13]

THE NURSING CODE OF ETHICS

The flavor of recent publications reflects some changes in the situation but also contains some threads of continuity from these earlier concerns. The ANA Code for Nurses outlined in Chapter 1[14] makes it clear that the nurse's primary commitment is to the patient's care and safety. To fulfill this commitment, the ANA maintains that the nurse must be alert to any instance of incompetent, unethical, or illegal practices by any member of the health team and must be willing to take appropriate actions, if necessary. As to fulfilling this commitment in his or her own nursing practice, the nurse has the personal responsibility of maintaining competence in practice throughout a professional career. In addition, if a nurse does not believe himself or herself to be competent or adequately prepared to carry out a specific function, the nurse has the right and responsibility to refuse in order to protect both self and client.

Any such professional code must, by its very nature, address the general and the ideal, but in doing that it brings to the attention of practitioners the areas of ethical responsibilities, possible areas of ethical conflict, and potential mechanisms for coping with such conflict. In dealing with the general and the ideal rather than the specific and the concrete, a code can only allude to the formal and informal social systems in which practitioners function. While most professionals believe codes to be essential since they are one characteristic of a profession, some individuals have raised questions about codes.[15]

Taking into account historical factors and present realities, four central questions underlie the discussion in the remainder of this chapter. First, can nurses, employed in the bureaucratic system of the hospital, and other health facilities, be ethical as outlined in the ANA Code for Nurses? Second, if they practice according to these ethical principles, do they run any risks, and, if so, what are they? Third, do nurses have the right as well as the obligation to provide adequate, if not excellent, nursing care and are they willing and able to exercise this right? Finally, what can nurses expect from nursing in the way of support if they take an ethical stance that disrupts some aspect of the work place norms? These questions will serve to weave together the ideas in the next section on possible constraints that can function at times to inhibit ethical behavior on the part of nurses.

ORGANIZATIONAL AND SOCIAL CONSTRAINTS

One of the most interesting dimensions of hospital nursing arises in the potential for conflicting moral claims on the nurse. All nurses from top administrators to staff find themselves in situations involving multiple obligations. Until around the time of the Second World War, many, if not most, nurses in hospitals worked as private duty nurses and received a fee for their services from the patient. A number of economic and sociological factors converged in the 1930s and 1940s, and this shift away from fee for service to hospital-employee status occurred. Whereas previously the nurse's obligation had been to the one patient and the patient's physician, with this shift came a change in occupational status, and the ethics of the situation became more complex. As a hospital employee, the nurse must now balance obligations to the institution, to the attending physician and the house staff, and to the patients themselves while attempting to practice nursing using the ethics code of the profession as a guideline.

Research in the past indicated that nurses believed that their first loyalty belonged to the hospital where they worked. By and large, the potential ethical issues emerging from this situation went without discussion. In the last 20 years, numerous members of the health professions and social scientists have described the roles, role expectations, functions, and status positions of those working in hospitals as well as the social network within which these workers function. Much has been said about the interpersonal and communication problems that arise, but a great deal less has been said about ethical dilemmas except indirectly as they spin off from organizational, interpersonal, and communication problems.

As far back as 1964, one such study, which examined baccalaureate students' images of nursing, reported that these students, influenced by faculty members, came to gravitate perceptibly toward individualistic innovative views of nursing and away from bureaucratic orientations.[16] In a collection of essays, a sociologist also writing in the 1960s described the physician as having a number of different positions that simultaneously provided him with multiple statuses and freedoms from organizational control; however, he did have a quasi-contractual relationship with the hospital. The sheer power that came from the free movement accorded to the physician within an otherwise formal bureaucracy sharply contrasted with the role of the nurse, which was profoundly affected by her obligation to represent continuity of time and place. Although the patient care unit was her turf, the nurse and the doctor both knew that in any direct conflict between them they would be subject to unequal privilege within the system. The implicit threat of the doctor's use of the free-flowing communication prerogative traditionally put the nurse in a position of having to use flattery, tact, or even subterfuge in her role of coordinator between the entrepreneur and the bureaucratic system.[17]

In another early essay, reflecting the 1960s but relevant in numerous places today, Esther Lucille Brown discusses the hospital organization as a deterrent to professional nursing. She notes a number of factors including the downward communication of frequent orders, rules, and prescribed procedures issued by persons in authority; the often inadequate channels for upward communication of plans, suggestions, and complaints originating on the lower hierarchic levels of nursing; and the problems of limited lateral communication and psychological isolation can decrease initiative and motivation and encourage dependency, feelings of powerlessness, and dissatisfaction.[18]

In the mid-1970s, the experiences of seven new nurses attempting to innovate inpatient care illustrated some of these problems. They found the nursing administration authoritarian and stifling to the extent that they seemed to hamper improvement in patient care rather than encourage it. These young women asked, "When will nursing administrators let nurses practice as legally indicated in their state's Nurse Practice Act?" [19]

The question for us here in this era of managed care, diminished fee-for-service, and downsizing are whether these sociological realities of only a few decades ago are still with us and if so, to what extent and in what degree? Importantly, what if any, differences do these changes make in the nurse's role and ethics?

Nurses traditionally have helped doctors in scientific tasks and also helped overcome inadequacies in the scientific method of practicing medicine. Essentially, the nurse has done this by helping to prevent knowledge concerning ambiguities, uncertainties, and errors from reaching the patient and the family. The nurse has been expected to react with moral passivity to knowledge of hospital events. If the nurses had been perceived as full-fledged professional peers of the physician they would, conceivably, have taken a more active moral stand, whereas they have served more as a sponge and a buffer in the system.

Professionals are part of a moral community. They have social links not only to their clients and colleagues in their own profession but also to other groups with whose activities their skills must dovetail. Furthermore, the legitimacy of their professional contribution must be acknowledged by these other groups. By comparison to the professions, semiprofessional groups, which some believe nursing to be, are more bureaucratic and subject to numerous rules governing not just the central work tasks, but extraneous details of conduct on the job. Semiprofessionals do not have a strong reference group orientation to colleagues and do not tend to see the generalized colleague group as a source of norms. Therefore, they become more willing to accept an administrative superior as such a source. One reason given for this pattern in the semiprofessions has been the prevalence of women, who have been seen to be more amenable to administrative control than men, less conscious of organizational status, and more submissive in this context than men. Such constraints do not tend to make for job satisfaction and can compound already existing ethical dilemmas.

A 1977 survey illustrates this point. Out of 10,000 nurses throughout the country who responded to this survey, 3,800 said that they would not want to be a patient in the hospitals where they worked.[20] Not only did these findings raise serious questions about the quality of hospital care, they shocked some leaders of the nation's hospital industry. Specifically, the survey reported that 18 percent of the respondents said that they knew of deaths caused accidentally by nurses, and 42 percent said that they knew of deaths caused by doctors. Of these nurses, 4 percent reported that they themselves had made mistakes that they believed had led to a patient's death. These findings raise a host of questions regarding the ethical issues in these situations. Such questions come to mind as: How were these situations dealt with ethically? Were formal or informal institutional mechanisms available to consider the ethical aspects of these problem situations? With today's emphasis on out-of-hospital care, the concerns remain, especially in light of the fact that in some instances people with less preparation are replacing nurses in hospitals and other care facilities for economic reasons.[21]

One typical situation reported by a nurse in this 1977 survey told of a shortage of nursing personnel on the evening shift in the intensive care unit, where the nurse had responsibility for six patients on ventilators in three separate rooms. This nurse spent about fifteen minutes with one patient who was hemorrhaging and then returned to another room where the patient had accidentally disconnected himself from the machine, arrested, and died. This incident raised the question of human resources and staffing in an area where, by definition, critically ill patients require close attention. What obligation does the nurse have to voice her concern regarding the ethical or legal aspects of this situation? Where would she go with such a concern? Does the nursing service leadership have a moral obligation to try to prevent such an occurrence? One central question basic to all the others has to do with the nature and extent of the professional colleagueship that nurses have with one another and with the nursing service hierarchy. If one nurse raises questions that examine the ethical issues involved in a given situation, whom, if anyone, can he or she rely on for support in the attempt to practice according to the ANA Code for Nurses? What formal channels need the nurse go through in order to have concerns heard and seriously considered? At the core of these questions lies the larger question of whether nurses have professional, collegial relationships with one another in the work place and whether such a social network can function to provide an arena in which ethical dilemmas can be discussed.[22] As part of this larger question, the role of the nursing leadership must be examined. Given the continuing bureaucratic structure of health care facilities, what can the nursing leadership in a given facility do to implement the ANA Code for Nurses? How does this leadership view the obligations and rights of the staff nurse? An important question that has not received sufficient attention asks: to whom does the nurse administrator owe a primary ethical obligation?

Another finding of this survey suggests that the doctor–nurse game, first described three decades ago in what is now a classic essay, continues to be a factor in the daily routine and decision making.[23,24] One nurse put it this way: "The conflict itself is not so upsetting as the fact that the patient may have to wait hours or a day before the doctor eventually gets around to ordering what the nurse suggested should be done." A lack of effective communication between doctors and nurses can be a significant factor in explaining poor patient care. Nurses have power when it comes to making decisions about their patients, but they must never seem to be giving advice to the doctor. Nurses sometimes pretend they never made diagnoses, although their diagnoses are crucial to the patients' lives.[25]

Numerous earlier studies indicate that nurses perceive physicians as more deficient in communication and participation-encouraging behavior than in directive behaviors. The desired change in physician leadership patterns appears to require change not only in interprofessional behavior but also throughout the health care system of hospital organization.[26] As a matter of fact, doctors have not enjoyed a good reputation in their relationships with co-workers. They have tended to regard others as working for them and not for the patient. Despite this delegation of tasks, doctors continue to feel a final medical responsibility, including ethical and legal aspects, for all that happens to their patients.

Considerable evidence has been gathered to indicate that the doctor–nurse relationship has been characterized by a fair amount of medical authoritarianism, on the one hand, and nursing's acceptance of dependence or even deference, on the other.[27] This led to the belief among many nurses that the most fundamental problem in nursing is its status as a woman's occupation in a male-dominated culture. Even the administrative positions in nursing generally are available only with approval of the male-dominated systems in medicine and hospital administration. Historically, the subordination of women and the sex segregation of nursing and medicine helped to establish interactional patterns between the two professions that included subordination of nurses as well as informal doctor–nurse games. Reinforced by hospital training schools and the state laws that restricted the roles of nurses, these patterns led to stereotyped communication and interaction between nurses and physicians, and this in turn has been a barrier to the full use of the knowledge and skills of nurses. In nursing, those with ambitions for advancement have historically left the bedside, since only by removing themselves from direct clinical involvement could they gain any feeling of autonomy. Certain practice patterns, such as primary care nursing, seem to be changing this drain from the bedside. In addition, there are magnet hospitals that draw and keep nurses because they experience job satisfaction. The study on these hospitals identified elements that drew and kept nurses. These elements were in the areas of management, professional practice, and education. Essentially, these hospitals were democratic and encouraged input from everyone including discussions of ethical issues.[28,29]

The health services industry has been unusual in that most of the skilled and unskilled workers are women, although the industry is largely controlled by men. Health service occupations are organized like craft unions, with rigid hierarchic separation and control by the top occupation. Conflicts occurring between men and women, between management and workers, often get played out as conflicts between occupations. Because this occupational and sexual segregation overlap, conflict usually revolves around the shape and structure of the occupation and can best be characterized as maneuvering for turf, or, put another way, for control of occupational territory. These conflicts can themselves have an impact on ethical problems. They can both create and obscure ethical issues.

A number of factors come together to maintain the situation referred to above. In the past, nursing has drawn into its ranks young women who have had a traditional view of the female role. The picture that emerged was that of conventionally oriented young women who were much more heavily invested in traditional feminine life goals than in career pursuits and reluctant to make more than incidental concessions toward professional involvement. Today some nurses still view nursing as a job and not as a career or a profession. But for many women in nursing and other professions as well, various factors emerge that make fully enacting a professional role problematic. The work world has been, for the most part, geared to men and not to women, who often have different and greater home responsibilities. This reminds us too that not only do we often lack good child care facilities, but men have been socialized to hold certain ideas about themselves and their wives regarding their respective roles both in the home and outside of it.

At a 1975 research conference, Hall reported on findings from a study in which she compared female nursing students with female medical students. Again, the study found the nursing students expressed a more traditional view of the female role and lacked a career commitment.[30] In short, up to that time, nursing had mostly attracted women with a traditional view of their role, and this has had serious consequences for nursing and has served to maintain the status quo in the decision-making arrangements within hospitals. Some earlier studies also make this point regarding maintenance of the status quo. Whether this continues to be the picture at the present time or not is difficult to say. However, the fact remains that many

1975 nursing students are still active in the work force today. Certainly more nurses have obtained more education in the last two decades. In addition, fewer nurses work in hospitals than previously reported. Advanced practice roles and many more clinical settings have become available and this is likely to increase with managed care. More nurses may work in community health or home health than in hospitals in the near future as a result of health care reform. All of these factors may mean that more nurses will develop more career commitments.[31]

The official view of the nursing profession has been that nurses will habitually defend the well-being of the patient as they see it and strive to maintain the standards of the profession. Early studies surely count among implications the idea that professional relationships between nurse and doctors may exert a limiting effect upon the nurses' resourcefulness and, in some cases, increase the hazard to which the patients undergoing treatment are exposed. The trust and efficiency that nurses demonstrate are qualities that, in their place, can be of inestimable value to physicians and patients. Obviously, the nursing and medical professions need to find ways in which these and other traditional values can be reconciled with nurses' fuller exercise of their intellectual and ethical potentialities.

Before completing this discussion on organizational and social constraints, special notice must be given to the concept of paternalism. In his essay *On Liberty*, Mill wrote that ". . . the sole end for which mankind are warranted, individually or collectively, in interfering with the liberty or action of any of their number, is self-protection. . . . He cannot rightfully be compelled to do or forbear because it will be better for him to do so, because it will make him happier, because, in the opinion of others to do so would be wise, or even right." [32] What Mill is essentially saying is that we cannot advance the interests of the individual by compulsion, or, if we attempt to do so, the evil involved outweighs the good done. Mill believed that the individual person could best serve as judge and appraiser of his own welfare, interests, needs, and so forth. Others, including fellow utilitarians, have vigorously attacked this claim on the grounds that little proof exists to indicate that most adults are well acquainted with their own interests.[33]

Paternalism can be thought of as the use of coercion to achieve a good that is not recognized as such by those individuals for whom the good is intended. Because coercing a person for his or her own good denies him or her a status as an individual entity, Mill strongly objected to paternalism and did so in absolute terms. To be able to choose is a good that is independent of the wisdom of what is chosen, or, as Mill put it, a person's mode of laying out his or her existence is the best, not because it is the best in itself, but because it is his or her own mode. Mill's position has some problems in it, which remain beyond the scope of this discussion; however, for him paternalism became justified only to preserve a wider range of freedom for the individual in question.

The concept of paternalism, as used in the health care ethics literature, most often refers to the attitudes and behaviors of the physician toward the patient. However, Ashley, in her historical study mentioned earlier, documented that paternalism on the part of doctors and hospitals has resulted in serious and systematic injustice against women in the health sciences that has been both morally indefensible and socially damaging. Medicine and nursing have not constituted a complementary pair of professional groups sharing common interests and goals.[34]

Although the two professions developed in close proximity, this has not often resulted in cooperative activity for the good of the patient. In large part, this situation resulted from the paternalism in medicine—paternalism, in this case, laced with prestige and power. During the 1980s, an example of medical paternalism can be found in the American Medical Association's attempt to create a new category of worker, the Registered Care Technician, to combat the impact from the nursing shortage. This action was undertaken in a unilateral fashion without consultation with the ANA. Such a situation placed the nursing association on the defensive and caused it to spend time, money, and energy on trying to defeat the establishment of this new worker in the clinical setting.

Until recently, the major factor that caused nurses to leave nursing was undesirable working conditions. Specifically, these undesirable conditions included a lack of administrative support by hospital and nursing service administrators. When conflicts arise between a nurse and a physician, the administrators frequently side with the physician and do not support nurses. Lack of autonomy, inflexibility of working hours, and being pulled from a familiar unit to be placed temporarily on a short-staffed unit are also indicative of the lack of administrative support. Other difficulties included child and family schedules, frequent overtime with no additional compensation, and low salaries. The important factor driving people out of nursing has been the tension of not having a say over their own actions and not having confidence that patients were receiving safe care.[35,36] In 1981, the National Commission on Nursing conducted public hearings and published a report. Four of the five problems most frequently mentioned were: (1) the status and image of nursing; (2) the effective management of nursing resources including staffing, scheduling, and salary; (3) the relationship among nursing staff, medical staff, and hospital administration; and (4) the maturing of nursing as a self-determining profession.[37]

These conditions that lead to job dissatisfaction for nurses raise many questions about the ethics of care, as well as questions about the ethical obligations of nurse administrators as mentioned earlier. At the base line, the central question has to do with the multiple ethical obligations that nursing administrators confront and how they deal with them. What are the administrator's ethical obligations toward the nursing staff and how can these be met in the hospital environment?[38,39] In addition, is there support not only from the administration but from nursing peers as well? This raises the question as to how nurses can work together professionally to deal effectively with ethical dilemmas that arise in their daily practice.[40]

This chapter has raised questions on the possible organizational and social constraints in hospitals and other facilities that may act to impede the ethical practice of nursing. Several interrelated themes have been developed and include the role and social position of the physician and the nurse in the facility's social system, the bureaucratic nature of that system, the role and power of the nursing leadership in the system, sexism, and paternalism. In addition, the traditional female sex role socialization, which may have been reinforced by some nursing school values, favors passivity in many matters, including those of an ethical nature. In the extreme, it leads to the Nazi mentality, where one does a good job by simply following orders. All of these factors combine to maintain the status quo.

The crucial questions for the nurse concerning ethical dilemmas are: Given these factors, can the nurse be ethical? Is one factor the task of becoming aware of the ethical, as well as the clinical, aspects of nursing situations? Does one need to think through one's own values and ethical stances? What in the system can help the nurses to act on their values and ethical stances? Would a formal mechanism of staff discussion help? Could some structural mechanisms be developed to provide colleagueship within the nursing ranks and between the staff and the leadership levels? Do nurses have a right as well as an obligation to attempt to practice according to the ANA Code for Nurses? Do they want to invest that much? The remainder of this book assumes that nurses do want to be guided by moral considerations in their professional activities, and to that end the following chapters discuss some central ethical dilemmas and nursing practice. But first, a brief discussion of advocacy and formal mechanisms as an arena in which ethical dilemmas can be discussed is useful.

ADVOCACY

Beginning in the 1970s, nursing began an extensive discussion focused on nurses as the patient's advocate. The ethical responsibility of this role is to see that the patient's rights and interests are protected in health care settings. The earliest articles on this topic suggested that advocacy means informing patients about their rights, providing facts about their health care situation, and supporting them in the decisions that they make.[41-43] This definition of the advocacy role has been further developed by several authors.[44-47] Two themes have commingled in these discussions. First, the protection of patients' rights, and second, advancement of the nursing profession, have come together and in so doing have raised some questions such as the following: Are nurses assertive enough to take on such a role? Do nurses provide organized support for the idea of patient rights and do students learn the act of advocacy in nursing schools? Does the power structures found in health care facilities prevent nurses from identifying unethical and unsafe practices by instilling a fear of reprisal?

Several models of advocacy have been noted in the literature.[48-49] The usual one referred to above essentially says that in order for the patient to act as an autonomous moral agent, the nurse must be autonomous also. All nurses and students preparing to be nurses need to think about this claim that nursing has made. Is it a useful model? Is "the good" for patients contingent on "the good" for nursing?

In this advocacy model a subtext is that of whistle blowing.[50-52] If nurses have the ethical responsibility to protect patients' rights then they must at times report the incompetent or unethical actions performed by colleagues.

In this era, professional autonomy for all health care professionals is being increasingly limited and more emphasis is being placed on the common good as opposed to the patient's autonomy. The challenge is to reach a balance between these two concepts. In addition, nurses may find themselves working more and more outside the traditional settings, which may dramatically change work place dynamics. An examination of such ideals as patient advocacy and whistle blowing are in need of extensive reexamination and a more sophisticated rendering or replacement to carry nursing into the 21st century.

MECHANISMS FOR DISCUSSING DILEMMAS

Ethics rounds are an excellent medium in which to discuss ethical dilemmas. These rounds are similar to any other nursing or medical rounds, except that the clinical data become background material necessary to focus on the ethical dilemmas. The various formats for and possible participants in ethics rounds have been discussed in earlier publications when this idea was new.[53] Every health care facility interested in having ethics rounds will need to work out the details to fit its particular situation.

Many hospitals and other health facilities have an ethics committee established to deal with those clinical ethical dilemmas that have not been worked out at the ward level. From observation of such committees, it is apparent that they function most effectively when a variety of people are members. Such categories of health professionals as hospital administrator, lawyer, nurse, physician, hospital chaplain, social worker, and bioethicist, if one is available, together bring a wealth of information and perspectives to the issue at hand. The extent to which an ethics committee will be effective will depend on the chair and members, whether the committee itself and others take the committee seriously, and how the committee meets its charge. Such a committee is one obvious place of interaction between the ethical and the political.

In addition to the development of a clinical ethics committee, some institutions have also established a nursing ethics group to address the ethical issues of nursing practice. Such a forum examines ethical problems that relate specifically to nursing and explores ethical choices nurses consider and make on a daily basis.

If your place of work does not have a clinical ethics committee or has one without nursing representation, you and some of your colleagues may want to change that. Also you may find a nursing ethics group a useful arena in which to discuss the nursing ethical dilemmas you confront.[54]

Suggested Questions for Discussion

1. Should an agitated psychiatric patient be given the maximum dose of a medication to calm him? He is keeping other patients awake and is disrupting the ward routine, preventing the staff from getting their work done.

2. Should the nurse call a physician in the middle of the night about a patient's complaint of severe gastric pain? The nurse knows the physician will be angry about being awakened.

3. Should an alert, frail, elderly woman who wants to walk in the busy hall be tied in her chair for her own safety? Last week she fell and the institution is vary wary of liability related to patient injuries.

4. Should the newly graduated nurse refuse to give a drug ordered by the medical chief of service? According to her information, the patient is receiving another drug that may interact with this one and possibly produce negative side effects.

5. Should the staff nurse report the charge nurse for what the staff nurse believes to be an infraction of confidentiality?

6. When a medical mistake is made in the operating room and the patient dies as a result, the family is told the patient died of the disease and that the surgical team did all it could to save the patient. What should the scrub nurse, who was in the sterile field when the mistake occurred, do?

7. The nurse does not like the patient because he is so difficult and acts in such a terrible way to his family and to the hospital staff. She finds it really hard to give him even basic nursing care and just wants to do as little as possible and leave his room. What should the nurse do?

8. The nurse is a member of a collective barganing unit who has called a strike against the hospital. The nurse disagrees with the unions approach and its issues. What should the nurse do?

9. A neurological intensive care nurse must care for a brain dead patient whose organs will soon be harvested for transplantation. What meaning does the nurse place on this caring experience?

10. The mother of an AIDS patient knows that her son is seriously ill but does not know the diagnosis. One day she asks the nurse if he is dying saying she is afraid he has leukemia. What should the nurse do?

REFERENCES

1. Murphy P: Clinical ethics: Must nurses be forever in the middle. *Missouri Nurse* 63(5):6, 16, 1994.
2. Davis AJ: The sources of a practice code of ethics for nurses. *J Adv Nurs* 16(11): 1358–1362, 1991.
3. Smith S: When ethics and orders conflict. *RN* 54(9):61–62, 64, 66, 1991.
4. Kuhn JE: A nurse's right to refuse a patient care assignment. *AORN J* 62(3): 412–414, 416, 418, 1995.
5. Bosek MS: Disregarding a physician's order: Insurrection or compassion? *Medsurg Nurs* 4(5):396–397, 400, 1995.
6. Grundstein-Amado R: Differences in ethical decision-making processes among nurses and doctors. *J Adv Nurs* 17(2):129–137, 1992.
7. Gallagher A: Medical and nursing ethics: Never the twain? *Nurs Ethics* 2(2): 95–101, 1995.
8. Ashley JA: *Hospitals, Paternalism, and the Role of the Nurse.* New York: Teacher's College Press; 1976.
9. Robb IH: *Nursing Ethics.* Cleveland: Koeckert; 1900.
10. Aikens CA: *Studies in Ethics for Nurses.* 4th ed. Philadelphia: Saunders; 1937.
11. Moore DTV: *Principles of Ethics.* 4th ed. Philadelphia: Lippincott; 1943.
12. McAllister JB: *Ethics with Special Application to the Medical and Nursing Professions,* 2nd ed. Philadelphia: Saunders; 1955.
13. Deloughery GL, Gebbie KM: *Political Dynamics: Impact on Nurses and Nursing,* St. Louis: Mosby; 1975.
14. American Nurses Association. *Code for Nurses with Interpretive Statements.* Washington, DC: American Nurses Association; 1986.
15. Tadd V: Professional codes: An exercise in tokenism? *Nurs Ethics* 1(1):15–23, 1994.
16. Davis F, Olesen VL: Baccalaureate students' images of nursing. *Nurs Res* 13:8–15, 1964.
17. Mauksch HO: The organizational context of nursing practice. In Davis F (ed): *The Nursing Profession: Five Sociological Essays.* New York: Wiley; 1966, pp 109–137.
18. Brown EL: Nursing and patient care. In Davis F (ed): *The Nursing Profession: Five Sociological Essays.* New York: Wiley; 1966, pp 176–203.

19. Genn N: Where can nurses practice as they're taught? *Am J Nurs* 74: 2212–2215, 1974.
20. Hospital nurses in a poll report needless death. *New York Times* Jan 9, 1977, p 21.
21. Bantz D, Wieske A, Horowitz J: Perspectives of practicing nurses on ethical issues in health care economics. *Nurs Economics* 13(6):362–366, 1995.
22. Girouard SA: An obligation to intra-professional ethics. *Am Nurse* 26(3):4, 1994.
23. Stein, LI: The doctor-nurse game. *Arch Gen Psychiatry* 16(6):699–703, 1967.
24. Marsden C: Ethics of the "doctor-nurse game." *Heart Lung* 19(4):422–424, 1990.
25. Caswell D, Cryer HG: Case study: When the nurse and physician don't agree. *J Cardiovasc Nurs* 9(3):30–41, 1995.
26. Bates B: Doctor and nurse: Changing roles and relations. *N Engl J Med* 283(3): 129–134, 1970.
27. Bates B: Chamberlin RW: Physician leadership as perceived by nurses. *Nurs Res* 19(6):534–539, 1970.
28. McClure ML, Poulin MA, Sovie MD, Wandelt MA: *Magnet Hospitals.* Kansas City, MO: Am Academy of Nurs; 1983.
29. Corley MC, Raines DA: Environments that support ethical nursing practice. *AWHONNs Clin Issues in Perinat Womens Health Nurs* 4(4):611–619, 1993.
30. Hall B: *Comparative study of female nursing students and female medical students.* Paper presented at Western Interstate Council of Higher Education in Nsg. Research Conference, Phoenix, AZ, Spring 1975.
31. Davis AJ: Dilemmas in alternative care settings. *West J Nurs Res* 13(5):650–652, 1991.
32. Mill JS: *On Liberty.* Indianapolis, IN: Hackett Publishing; 1978.
33. Hart HLA: *Law, Liberty & Morality.* Stanford, CA: Stanford University Press; 1963.
34. Liaschenko J: Artificial personhood: Nursing ethics in a medical world. *Nurs Ethics* 2(3):185–196, 1995.
35. Kendrick K: Accountability in practice. *Prof Nurse* 10(7):1–4, 1995.
36. Hardingham LB: Ethics in the workplace. Soul and spirit: Where should moral leadership in nursing come from? *AARN News Letter* 51(4):21, 1995.
37. National Commission on Nursing: *Initial Report and Preliminary Recommendations.* Chicago: Hospital Research and Educational Trust; 1981, p 10.
38. Aroskar, MA: The challenge of ethical leadership in nursing. *J Prof Nurs* 10(5): 270, 1994.
39. Cassells JM: Administrative strategies to support staff nurses as moral agents in clinical practice. *Nurs Connections* 3(4):31–37, 1990.
40. Hardingham LB: Ethics in the workplace. Professional autonomy: Nurses as autonomous agents. *AARN News Letter* 51(3):10–11, 1995.
41. Kohnke MF: The nurse as advocate. *Am J Nurs* 80(11):2038–2040, 1980.
42. Annas GJ: The patient rights advocate: Can nurses fill the role? *Supervisor Nurse* 5(7):20–25, 1974.
43. Trandel-Korenchuk D, Trandel-Korenchuk K: Nursing advocacy of patients' rights: Myth or reality? *Nurse Practitioner* 8(4):37, 40–42, 1983.
44. Morrison A: The nurse's role in relation to advocacy. *Nurs Stand* 5(41):37–40, 1991.

45. Rushton CH: Creating an ethical practice environment: A focus on advocacy. *Crit Care Nurs Clinics North Am* 7(2):387–397, 1995.
46. Gaylord N, Grace P: Nursing advocacy: An ethic of practice. *Nurs Ethics* 2(1):11–18, 1995.
47. Oddi LF, Cassidy VR, Fisher C: Nurses' sensitivity to the ethical aspects of clinical practice. *Nurs Ethics* 2(3):197–209, 1995.
48. Bernal EW: The nurse as patient advocate. *Hastings Cent Rep* 22(4):18–23, 1992.
49. Sellin SC: Out on a limb: A qualitative study of patient advocacy in institutional nursing. *Nurs Ethics* 2(1):19–29, 1995.
50. DiMotto J: Whistle blowing: Seven tips for reporting unsafe conduct. *Nurs Quality Connection* 4(4):8, 12, 1995.
51. Haddad AM: Whistle blowing in the OR: The ethical implications. *Today's OR Nurse* 13(3):30–33, 1991.
52. Bosek MS: Whistle blowing: An act of advocacy. *Med Surg Nurs* 2(6):480–482, 1993.
53. Davis AJ: Helping your staff address ethical dilemmas. *J Nurs Admin* 12(2):9–13, 1982.
54. Pence T, Cantrall J (eds): *Ethics in Nursing: An Anthology.* New York: National League for Nursing; 1990.

6

Rights, Responsibilities, and Health Care

Rights *and* responsibilities of both patients and nurses are of concern to nurses as they seek to meet individual needs and to act as patient advocates in health care organizations where cost containment is currently a major goal. One dimension of cost containment that is not yet widely recognized is that taking patient rights such as self-determination seriously through patient involvement in treatment decision making gives better patient outcomes while using fewer resources.[1] Nurses and nursing services are key players in such efforts.

The focus for the past two decades has been on patient rights, with little attention paid to patient responsibilities. An increasing emphasis on patient responsibilities and obligations in policy proposals has caused this focus to shift to some degree. One example is the emphasis on personal responsibility for one's health and for moderation of health risks that can be changed through choices of healthy behaviors and life styles. More attention is also being paid to the rights, as well as responsibilities, of nurses and how they are linked with the enhancement of quality patient care and a sense of moral adequacy in practice.[2]

The ANA Code for Nurses with Interpretive Statements (1985) uses the language of rights. These include safeguarding "the client's right to privacy," a major value in our individualistic society. This right is interpreted as an inalienable right of all persons and is considered to be a basic human right in health care. Several client rights are mentioned in the interpretation of Statement I in the Code, which addresses nurses' obligations to provide client services based on respect for human dignity and the uniqueness of the client. Clients as individuals have moral rights to determine what will be done with their own bodies, to be given information that is necessary for making decisions, to be told the possible effects of care (including nursing care), and to accept, refuse, or terminate medical treatment. Nursing views of rights are far reaching. They have implications for nursing interventions and for the advocate role claimed by nurses. They must also be considered in the wider context of "rights" discussions, a focus on primary prevention, and the increasing emphasis on personal responsibility for one's health, recognizing that the use of "rights" language is often confusing because there are many ideas about "rights."

CONCEPTS OF RIGHTS

Rights and obligations of individual persons emerge within the relationships of a human community. Our society has changed dramatically during the past two centuries from a society that emphasized the obligations of citizens to one that has focused more recently on the rights of citizens and the protection of these rights. The list of individual rights claimed in today's world is almost endless. *Rights*, as entitlements, are claimed to privacy, to life, to death, to a healthy environment, and to health care. Special rights *of* various groups, such as children, the poor, the dying, and the elderly are also claimed. One explanation for more emphasis over the past few decades on rights in health care derives in part from an atmosphere in health care delivery organizations that is often intimidating, paternalistic, and disrespectful of patients in the decision-making process. Rights language may also be used to indicate areas in our society where social change is needed in order to move toward a more just system, as in claims of rights to health care.

There are many views about what constitutes a right and about different types of rights. Yet, the underlying notion of rights is grounded in respect for persons within a social context. Philosopher Bertram Bandman, in writing about human rights, said that they are moral rights of fundamental importance. They are more important than any other rights and are shared equally by all human beings. If one is deprived of human rights, there is a grave affront to justice.[3] Many human rights are stated in the negative rather than as positive rights to something. An example of a negative right is the right not to be tortured. The claim of a right to the benefits of health care is stated as a positive right. Negative rights, such as the right not to be interfered with, are generally considered to be stronger than claims of positive rights.

Another view of rights says that individuals derive rights from natural law, which has its source in the Greek tradition of justice—that is, the law of the cosmos as necessary, inevitable, and eternal to be discovered through reasoning. This divinely ordered Platonic universe eventually merged with the Judaic concept of the world where natural rights are created by God, the lawgiver. Natural law as a source of rights says that there are universal, and inalienable rights of persons as part of nature.[4] The origin of rights in this tradition is grounded in metaphysics and theology. Some authors claim that the only way to know what these alleged natural rights are is through the use of human reason. Others appeal to divine revelation. Both appeal to the idea that rights are discovered rather than created by human beings in a social context.

A more modern world view maintains that rights are derived from the state and created by law—a more limited and legalistic view of rights. While documents such as the United Nations Declaration of Human Rights claim that there are fundamental human rights, including health-related rights, which all people should enjoy, the assertion of rights does not mean they exist automatically in the legal sense or that they are exercised in a society. Many concepts of rights such as women's rights or rights to health care are entwined with a given social system and its legal subsystem, since rights may be defined as legitimate claims to something, such as protection of privacy, and claims against someone or something. An example is that the claim to protect privacy could be made against a health services organization or an individual within that organization.

RIGHTS AND OBLIGATIONS IN HEALTH CARE

Legally, a right has to do with the power of an individual to change something or to keep it the same, such as a contractual relationship for health care benefits in a managed care organization. Distinguishing rights from claims, because they are often confused, William Curran, an expert in health law, suggests that a claim is a right governing the actions of another person in relation to one's person or property. An example of such a claim is an individual's right not to be assaulted by a physician while receiving medical care and treatment.[5] The other side of a claim is a duty or an obligation. In the example given, the physician has the obligation not to assault the patient and a duty to avoid harm; a patient has a right to safe nursing care while in the hospital and the nurses employed by the hospital have a corresponding legal and moral obligation to provide safe care. This notion of rights is distinct from a privilege, which is a benefit or advantage given to you by someone else such as membership in an exclusive club. In claiming a legal right, one must seek an answer to questions of whether or not something is actually endangered, such as one's person or property, and who, if anyone, has an obligation to honor the claim.

The Constitution of the United States sets forth what people may generally expect from the federal government, such as the purposes and functions of government, the relationship with state governments, and some notion of what individuals must give up in order to preserve the interests and safety of everyone. Constitutional amendments speak more distinctly to rights or protection of individuals or groups from governmental interference. While constitutional amendments provide citizens with a very broad sweep of rights, there is no constitutional amendment specific to health or health care. Ruth Macklin, philosopher and bioethicist, discusses views on special and general rights of philosopher H.L.A. Hart.[6] He says that special rights are those that arise out of particular transactions or relations between persons in a transaction. In these transactions, rights and duties exist only between the participants, as in health professional–patient relationships or child–parent relationships. General rights, according to Hart, are those that arise out of a principle of equity, that all persons equally have the right to be free—that is, a person may not be unjustifiably coerced to submit to medical treatment. On the other hand, when a conflict of individual rights occurs, such as in a nursing home where two roommates claim a right to privacy and demand a private room, residents do not have an automatic right to a private room on demand. Hart's discussion of special and general rights still does not provide us with sufficient justification for making claims about individual rights. One could, however, review policies of a health care organization or treatment of nursing home residents in light of whether they include adequate protection of individual autonomy and safety as special rights of residents and patients as a class. In addition to moral and legal rights, there are intermediate rights. These are rights that, if taken into a court of law, would in all likelihood be recognized as legal rights. Some think that access to the benefits of health care might fall into this category of intermediate rights.

Macklin maintains that some of the debates and uncertainties about rights would be resolved if we had a framework provided by an overall theory of justice within which such debates could be decided. One example might be Rawls' theory of justice as fairness, whereby the least advantaged in our society must receive some benefit from social and health policies that are developed. The impact of governmental policies on society's most vulnerable would have to be considered in all policy development, and the burdens of a policy could not fall solely on the least advantaged, such as the elderly, poor, or children. Lacking a social consensus on an overall concept of justice, it is difficult to justify specific rights in our society such as a right to health care. However, claims to rights may still serve "as expressions of moral outrage or as demands for social and legislative reform." [7] This use of rights language is implicit in the federal Patient Self-Determination Act related to the use of written advance directives for medical treatment and in state mandates for 48-hour maternity stays after normal deliveries.

In asserting certain rights in health care, one should recognize that this is only one way of placing issues within an ethical framework. Framing an issue solely in terms of rights, with no consideration of corresponding obligations or responsibilities, often leads to adversarial confrontations rather than resolution. One may also consider a Kantian approach, which stresses duties and obligations such as respect for persons, or the utilitarian approach, which looks at consequences of actions in terms of utility and the greatest good or the least suffering for the greatest number of people. Limitations of using a rights approach to deal with conflict is evident when individual rights to health care are claimed. Such claims may have moral standing but no legal standing. Another difficulty is that a person can justifiably claim to possess a right even though that claim is currently unprotected by law or social custom. This is an example of an unrealized right. Unrealized rights are claims to something not recognized as a right by society. This is the case with claims of rights to health care. If there were a realized right to health care, it would imply that health care organizations and professionals should provide care to those who need or want it.[8] This is an example of a corresponding obligation.

Macklin warns that there are many moral and philosophical problems in the attempt to discover where rights come from and in whom they reside, even though they are so often appealed to in public debate and in making demands for action of a particular kind, such as equitable access to health care.[9] In attempting to translate rights into correlative obligations, she says that not all of the health care obligations derived from the rights claimed by some persons or groups can be delivered.[10] Macklin's point is well taken when one considers issues such as health care rationing and equitable access that arise when claimed rights to health care of particular groups and individuals come into conflict or are simply not realized in our society. Should the latest medical technologies be provided for a middle class child covered by health insurance and little or no primary care be provided to the child whose parents are working at a minimum wage job with no health insurance coverage? Can an obligation to provide care be derived solely from a child's needs for health care? One could argue in the affirmative if one uses a notion of distributive justice grounded in individual needs for medical care, that is, the criterion of medical necessity.

Another example of obligations arising from sources other than rights of individuals or groups is the obligation of nurses to provide competent nursing care. These obligations arise for the individual nurse who has the knowledge base of a profession that provides a socially valuable service. Nurses, as providers of a socially valuable service, are in a special relationship with their patients. This relationship carries with it explicit obligations and responsibilities for nurses to act in particular ways, such as performing nursing procedures safely and treating patients with respect for their individual dignity. Later, it will be argued that nurses' special rights could be derived from the special relationship of nurses with persons who are vulnerable by virtue of their health or sickness problems.

For purposes of this chapter, following Macklin's thinking, the concept of rights will be used to indicate some legitimate expectations of persons in an identified society at a given time. It may be more useful to think of claims about rights not as things to be discovered as true or false but as language used to promote change and social legislative reform. Rights do not assert anything about the moral order *per se*, but the idea that jeopardizing human rights is an affront to justice is compelling. Many would agree that human rights include a right to health care as a necessary means to carrying on one's life. If this is the case, the fact that not all people have access to health care is ethically unacceptable. One challenge for individual claims of rights to health care is to whom does one present the claim—Physicians? Nurses? Government? Insurers? Are there corresponding moral obligations or responsibilities on the part of some individuals or institutions to provide persons with needed health care? What role should individual responsibility for health play in development of health policy, financing, and delivery of health services? Part of the problem in responding to such a claim lies in our definitions of health itself. Health is a slippery term, even when one thinks of it as absence of illness or the ability to carry on daily activities. The World Health Organization's (WHO) concept that health is a "state of complete physical, mental, and social well-being" does not give much direction when considered in the light of rights claims, development and implementation of organizational and public policies, and the limitless economic burdens that an attempt at its realization would entail for society. It provides no boundaries within which to consider moral or legal obligations to provide health care. Health per se is not always a top social priority, even as the means to other ends. The concept of a right to health care also runs into difficulty when one starts talking about individual choices and responsibility for one's health, especially when those choices involve identified health risk factors and unhealthy life styles.

The 1980s saw a shift to a focus on obligations in health care as illustrated in the report entitled *Securing Access to Health Care*, issued by the President's Commission for the Study of Ethical Problems in Medicine and Biomedical and Behavioral Research (1983). This report concludes that society as a whole has an ethical obligation to ensure equitable access to health care. The focus in this document has shifted from the general right to medical care orientation as found in Medicare and Medicaid policies. Equitable access, as discussed in the Commission report, refers to everyone having access to some level of health care, that is, "enough care to achieve sufficient welfare, opportunity, information, and evidence of interpersonal concern to facilitate a reasonably full and satisfying life." [11] Inherent in these societal obligations is the notion of the special importance of health care in relieving suffering and in demonstrating mutual empathy and compassion for all citizens. This shift may reflect the renewed concern for our interdependence and interconnectedness in community.

The reality of our interrelatedness as human beings has been largely neglected in the societal emphasis on the value of individualism, which is only one side of the many faceted coin of our lived experience. Individuals, groups, and families are not absolutely autonomous and isolated. Even the idea that the exercise of individual rights includes corollary obligations and responsibilities negates a perspective of radical individualism that was more evident in earlier bioethics and nursing ethics literature. The document "Nursing's Agenda for Health Care Reform" (1992) reflects the changing emphasis from rights to responsibilities in urging creation of a health care system that fosters consumer responsibility for personal health and self-care.[12] Philosopher Daniel Callahan suggests that the "right to health care" as a social obligation might be undertaken by a society in terms of equal access to available health care and facilities.[13] While this seems reasonable on the face of it, such a concept has difficulties because of the competition of health with other welfare rights and with other societal needs such as publicly supported education and defense. Debates still rage as to whether children and the elderly have the same rights to health care and whether or not those who have life styles that put them at risk should have equal access to health care especially at public expense. Drug abusers and smokers come to mind. An added complexity in dealing with the latter issue is that we cannot yet explain *why* individuals have undesirable health habits. Since there is little empirical data available to help in the resolution of these issues, there is no empirically established foundation that serves to guide development of health policy on the relationship of individual and collective responsibility for health. Additionally, we have multiple and often conflicting societal goals for health care. One goal is to contain costs and another is to provide needed care. One possible resolution to the dilemmas involved in rights arguments for health care is embodied in the concept of legislating universal health insurance or a national health plan for the United States. The latest effort to legislate a national health security plan in the 1990s during the Clinton administration focused on the language of responsibility rather than rights, which again suggests that the language of individual rights makes only a limited contribution to the development of public policy that focuses on the common good and recognizes our interdependence in modern society.[14]

Questions of rights to and obligations in health care are by no means settled as various efforts are made by federal and state governments and health care organizations to control costs and to devise ways to provide health care to the uninsured and underinsured in health care reform efforts and managed care arrangements. An argument could be made that if it is the obligation of both the public and private sectors to assure equitable access to health care, with the federal government as ultimately responsible, then individuals have corresponding obligations to consider the influence of life style choices on their personal health and the interests of others. We have yet to see how successful this argument will be.

The assumption that honoring claims of rights to medical care will deal with health problems in our society such as violence and AIDS is not an adequate response. Availability of and access to medical care must still be balanced with considerations of individual responsibility for health protection and maintenance. Furthermore, debates about rights to and responsibilities in health care suggest that these debates should include attention to such "preconditions" of health as general environmental conditions, for example, clean air, clean water, adequate housing, and income adequacy, all of which contribute to health status.[15] These are the life support systems to all of us. They may be even more significant as factors in determining health status for many individuals and communities than in building more medical care facilities or developing reimbursement schemes that pay for more medical care. This is an argument for both societal and individual responsibility for health and the environmental conditions that affect health.

The report of the President's Commission on *Securing Access to Health Care* concludes that society has an obligation to provide all citizens with an adequate level of care without excessive burdens.[16] It goes on to state that the costs of achieving equitable access ought to be shared in a fair way. Efforts to contain rising health care costs, while important, should not focus on limiting access for the least well-served people or the most vulnerable. Taking such a concept seriously means that a state effort, such as the initiative in Oregon to set priorities for Medicaid funding, is ethically questionable because of the impact solely on the poor who are dependent on public funds for their health care. Efforts to control health care costs that are driving policy development and decision making do impact claims of patient rights to health care and obligations of individuals, health care organizations, and government. As our society struggles to control health care costs and to meet health care needs of the uninsured or underinsured, we are reminded of Macklin's point that we have difficulty in determining what rights are and how they originate because we have no overall theory of justice to provide a societal framework in which legitimate rights can be claimed.

Another challenge remains. That challenge is to determine what constitutes an adequate level of health care benefits. This is complicated by claims of "needs" that would have been considered luxuries a generation ago in our society and public expectations of medical care. If one does appeal to needs as a standard for making medical care available, whose definition of needs serves as the criterion? Needs and demands represent two very different concepts in looking at claims of rights to care. Is the health care system obligated to meet insured individuals' demands for use of all available health care technologies even if the medical benefits to be obtained are questionable? How should health care professionals and consumers decide what needs are to be met in providing an adequate level of health care benefits for all in need?

Callahan claims that in order to make such determinations, we must, as a society, consider what are the appropriate goals of health and priorities for health care.[17] He suggests that the first priorities should be activities such as care for the chronically ill with physical or mental health problems and broad public health measures that include prevention and decreasing morbidity. Curing diseases of all individuals and use of all available high tech care at the end of life would not be the top priorities in health care in his view. Instead, there would be an assurance that individuals would receive needed care and not be abandoned by the community when they need continuing care. The issue of individual patient abandonment has been met, at least in crisis situations, with federal legislation that forbids the "dumping" of medically unstable patients or women in active labor from one hospital emergency room to another due to lack of a source of reimbursement. Such a response still does not address the health care needs of the uninsured or incompletely insured regardless of the rhetoric about rights to health care.

One way to have enforceable rights to medical care is through a private contract for reimbursement in the form of health insurance. Unfortunately, even if one has health insurance or belongs to a managed care plan such as a health maintenance organization (HMO), all costs associated with medical care are not covered and often one's choice of provider is limited by one's employer. HMOs have achieved varying degrees of success in delivering cost-effective health care. Some have floundered and failed whereas others are meeting their goals to provide cost-effective quality care to their members. Some insurance plans such as Medicare still provide incentives for hospitalization rather than ambulatory care or preventive health services. With downsizing of health care organizations, growth of managed care, and more acutely ill patients being discharged from hospitals now than in the past, there is an enormous need to develop and finance long-term care and home care services in efforts to provide needed continuity of care that does not simply shift the financial and human energy costs of care to family members and loved ones.

PATIENT RIGHTS AND OBLIGATIONS IN HEALTH CARE

The overall goals of what has been called the Patients' Rights Movement of the past three decades were concerned with quality of health care, enhancement of patient decision making, and having some impact on behavior of health care providers to make the system more answerable to patient needs. More specifically, individuals were to be assured more self-determination and control over their own bodies when using health care services that are often characterized by professional and payer dominance, complicated bureaucratic structures, endless red tape, and authoritarianism. In this area, one sees clearly the pressures and tensions between what professionals consider to be their obligations to provide care in the way they feel would be most beneficial to patients, patients' rights to self-determination in medical care and treatment, and managed care capitated system arrangements that sometimes prevent physicians from providing comprehensive information for patient decision making. Issues of confidentiality, patients' informed consent and decision making, and rationing of health care reflect the conflict that often exists between the respective rights and obligations of consumers and providers.

Patients are protected against assault and battery by the law of torts (injury or wrongful acts) through the legal doctrine of informed consent. But ethical issues continue in operationalizing informed consent and decision making when it comes to patient care situations that are complex and dynamic. For example, how does one provide adequate information for informed patient decision making when the patient is confused? What does one tell a patient about the risks of a particular medical procedure? The standard in current use is what the reasonable patient needs to know to make a decision about accepting or refusing medical treatment; it is a process of education. Informed consent is not simply a matter of having patients sign forms. The rights of patients to participate in decision making are particularly difficult to honor with some classes of patients such as young children and patients with limited decision-making capacity. The President's Commission discussed the assessment of decision-making capacity as a responsibility of health–care providers, since the determination of legal competence is not an issue in most patient decision-making situations.

A further problem to be considered in claiming patient rights in health care is the imbalance of power in patient–physician, nurse–patient, or patient–provider–payer relationships. Patients traditionally are in a dependent relationship vis-a-vis payers and health care professionals with the sick role generally legitimized by the physician. In most instances, it is still the physician who serves as the gatekeeper in health care systems including access to specialists, although this is changing in some areas of primary care and in managed care systems where nurses often perform a triage function. In many of our current health care settings, patients have access to services only with the sanction of both providers and payers.

The patients' rights movement originally sought a new model for provider–patient relationships in which the traditional relationship based on provider beneficence becomes more of a cooperative partnership in attaining and maintaining health utilizing a shared decision-making process. The original AHA Patient's Bill of Rights is presented here in its entirety because it still serves as the basis for patient bills of rights established in hospitals, nursing homes, home care, and other health care organizations. Current patient, resident, or member (as in HMOs) bills of rights generally incorporate responsibilities and obligations as well as rights and are legislated in some states.

American Hospital Association

Statement on a Patient's Bill of Rights*

1. The patient has the right to considerate and respectful care.

2. The patient has the right to obtain from his physician complete current information concerning his diagnosis, treatment, and prognosis in terms the patient

---

*Reprinted with permission of the American Hospital Association, 840 North Lake Shore Drive, Chicago, Illinois 60611, 1970.

can be reasonably expected to understand. When it is not medically advisable to give such information to the patient, the information should be made available to an appropriate person in his behalf. He has the right to know by name the physician responsible for coordinating his care.

3. The patient has the right to receive from his physician information necessary to give informed consent prior to the start of any procedure and/or treatment. Except in emergencies, such information for informed consent should include but not necessarily be limited to the specific procedure and/or treatment, the medically significant risks involved, and the probable duration of incapacitation. Where medically significant alternatives for care or treatment exist, or when the patient requests information concerning medical alternatives, the patient has the right to such information. The patient also has the right to know the name of the person responsible for the procedures and/or treatment.

4. The patient has the right to refuse treatment to the extent permitted by law, and to be informed of the medical consequences of his action.

5. The patient has the right to every consideration of his privacy concerning his own medical care program. Case discussion, consultation, examination, and treatment are confidential and should be conducted discreetly. Those not directly involved in his care must have the permission of the patient to be present.

6. The patient has the right to expect that all communications and records pertaining to his care should be treated as confidential.

7. The patient has the right to expect that within its capacity a hospital must make reasonable response to the request of a patient for services. The hospital must provide evaluation, service, and/or referral as indicated by the urgency of the case. When medically permissible, a patient may be transferred to another facility only after he has received complete information and explanation concerning the needs for, and the alternatives to, such a transfer. The institution to which the patient is to be transferred must first have accepted the patient for transfer.

8. The patient has the right to obtain information as to any relationship of his hospital to other health care and educational institutions insofar as his care is concerned. The patient has the right to obtain information as to the existence of any professional relationships among individuals, by name, who are treating him.

9. The patient has the right to be advised if the hospital proposes to engage in or perform human experimentation affecting his care or treatment. The patient has the right to refuse to participate in such research projects.

10. The patient has the right to expect reasonable continuity of care. He has the right to know in advance what appointment times and physicians are available

and where. The patient has the right to expect that the hospital will provide a mechanism whereby he is informed by his physician or a delegate of the physician of the patient's continuing health care requirements following discharge.

11. The patient has the right to examine and receive an explanation of his bill regardless of source of payment.

12. The patient has the right to know what hospital rules and regulations apply to his conduct as a patient.

These proclaimed rights are legally enforceable only in those states that have legislated the Patients' Bill of Rights and where they are already found in some hospital charters.Even if many of these rights are legally unenforceable, they have moral standing and provide patients, families, and providers with knowledge of rights that consumers might expect and demand as an expression of respect for the dignity of the individual. A declaration of patient rights and responsibilities is even more important in today's health care environment, in which cost-containment efforts so often seem to be driving organizational decision making and recommendations for patient care.

Some states, such as Minnesota, have legislated a patient bill of rights, advance directives, and durable power of attorney for health care so that patients' rights and their choices and directions for care do have legal as well as moral standing. The advance directive is an effort to further ensure patient rights to receive or refuse treatment and to direct treatment decisions when the patient is unable to do so. The federal Patient Self-Determination Act (1991) legislates that patients in health care institutions that receive federal funds such as Medicare must inform patients of their rights to complete advance directives. Patients are not and cannot be required to complete advance directives as a condition of receiving medical care and treatment. Such legislation serves one of the purposes that Macklin points to in her comments that "rights" language and the proclamation of those rights can be used to generate action and appropriate policy development by health care organizations that might not occur otherwise.

The reader may be wondering "why all the discussion about legally enforceable rights"? Are there any rights and obligations that are granted for "humanitarian" or moral reasons based on one's membership in the human community? Talk about legal rights seems to reinforce Macklin's perception that the language of rights does not seem to help us much in dealing with specific ethical issues and dilemmas in health care. And, indeed, when attempting to honor patient rights, we must also consider ethical principles and values such as respect for persons, avoiding or preventing harm while benefitting patients, and justice as fairness in an environment of health care rationing.

Some health care organizations have created other mechanisms for taking patient rights more seriously by employing patient representatives, that is, individuals who are skilled in patient relations. Most often, patient representatives deal with nonnursing and nonmedical matters related to patient comfort and convenience during hospitalization and are more accurately described as management's representative to patients. George Annas, an expert in health law, argues that patient advocates should have medical care and treatment as their major concern. In that context, the advocate should have the following powers in order to fulfill the duties of patient advocate: access to all the patient's hospital records; active participation in hospital committees monitoring quality of patient care; power to present patient complaints directly to hospital administrators and the hospital's executive committee; access to all chiefs of service; access to patient support services; and, the ability to delay discharges. Existing patient advocate systems do not generally follow this model.[18] While Annas agrees that the patient advocate's function is no panacea, it does provide a mechanism for taking patient rights more seriously in health care bureaucracies where paternalistic practices still occur, vulnerable individuals feel intimidated, and physician decisions are often scrutinized for impact on the institution's or managed care plan's "bottom line." Nursing claims to the role of patient advocate require scrutiny under the Annas concept of advocacy.

FURTHER THOUGHTS FOR NURSING PRACTICE

Nurses claim that they serve as patient advocates. What nurses mean when invoking the term is often not made explicit although advocacy is commonly understood to mean identifying and respecting the patients' wishes. This meaning is hardly adequate for nurses, however, because the idea has the potential to make nurses a means to patient ends and to negate nurses' autonomy as moral beings. Winslow, a professor of religion, argues that for nurses to serve successfully as patient advocates, there must be further clarification of the meaning of advocacy in nursing practice, review and revision of states' nurse practice acts, public education in order for patients and families to understand the advocacy role of nurses, an understanding by nurses of the difficulties and challenges surrounding the practice of patient advocacy, and preparation of nurses to deal with controversy surrounding advocacy for patients in complex bureaucratic structures.[19]

Many nurses are employed in health care organizations in states where it is necessary to legislate patients' bills of rights in order for patients' rights to have legal standing as discussed earlier. One might ask who, then, does advocate for vulnerable patients and their rights to make treatment decisions for themselves in what is generally an intimidating environment or what Annas graphically describes as "a human rights wasteland." [20] An example is use of all available technologies that merely prolong dying thus perpetuating the traditional medical ethic of doing everything possible for the individual patient. Often these interventions are used without taking the patient's perspective and values into account. The patient's perspective may well differ from that of the provider; the patient may wish to refuse certain types of recommended treatments or automatic use of all available technologies in an effort to stave off death when comfort care is the more appropriate mode for that patient. It has also been pointed out that nurses cannot advocate for patients in the sense of ensuring their rights because nurses, as employees, are not accountable solely to patients even though this is a stance of the ANA Code for Nurses. Nurses are accountable to numerous others such as employers, physicians, and to themselves as moral agents and professionals.

Nurses, in all health care settings, must look at the specific ways in which they encourage or discourage patient or client autonomy within the limits of safety and standards of nursing care. Nursing interventions that are appropriate for the comatose patient change, or should change, dramatically when care is being provided for a conscious patient with decision-making capacity. While there is always a general obligation to respect patients in decision making about treatments, it can be argued that there are more specific obligations to respect patient self-determination in decision making with and for patients with decision-making capacity. As patients or their surrogates expect or demand that patient rights be honored in health care settings, what is nursing's response? Is the individual simply labeled as another "difficult" patient or family member? The nursing obligation and responsibility to assist patients in obtaining and deliberating about the information necessary to informed decision making about care and treatment holds tremendous implications for practice. It should be a key concern for nurses who plan for continuity of care in the context of shorter hospitalizations for many patients than in the past and the reality that many procedures formerly done in the hospital are done on an outpatient basis in an ambulatory care setting. Recognition of such moral obligations are critical for nurses in any setting—patient care, education, research, or policy development.

In order to fulfill nursing obligations of patient advocacy, there must be supportive organizational environments for this kind of practice and a more collegial system of nursing care—the domain of organizational ethics. Without such environments, ethical nursing practice is often compromised by fear and lack of colleague support. Profound changes are required in many health care organizations, including managed care organizations, in order to create environments in which patients can make better informed decisions and choices related to their health and environments in which patient goals and values would always be considered in decision making when patients are unable to do this for themselves. One way in which patient goals and values can be considered in circumstances in which patients are unable to make their own decisions is for patients to complete advance directives or name a durable power of attorney for health care decisions. The ANA Code for Nurses and ANA Standards for Nursing Practice identify and support ethical nursing practice. They can be used to support positions on advocacy for patient care and organizational environments for professional nursing practice. Nurses, as members of a special moral community, can form coalitions and actively work together to create such organizational environments even in a time of restructuring and cost containment.[21] Integrity of nurses and nursing service as well as patient safety and welfare are at stake.

Other mechanisms to assist nurses in a patient advocacy role include: learning to identify situations in which ethical principles and values are at stake; incorporating identified ethical considerations in decision making with and for patients and in policy development and implementation; active participation on multidisciplinary and nursing ethics committees; initiating and conducting ethics rounds on patient care units. Annas' requirements for patient advocates presented earlier further enrich the concept of advocacy to be considered in order for nurses to adequately fulfill such a role.

Two decades ago, nursing leader Claire Fagin asserted that achievement and exercise of nurses' rights is a prerequisite to nurses helping patients achieve their rights.[22] Nursing's tradition and history have focused on responsibility and service of the nurse as a helping professional rather than autonomy and nurses' rights. Fagin sees nurses' rights emerging out of human rights and women's rights, since the majority of nurses are women. One's human rights ought to encompass the creation of situations that will enhance "humanness," for example, feelings of compassion, sympathy, and intelligence. Involved in women's rights are freedom of choice, equality, and respect for the individual person. This does not mean asking for special privileges but for the right to equal and full participation in such areas as decision making that affects one's practice, the right to the type of environment that allows for professional nursing practice and professional economic rewards, rights to a work environment that minimizes physical and emotional stresses, the right to set standards for excellence in nursing practice, and the right to participate in development of policy that affects nurses and nursing care. One can argue that it is the obligation of professional nursing to exercise such rights. Why? It is in order that nurses' special rights not be permanently lost in depersonalized bureaucracies, where physicians provide care perceived by the public as valuable but where the direct care provided by nurses is often attributed to the physician's orders and is an unidentified aspect of hospital or institutional services—nurses as invisible providers of care.

Assertion of special rights for nurses in their practice is not an end in and of itself but is the means to improved services for patients and clients and more ethically adequate nursing practice. While the ANA Code for Nurses (1985) addresses itself primarily to nursing obligations, it also provides a framework for consideration of special rights of nurses derived from the special relationship of nursing to society as an essential service to those in need of nursing care and expertise, such as individuals who are critically ill and at-risk population groups. Integral to the concept of nursing responsibilities and obligations is the authority or right to fulfill one's responsibilities as a professional person, that is, as a nurse in this instance. Responsibility without the corresponding right or authority to discharge one's professional obligations as a nurse leads to feelings of powerlessness and a sense of moral inadequacy in one's practice. The nurse's sense of integrity is in jeopardy under such circumstances, with profound implications for the individual nurse, for patient care, and for the nursing profession. Philosopher Nel Noddings expressed this idea powerfully in her comment: "There can be no greater evil, then, than this: that the moral autonomy of the one-caring be so shattered that she acts against her own commitment to care." [23]

Some would argue that nurses as professionals have no special rights, only obligations or responsibilities. Generally, rights of health care professionals are considered as privileges that can be derived from patient or client rights. We argue that nurses do have special rights that can be considered as derivative from nursing responsibilities to and relationships with clients as well as nursing's social contract with the society of which it is an integral part. It is possible to argue that if nursing care is considered to be a societal necessity and right of those in need, then nurses have a corresponding responsibility *and* special right to provide nursing care to clients, care without which clients would suffer. While rights of individuals to nursing care are of great importance, they are not absolute in the sense of overriding all other considerations. For example, patients do not have a right to insist that nurses provide services that violate the bounds of acceptable practice or a nurse's own deeply held moral beliefs such as providing the means in an assisted suicide at a patient's request.

How do nurses' rights and obligations fit with situations where nurses question whether to accept or reject care of a particular client or group of clients? It can be argued that health care professionals have a duty to accept some personal risk of disease if in doing so another's life can be prolonged or suffering decreased. This is even a societal expectation. At the same time, nurses are not morally required to put themselves at serious personal risk, though they (and others) have and may choose to do so. Nurses have the right to knowledge necessary to make informed decisions about provision of nursing care in such situations of identified personal risk. Adequately informed decison making is essential for both clients and nurses and might be viewed as a fundamental human right. While putting one's self at serious personal risk can be understood as above and beyond what can be reasonably expected or required, nurses have an obligation not to abandon their patients. Individual *and* collective nursing actions may be required to assure that identified patients are not abandoned.

Professional standards of nursing practice, the ANA Code for Nurses, and nursing's social contract with society support the idea that nurses have special rights. It is an obligation of nurses individually and collectively to work together in using these documents and mandates to support their efforts to change inadequate or unsafe conditions of patient care in health care systems. Actualizing nurses' special rights can help patients to exercise their rights and responsibilities and to reduce financial and other costs of care, such as patient infections, complications, and injuries to nurses.[24] An early example of patients exercising their rights is when nurses worked together in the 1970s to achieve an environment for professional practice at the Iowa Veterans Home in Marshalltown, Iowa. The residents became more active collectively in developing mechanisms for participating in decision making that affected their welfare.[25] While some activities may not be realistic in short-term acute care settings, nurses still have an obligation (even a right) to consider the consequences for the welfare of patients and the provision of needed nursing care even if such environments cannot always be achieved completely. Nursing obligations to patients do not simply end when a patient leaves an acute care setting. Florence Nightingale argued more than a century ago that a nursing obligation was the development of healing environments for patients. One can take this a step further to incorporate aspects of a healing environment in any care setting to assure that patients and nurses are heard and respected as self-determining individuals and as members of the human community.

Nurses can claim both obligations and special rights to ensure patient care environments for the public where standards of practice and the Code for Nurses are explicitly used to guide nursing practice. Achievement of more ethical nursing practice that ensures the integrity of nurses and the nursing care received by the public is another example of a responsibility and special right. These responsibilities and special rights of nurses require a new mindset, ethical reflection, decision making, organizational policy development, and action, often political action. To talk about nurses' and patients' rights without working to make them a reality is to surrender to passivity and continuing dependence on others. This is not the vision of what professional nursing can and should be for nurses as moral agents and for patient care. Nurses can, do, and should promote and protect patient welfare at the bedside, in homes, schools, the workplace, and at policy-making levels of organizations and government.

Issues of rights, responsibilities, and obligations do not have to automatically remain in the realm of unresolved ethical dilemmas. Nurses can take individual and collective action to make patients' rights and nurses' special rights become realized rights by working to create environments in which patients' and nursing values are an integral part of the decision-making process in shared decisions about treatment and to assure more adequate access to necessary health and nursing care through organizational and public policies.

■ CASE STUDY I.

The home health nursing service in your hospital is facing budget cuts and staff limitations. In order to accommodate the patients who are being discharged earlier with more acute nursing needs in the home, your manager has proposed limiting visits to some chronic patients. She has proposed closing cases of "non-compliant" patients, and patients who show no improvement in spite of visits from the home health nurse for several months.

One such patient is Mrs. Lombardi. She is a 76-year-old woman with a stasis ulcer on her right ankle. You have been visiting her twice a week for the last 7 months, doing dressing changes on the wound and monitoring her diabetes. She has very brittle diabetes, is overweight, and lives alone. The wound is clean but has shown no sign of healing. Mrs. Lombardi is a heavy smoker with a 55-year history of smoking two packs per day. You have counseled her regularly about the risks of smoking but she says she has no interest in stopping at this late stage of her life and besides, she has tried many times to quit using many different methods and has never been successful. She is aware that her ability to heal the ulcer may be compromised by continuing to smoke.

Your manager now says that, because Mrs. Lombardi continues to smoke, she is noncompliant with her treatment. He recommends, additionally, that you close her case and stop the home visits since the wound shows no evidence of healing.

Further Questions for Discussion

1. Is Mrs. Lombardi acting irresponsibly regarding her health by continuing to smoke?

2. Does she have a right to expect continued treatment given the fact that the ulcer is unhealed?

3. What is your responsibility as her visiting nurse in this situation?

■ CASE STUDY II.

Mr. Washington is a 68-year-old man with metastatic exophageal cancer. He has been treated for the last 3 years, first with brachiotherapy and later with chemotherapy. The cancer has continued to metastasize in spite of these therapies. He is admitted to the intensive care unit for treatment of pneumonia and placed on a ventilator. After the pneumonia has been successfully treated, however, he is unable to be weaned from the ventilator. Continued tumor growth has completely occluded his airway. The tumor has invaded the brain, he is paralyzed on the right side, and shows no sign of recognizing anyone. He withdraws from stimuli, grimaces as if in pain, and tries to pinch or hit the nurses with his left hand. He has developed a seizure disorder requiring heavy medication. Cancerous nodules extrude from his neck and his left eye and ear have become completely consumed by tumor as has his tongue, which now extends from his mouth about 5 inches and is about 3 inches thick. He receives tube feedings and morphine and fentanyl for pain. His nursing care is quite challenging and his left hand has to be kept mitted to prevent him from harming the staff. Great care has to be taken to keep his tongue moist and clean. His teeth cut into his tongue and careful oral suctioning frequently results in heavy bleeding from his mouth. The stench from the many tumors is overwhelming and difficult to mask or control. He has been in this situation for 4 months.

His wife, Mildred, holds his Durable Power of Attorney for Health Care and says that he wants everything to be done to keep him alive in any condition. She will not consider withdrawing any therapy and wants very aggressive care continued. Additionally, she demands that his pain medication be kept at a low level so he will be more responsive when she comes to visit. She is very demanding about his care and is frequently abusive to the staff. The nursing and medical staff are quite concerned about continuing to provide aggressive care. They feel that his existence is filled with suffering and that they are merely prolonging a horrible death. The nurses are particularly concerned as to whether or not his pain is adequately treated. Many nurses refuse to care for him at all and others have nightmares about torture. They complain that they are being held hostage by his wife's demands for care and fear they are compromising their personal integrity as well as that of the nursing profession.

Further Questions for Discussion

1. Does a patient have a right to total control over what care will be provided in every instance?

2. Do the nurses have any right to refuse to care for Mr. Washington? Is there any place for consideration of ideals of personal or professional integrity in this type of situation?

3. Is there a responsibility to honor a patient's or surrogate's wishes when doing so contributes to considerable suffering and a prolonged death for the patient?

REFERENCES

1. Summers J: Take patient rights seriously to improve patient care and to lower costs. *Health Care Manage Rev* 10(4):55–62, Fall 1985.
2. Report of American Nurses Association Committee on Ethics to House of Delegates: *Enhancing Quality of Care Through Understanding Nurses' Responsibilities and Rights.* Kansas City, MO: American Nurses Association; June 1986.
3. Bandman B: The human rights of patients, nurses, and other health professionals. In Bandman EL, Bandman B (eds): *Bioethics and Human Rights.* Boston: Little, Brown; 1978, pp 321–322.
4. Macklin R: Moral concerns and appeals to rights and duties. *Hastings Cent Rep* 6(5):31–38, 1976.
5. Curran WJ: Notes from lecture given in Human Rights and Health, Harvard School of Public Health, October 5, 1976.
6. Macklin R: *op. cit.,* p 37.
7. *Ibid.,* p 31.
8. Gorovitz S, Jameton AL, Macklin R, et al (eds): *Moral Problems in Medicine.* Englewood Cliffs, NJ: Prentice-Hall; 1976, pp 426–427.
9. Macklin R: *op. cit.,* p 32.
10. *Ibid.,* pp 35–36.
11. President's Commission for the Study of Ethical Problems in Medicine and Biomedical and Behavioral Research: *Securing Access to Health Care. Volume One: Report.* Washington, DC: U.S. Government Printing Office; 1983, p 20.
12. American Nurses Association. *Nursing's Agenda for Health Care Reform.* Washington, DC: American Nurses Association Publishing; 1992.
13. Callahan D: Health and society: Some ethical imperatives. *Daedalus* 106:23–33, Winter 1977.
14. Bellah RN, Madsen R, Sullivan WM, Swidler A, Tipton SM: *The Good Society.* New York: Vintage Books; 1991.
15. Sparer EV: The legal right to health care. *Hastings Cent Rep* 6(5):39–47, 1976.
16. President's Commission: *op. cit.,* p 4.
17. Callahan D: *What Kind of Life?* New York: Simon & Schuster; 1989.
18. Annas GJ: *Judging Medicine.* Clifton, NJ: Humana; 1988.
19. Winslow GR: From loyalty to advocacy: A new metaphor for nursing. *Hastings Cent Rep* 14(3):32–40, 1984.
20. Annas GJ: *op. cit.,* p 4.

21. Aroskar MA: Envisioning nursing as a moral community. *Nurs Outlook* 43(3):134–138, 1995.
22. Fagin CM: Nurses' rights. *Am J Nurs* 75(1):82–85, 1975.
23. Noddings N: *Caring: A Feminine Approach to Ethics and Moral Education.* Berkeley, CA: University of California Press; 1984.
24. American Nurses Association: Written Testimony of the American Nurses Association before the Institute of Medicine Commission on the Adequacy of Nurse Staffing. Washington, DC: American Nurses Association; September 1994.
25. Maas J, Jacox AK: *Guidelines for Nurse Autonomy/Patient Welfare.* New York: Appleton-Century-Crofts; 1977.

7

Ethical Principles of Informed Consent

Informed consent is a cornerstone of contemporary health care practice. Because informed consent is grounded in the ethical principle of autonomy, it is important to review briefly what is involved in the complex idea of autonomy. Miller discusses the four senses of autonomy used by contemporary philosophers.[1] These include free action, authenticity, effective deliberation, and moral reflection. Autonomy as free action means that a given action is voluntary, that is, not coerced and intentional meaning conscious. Autonomy as authenticity means that an action is in keeping with one's beliefs, values, and life plans. Autonomy as effective deliberation means that an individual defines himself or herself as in a situation where a decision must be made, that alternative courses of action and their consequences were evaluated and that a given action was chosen on the basis of that evaluation. Finally, autonomy in the sense of moral reflection means that one accepts the moral values on which one acts. All of these senses are important in bioethics and contribute to the practice of informed consent in various ways depending on the context.

Generally speaking, within bioethics, autonomy means that individuals have the right to information and, on the basis of this input, the right to agree or to refuse to participate in research or to undergo the treatment being proposed. Autonomy means that persons have the right to determine their course of action on the basis of a plan that they have developed for themselves. This does not mean that no limits on autonomy exist. Some individuals, because of their physical or mental conditions, have diminished autonomy. Others, such as institutionalized populations, also tend to have less autonomy in their daily lives because of their social situation. In addition, autonomy does not mean that individuals can do anything they want. The reasons people have for their autonomous actions are their own reasons, but they must be principled and not arbitrary reasons.[2] Although the complexities of the concept have led to much discussion in bioethics as well as moral and political philosophy, particularly around the limits of autonomy, autonomy remains central to informed consent. This autonomous person status is the reason we obtain informed consent even when there is no risk to the patient or research subject and when no immediate social utility occurs.

When patients make decisions based on necessary and clear information, they are acting as autonomous agents. From an ethical perspective, health professionals have the obligation to respect their decisions, even in those situations where they disagree with the patient. There are complex exceptions to these general situations, such as when parents decide on a course of action for their child that is harmful and might even lead to death. Another exception can be found in emergency situations where time and urgency preclude the usual process and health professionals have the primary obligation to treat in order to save life.

Informed consent also acts to safeguard patients by preventing harm being done to them. This involves the ethical principle of nonmaleficence, or the responsibility to do no harm. It is possible that patients may choose to be involved in research that includes substantial risk for them. In these cases, patients exercise their autonomy by choosing a potentially greater risk than might be chosen for them by someone else. Because they decide for themselves, with an understanding of what is involved, harm is not done and autonomous actions occur.

In addition to the ethical principles of autonomy and nonmaleficence, informed consent can also serve to protect all of society by encouraging self-scrutiny among health professionals and researchers and by involving the public in these matters.[3] This is the ethical principle of utility. It is useful in a democratic society to have informed, involved people.

Because people can give informed consent only if they have sufficient information on which to base a decision, an ethical principle guiding the giving of information is veracity, or truth telling. Trust in professional relations with clients and patients comes in part from veracity. The ethical question is when, if ever, it is ethically justified to withhold the truth as we know it from the patient.

RESEARCH AND INFORMED CONSENT

The idea of informed consent is relatively new to the practice of health care, arising in response to increases in medical knowledge and from abuse of human beings, largely prisoners, the poor, and the mentally disabled, in the pursuit of that knowledge.[4,5] Therefore, any discussion of informed consent must be placed within the larger context of the moral justification for conducting research using human subjects. In much, if not most, biomedical research with human subjects, we usually assume that previous trials have been conducted on animals and that there has been careful assessment of predictable risks in comparison with foreseeable benefits. Although the moral issues of using animals in research to better the human condition are worthy of our close attention, they remain outside the present discussion.[6-12]

In order to proceed with a discussion of why and whether we should conduct research using human subjects, some definitions will be helpful. Therapy refers to a class of activity intended to benefit an individual or member of a group. The person giving therapy has the intention of benefiting the recipient of the activity. Research, on the other hand, refers to scientific activity intended to contribute to the general knowledge in a field. Two subtypes of research can be identified. First, scientists conduct therapeutic research mainly for the benefit of the subject while also gaining knowledge. For example, giving a new drug to a cancer patient can be basically for therapeutic purposes while at the same time it can be a trial test for the drug. Second, scientists also engage in nontherapeutic research using human subjects to gain new knowledge. An example is an experiment that deliberately introduces change into a given situation and then measures and compares the respective effects on the control group and the experimental group. The control group does not usually benefit in any therapeutic way from the research. The motivation to participate of those in the control group is not therapeutic benefit but for the rewards from or the advancement of science.

Conducting research using human subjects can be morally justified on the basis of the ethics of good consequences. We all derive social benefits from research, whether that benefit is immediately therapeutic to us personally or whether it affects us indirectly by affecting resources. Eventually a procedure or a drug, after being tested on nonhumans, must be tested on some humans so that the knowledge gained can be used for the larger social good. Furthermore, serious harm would develop from not conducting research using human subjects, since scientific advances would be greatly limited. We can morally justify using human subjects by arguing from a utilitarian position that the practice produces good consequences for the greater number of people.

Using the concept of justice, one can also develop a nonconsequential argument to support and morally justify nontherapeutic research. We, as a society, benefit from the risks that others have taken in previous experiments; therefore, is it just for us to reap these benefits without reciprocal action? The fact that in biomedical research a time arrives when only human subjects can provide the data needed must neither overshadow nor obscure the ethical dilemmas involved.

Morally justifying the use of humans in experimentation does not resolve all of the possible ethical issues that can confront the researcher once such research gets under way. Such considerations as freedom of choice and coercion, the problem of uncertainty in determining the risk–benefit ratio, rights of the individual and needs of society, and the meaning of "the good" represent some of the more obvious dimensions of these ethical issues. The latter is of special interest because until recently, biomedical research has largely been thought of as an unquestioned good. Yet the advancement and power of medical knowledge has created problems to the extent that this unquestioned good is being increasingly challenged from many perspectives including, among others, nursing,[13-15] feminist scholars,[16-17] social critics,[18] philosophers,[19-20] and physicians.[21-22] One important example is from Renee Fox and Judith Swazey, the country's foremost scholars of organ transplantation, who followed the developments in this field from its inception. In a published farewell to the health care community,[23] the authors poignantly explained that they found the practice of organ transplants to be so troublesome morally that they could no longer chronicle it. Others have noted that when looking at the health care system as a whole, research frequently takes precedence over patient care.[24] While these issues may seem far removed from informed consent, they are not, as the history of informed consent is intimately tied to particular social factors in the history of research.

Research experimentation using humans as subjects can be traced back to the beginning of recorded history. This early research, mainly conducted in an unsystematic fashion within the clinical practice context, lead to instances of patients receiving treatments whose value had not been established by controlled, well-designed clinical investigation. Few questions arose over the years with regard to these practices, since it was assumed that the individuals being used for research purposes also benefited as the recipients of the knowledge gained in these experiments. Although the late 19th century saw an acceleration in the systematic use of human subjects for research purposes, this activity did not lead to an exploration of the need for safeguards protecting these individuals. One notable exception can be found in Bernard's 1865 publication, in which he demonstrated the need for research using human subjects and began to develop rules of ethical conduct to govern such an enterprise.[25]

Along with medicine, the law gave little attention to the rights of human subjects in experimentation. In the mid-1930s, the Michigan Supreme Court stated that experimentation, although important and necessary, must be undertaken with the knowledge and consent of the patient or someone responsible for him and such procedures must not vary too radically from accepted practice.[26] This broad generalization that the Court used to distinguish between rash experimentation with humans and systematic and ethical scientific research practice did not anticipate the grave concerns that arose in a few years from the Nuremberg disclosures. The atrocities perpetrated by German physicians in the name of clinical research during the Nazi regime demonstrated to the world the power of medicine, a power that is not neutral. This recognition disturbed many scientists, who then wanted ethical standards established on a world-wide basis to protect human subjects. There is important scholarship exploring the role of medicine[27-28] *and* nursing[29-31] in the Third Reich.

REGULATIONS AND HUMAN SUBJECTS

The Nazi experiments, so far outside the limits of what anyone would consider accepted medical and research practice, tended to be viewed by some as a terrible and tragic moment in history but separate from the general problem of protection for research subjects. Such a view obscured the fact that in principle, although perhaps not in the same magnitude, many similar moral issues had characterized research since the beginning of experimentation. The Military Tribunal that tried the Nazi physicians formulated a code of ethics that has shaped the ethos of the experimental aspects of post-World War II biomedical research. The major contribution of the code was to make the voluntary consent of the human subject absolutely essential. Furthermore, the duty and responsibility for ascertaining the quality of the consent rests upon each individual who initiates, directs, or engages in the experiment. This personal duty and responsibility may not be delegated to another with impunity. The code also says that the experiment should be such as to yield fruitful results for the good of society unprocurable by other methods or means of study and not trivial or unnecessary in nature. Furthermore, the degree of risk to be taken should never exceed that determined by the humanitarian importance of the problem to be solved by the experiment. During the course of the experiment, the human subject should be at liberty to end his participation in the experiment if he reaches the physical or mental state where continuation seems to him to be impossible. In addition, the scientist must be prepared to terminate the experiment at any stage if he believes that a continuation of the experiment is likely to result in injury, disability, or death for the experiment's subject.

The promulgation of other codes of ethics, such as the World Medical Association Helsinki Declaration of 1964, the American Medical Association Ethical Guidelines for Clinical Investigation of 1966, the American Nurses Association Human Rights Guidelines for Nurses in Clinical and Other Research of 1975, focused attention not only on the ethical dilemmas inherent in research activities but also on the limitation of codes. Succinctly worded and devoid of commentary, codes, although useful as general guidelines, cannot cover every possible eventuality and thus remain limited and subject to interpretation. These codes of ethics made it clear, however, that the professions recognized that self-regulation by investigators could not be relied on solely to safeguard the rights of human subjects in experiments. This realization, coupled with the growing awareness of the limitations of codes, led to the development of procedures to apply the general moral principles contained in the codes.

The procedures took the form of formal evaluation of research projects by institutional review committees. In 1953, the National Institutes of Health developed procedures to regulate research conducted at its clinical center.[32] In 1971, the Department of Health, Education, and Welfare formulated its policy for the protection of human subjects, and at present these policies vest basic responsibility for the protection of human subjects in institutional review committees.[33] Because of the prominent role that the federal government has in funding biomedical research, any institution engaged in research must have one. These committees are called Institutional Review Boards (IRBs). Such institutional committees in hospitals, medical centers, and other such facilities around the country are in charge of initial review of all research proposals and periodic re-review in order to ascertain that each researcher has outlined the risks and benefits and that the subjects have given their informed consent to participate in the study. Essentially, the IRB must determine that the rights and welfare of the subjects are protected, that the risks to an individual are outweighed by the potential benefit to him or her and society, and that informed consent will be obtained by adequate and appropriate methods. These governmental review standards, although worded in general terms, do detail the basic elements of informed consent, thereby drawing attention to its importance.

In spite of these important, substantive attempts to promote the conduct of research in such a way that protects human subjects, marked abuses continued. In 1966, Harvard anesthesiologist, Henry Beecher, published a list of research being conducted in which concern for the welfare of the subjects was completely sacrificed for medical knowledge.[34] Many of these studies are now common knowledge and bear an infamous notoriety: the cancer immunology experimentation at the Jewish Chronic Disease Hospital in New York, the hepatitis experiment on mentally retarded children institutionalized at Willowbrook, and the Tuskegee syphilis research on African Americans in the South. Although the Tuskegee experiment was initiated in the first half of the century, it continued into the early 1970s, long after the effectiveness of penicillin in treating syphilis had been established. The latter has been explored in detail,[35–39] including, in the contemporary play, *Miz Ever's Boys*, in which physician–playwright, Lawrence Feldshul, examines the complex relationships between the worlds of scientific medicine, the men, and the African American nurse, Miss Ever, who cared for them.

Although 30 years have elapsed since Beecher's indictment, we might wonder if the concerns raised by his disclosure have been adequately addressed. The answer seems to be mixed. On one hand, since research proposals must go through IRB committees, one can safely conclude that a study such as Tuskegee or Willowbrook would simply never be approved today. The harm to vulnerable people is too great and too explicit. On the other hand, there is evidence that misrepresentation and abuse persist.[40] But the fact that proposals must go through IRBs might give the impression that they provide more protection than they do. However, IRBs review research protocols at the local level and as Annas has noted, "IRBs as currently constituted do not protect research subjects but rather protect the institution and the institution's investigator."[41]

An interdisciplinary group, the National Commission for the Protection of Human Subjects of Biomedical and Behavioral Research, was established in 1974 to advise the then Department of Health, Education, and Welfare (HEW). This group was charged to investigate the ethical principles of human experimentation and develop guidelines for it on the national level. The Commission has published a number of important books that developed from its work. One such book addresses ethical issues surrounding informed consent.[42] In spite of the important contributions of this commission, an attempt to create a permanent commission for protection of human subjects failed. Following the Tuskegee scandal, Katz recommended that a National Human Investigation Board be formed, which would have the mandate to monitor, at least, all federally funded research.[43] Senator Edward Kennedy included this in a bill but the bill was never passed. According to Katz, "a major reason why this bill was never enacted may have been the Senate's reluctance to expose to public view the value conflicts inherent in the conduct of research."[44] This shows that the establishment of these commissions and councils and the development of guidelines and regulations are viewed by some professionals as onerous and even dangerous, because these activities may interfere with scientific advancement. Others, however, believe we require even more social control in these matters. They do not believe the present devices, including informed consent, protect human subjects enough from the ever-present potential for abuse.

INFORMED CONSENT AND THE RESEARCH SUBJECT

Informed consent implies a joint adventure in a common cause, a partnership between subject and investigator, or a process of coinvestigation. It is the propensity to overreach this joint adventure, even in a good cause, that makes consent necessary. The scientist has the ethical obligation to provide disclosure of information that includes the proclamation of benefits, the warning of risks, and the discussion of quandaries in order to obtain consent from the potential research subject. This consent must be based on the subject's understanding of the information to the greatest extent possible in order for him or her to be considered properly informed.

Although the concept of informed consent is commonly understood to have its origins in ethical thought, it actually originated in malpractice litigation of the 1950s such as *Canterbury v Spence*, mentioned in Chapter 1. More specifically, it arose from legal cases in which the patient's attorney had difficulty proving a physician's negligence when the usual community standards of medical practice were used for comparison. The informed consent approach shifted the legal claim from a charge of negligence to one of battery, because the patient would not have consented to the procedure had he or she known of the possible risk. If the doctor had not completely informed the patient as to the possible risks and alternatives, the patient could not be considered to have given his or her informed consent. Without effective consent, the physician had treated or operated upon the patient in an unlawful manner. This use of informed consent theory helped the patient's lawyer in these types of cases, because other doctors did not have to testify as to community standards. Later, however, the courts determined that the requirement of informed consent would be measured by the community standards of medical practitioners. The concept of informed consent had by that time gained acceptance both in medical practice procedures and in research experimentation but the idea was first used to protect physicians from legal liability.

Two early studies that have become classics, published 10 years apart, provide some insights into the ethical dilemmas involved in informed consent. We have already mentioned Beecher but his work is worthy of further discussion.[45] Beecher maintained that codes of ethics made the bland assumption that meaningful or informed consent was available for the asking, whereas in reality this very often was not the case. Although he conceded that consent in the fullest sense may not be obtainable, he said that it remains a goal toward which every researcher must nevertheless strive. With this in mind, he reviewed 50 studies in which he found only 2 mentions of informed consent; 12 studies seemed unethical, and generally his data suggested widespread ethical issues, especially with regard to informed consent. Following the position of the British Medical Research Council, Beecher said that not only should all investigations be conducted in an ethical manner, but in the publications it should also be made unmistakably clear that proprieties have been observed. He believed that journals have a moral obligation not to publish unethical research, even when those studies present very valuable data. Beecher believed that such a policy would discourage unethical experimentation. It is interesting to note that there has been discussion in the public domain about the ethical implications of using the data obtained through Nazi experimentation.[46-50] Beecher concluded by pointing out that the ethical approach has two important components, informed consent and the presence of an intelligent, informed, conscientious, compassionate, and responsible investigator.

The other study, by Barber, published in 1976, made note of the fact that in the previous decade we had increasingly perceived a social problem in the abuse of human subjects in medical experimentation.[51] Two major reasons have led to this general recognition that experimentation with humans is a subject for concern: the increased power, scope, and funding of biomedical research and changes in values that have increased the emphasis on equality, participation, and the challenging of arbitrary authority. Briefly, Barber and his colleagues conducted a survey in which they found investigators who were "permissive" regarding both informed consent and the risk–benefit ratio they were willing to accept. These data raise the question of how it happens that the treatment of human subjects is sometimes less than ethical, even in some of the most respected university hospitals.

Barber answered this question by saying that these abuses can be traced to defects in the training of researchers, to defects in the screening and monitoring of research by review committees, and to a fundamental tension between investigation and therapy. Barber's first answer may have been the case in 1976 but it is no longer a plausible answer to why, in Katz's assessment, informed consent has failed.[52] We have had more than enough time to train researchers. Nor is his second answer entirely sound given what has been stated earlier in reference to IRBs. His third answer seems closer to the mark because it points to the tension between research and therapy, which may be internal to the practice of scientific medicine. We discuss this idea further in a subsequent section.

In another early study, Gray interviewed 51 women who were, or had just been, subjects in another study to determine the effects of a new labor-inducing drug. His findings indicated that although all 51 women signed a consent form, 20 of them learned only from Gray's interview that they were research subjects. Of this group of 20, most of them did not understand that there might be hazards, that they would be subjected to special procedures, or that they were not required to participate in the study. Indeed, four of the women made it clear that they would not have participated had they understood and realized that they had a choice.[53] This points to an important aspect still relevant today: a signed form does not necessarily mean that *informed* consent has been obtained.[54] As Curtin indicated, "although the legal doctrine of informed consent arose to protect patients, the consent form arose to protect providers." [55] In the long run, all the regulations, reviews, and informed consent forms will serve a limited function unless the clinician and researcher bring their ethical reasoning and integrity to bear on these complex issues.

For most authorities on the matter, the core of the informed consent process from the beginning of the discussion was the balancing of risk to the human subject against possible benefits to the individual and society. However, Jonas, an early critic of this conception, voiced resistance to this "merely utilitarian view." He raised the issue of the peculiarity of human experimentation quite independent of the question of possible injury to the subject. According to him, the wrong involved with making a person an experimental subject is not so much that we make that person a means to an end, since that happens in social contexts of all kinds, but that we make the person a thing. He accused this approach of reducing the person in human experimentation to a passive thing or token, or a "sample" merely to be acted on.[56] The fact that this penetrating argument has been made again by Katz[57] should be a call to researchers to rethink the ethical issues in their deliberations of means and ends, the individual good and the common good, and the private and the public welfare, all of which must be considered in informed consent.

Ideally, informed consent can be thought of as a collaborative endeavor involving truth telling on the part of the researcher and free choice on the part of the subject within a context of some degree of uncertainty. If we already knew all the possible risks and benefits of a given procedure or drug, we would not need to undertake the research. In determining the most accurate risk–benefit ratio, we need a thoughtful, humane, and best-educated opinion. The Helsinki Declaration says that research involving human subjects cannot legitimately be carried out unless the importance of the objective is in proportion to the inherent risk to the subject. Such inherent risks may be easier to measure and weigh in the risk–benefit calculus with biomedical research than with research focused on psychological or social aspects. Nevertheless, the Helsinki Declaration does say that every precaution should be taken to minimize the impact of the study on the subject's physical and mental integrity and on the personality of the subject.

It has been documented that the social sciences differ from the natural sciences in some fundamental ways. Although uncertainty exists in the natural sciences, the difficulty in observing and analyzing social reality presents other very complex social science problems. The objects of social science research are living conditions, institutions, or human attitudes that combine changeability and rigidity in an unstable and, to some extent, an inscrutable pattern. Some social scientists have attempted to emulate the methods of natural sciences and this has at times led to a dangerous superficiality in approach. Such an analysis, regarded as strict or rigorous by natural science standards, may in social science research be lacking in both logical consistency and adequate reflection of reality.

Qualitative research is the generic descriptive term for social science research that does not model the natural sciences but rather, seeks to understand a given phenomenon from the perspectives of the subjects. Herein lies a major difference between these two approaches to the development of knowledge. Most qualitative research involves talking to research participants in which narrative data are generated in contrast to the numerical data of most natural science research, including biomedical research.[58] Anthropologists, sociologists, and nurses conduct a great deal of qualitative research. In contrast to biomedical research, qualitative research does not involve invasive bodily procedures and because the data are produced by talking, this research implies a different relationship between the investigator and the research participant. Nonetheless, there are several ethical issues involving protection of research participants.[59] Central among these are deception, mentioned below, trust, and confidentiality. Confidentiality is particularly important because the participants could be easily identified and given the often sensitive nature of the topic under study, there could be grave consequences to participants if confidentiality were violated.

In the research projects of both natural science and social science, the importance of the research also becomes a factor. Some research may have minimum risk but also minimum benefits to the subject and society. Should such research be done? How could we either support it or not on moral grounds? If such research includes inconveniences rather than risks to the human subjects, are there ethical considerations nonetheless? A more serious problem arises in the instance in which there is possible risk but minimum benefit involved in the study. In some research, the procedure is so intrusive that the possible risks become more obvious, whereas when the procedures are less intrusive, the possible risks may be overlooked. In each experimental situation, such dimensions of the risk–benefit ratio need reviewing with the potential human subject before an informed consent is obtained.

The dilemma inevitably arises as to the extent of the disclosure necessary to obtain a truly informed consent. In the past, when a patient engaged a physician or entered a hospital, these actions themselves often served as a blanket consent to such treatment as the physician or hospital staff, in the exercise of their professional judgment, deemed proper. Now the extent and the content of the disclosure for treatment purposes has expanded, taking into account the patient's rights and the professional's obligations.

The similar problem in research, noted nearly 50 years ago, results from the combination of helplessness, lack of technical competence, and the emotional disturbance experienced in the sick role that make the patient a peculiarly vulnerable object for exploration.[60] While this view of the totally passive and helpless patient as put forth by the sociologist Parsons has raised questions, the inequalities of knowledge and power between the person obtaining informed consent and the person giving it has been a major concern of feminists. Physicians have only just begun to address the power inherent to the practice of medicine.[61] But it is precisely this power differential, combined with the argument that patients do not want to know or cannot understand, that has made informed consent a necessity.

In these earlier discussions of informed consent, Baumrind made one of the more profound observations in discussing the issue of human experimentation. She maintained that subjects are less adversely affected by physical pain or psychological stress than by experiences that result in loss of trust in themselves and the investigators and, by extension, in the meaningfulness of life itself. The researcher violates the fundamental moral principles of reciprocity and justice when he, using his position of trust, acts to deceive or degrade those whose extension of trust has been granted on the basis of a contrary role expectation. He behaves unjustly when he uses naive (trusting) subjects and then exploits their naivete, no matter if the direct resulting harm is small. The harm becomes cumulative both to the individual and to society.[62] It is worth noting that within contemporary society there is widespread mistrust of experts, that is, those with special knowledge such as physicians, attorneys, business leaders, scientists, and to a lesser extent, academics. Historically, these groups have been granted enormous social privilege, including the pursuit of self-interest precisely because they have been charged with and thought to be serving a larger, social good. Flagrant abuse in research is one reason some of these groups have lost status in the public eye. There are classic examples of research that relied on deception to obtain their findings.[63–66] None of these studies, with publication dates ranging from 1965 to 1973, would today be approved by an IRB. Some argue that they are important studies and give us knowledge and insights that we would not otherwise have. While this may be true, our ethics has developed around obtaining informed consent to safeguard the human subject. Research that relies on deception makes that obligation difficult to meet. Regardless of the importance of the findings in these and other such studies, a serious ethical dilemma underlies the entire research structure. To rely on deception means that the researcher totally violates the ethical principle of truth telling and dupes a subject who cannot give his informed consent in a situation in which he has not been told the real nature of the research or indeed that he is participating in research at all. The question is usually raised as to whether this means that some research cannot or should not be performed. Yes, it does possibly mean just that. Although we have been concerned with deception in the practice of research, it is not limited to research. Deception can be used for the ostensible good of reassuring patients.[67] But trust is always violated when deception is used and it is therefore ethically unacceptable.

Another question raised relates to the problem of biasing the research by giving the subject too much detail. In this case, at least two solutions to the issue of informed consent exist. First, it may be possible to redesign the research so that disclosure will not bias the study. Second, it may be possible to tell the subject some details and also discuss the fact that to go into more details would make the research findings less reliable. The latter solution has possible problems, since, although the subject knows information is being withheld, he is not aware of the nature of the information.

While the actual practice is imperfect, the idea of informed consent does accord the patient the status of a person, not an experimental object, and provides a degree of assurance that he or she is being considered as an end and not merely as a means. Insofar as every treatment procedure and every involvement in research carry with them potential risk, it must be the patient or his or her guardian who has the right to decide not only whether to participate but also what factors are or are not relevant to his or her consent.

INFORMED CONSENT AND SELECTED HUMAN SUBJECTS

The concept of informed consent rests on the assumption that the researcher will adequately inform the potential research subject, in language he or she can understand, so that the individual or appointed guardian will in fact understand the risks and benefits and will be in a position either to agree to participate or to refuse to do so without negatively affecting the relationship with the researcher or the institution providing the service. Competent people have the right to decide whether to accept or reject proposed treatment and this includes being in a research protocol. The concept of competence, simply put, means that the patient has the ability to communicate choices, can understand relevant information, can appreciate the situation and its consequences, and can manipulate information rationally.[68–72] Other work on competence adds the important dimension of making decisions in keeping with one's values or how one lives their life.[73] Certain groups present special ethical problems and raise questions regarding the adequacy of informed consent. Research using students, prisoners, minors, the mentally ill, the mentally retarded, the elderly, especially those in an institution, and fetuses can and do raise many ethical dilemmas.

The problem of restricted choice is central to informed consent. Simply stated, the problem of restricted choice asks the question: What are the moral limitations of consent in situations or settings where choices are limited, and indeed, what counts as informed consent in such instances? Restricted choice can arise in a number of situations ranging from research with students to that with prisoners and other institutionalized persons. For example, when the instructor in a classroom asks the students to volunteer for research purposes, there exists at least the implied threat of loss of affection and possibly poorer academic grades if the student does not volunteer. This becomes a situation of restricted choice for the student, with ethical dilemmas involved. Previously some institutions granted students credit for participating in research. This procedure raised the issue of infringement of the rights of those who did not volunteer or were not chosen after volunteering.

There are more serious ethical implications that can arise in research using prisoners as human subjects. Regarding informed consent, the underlying ethical issue is: To what extent can prisoners exercise freedom of choice in giving consent or refusing it? The issues of restrictive choice and possible coercion have been weighed against the benefits to the individual prisoner, usually remuneration and better living conditions for research subjects, occasionally reduced sentences, benefits to society, and the obligations, if any, that the prisoner has to society. Many people concerned with this area of human experimentation believe that it may not be possible to overcome these serious ethical dilemmas. The fundamental ethical concepts embodied in the informed consent process can easily be violated in these circumstances.

A similar situation arises with the committed mentally ill patient, and the same ethical concerns may lead to the conclusion that informed consent is not a possibility. With voluntary patients in institutions, informed consent may be an adequate safeguard because of their legal status; however, that status can change and their choices can become restricted. Moreover, in either case, the patients' mental status caused by illness or by drugs and their ability to give consent must be viewed as the basis for a potential ethical dilemma. Laws in some states have addressed the informed consent issue for both involuntary and voluntary patients with regard to the right to refuse drugs. However, the question has been raised as to whether such legislation really provides a useful safeguard for the protection of the psychiatric patient's civil rights.

With the mentally retarded, the problems are the result of the individual's mental status—being institutionalized and dependent—and, who speaks for and safeguards the rights of the individual being asked to serve as a human subject. If someone else consents for him or her to act as a subject, then that person must be informed and give consent with the best interest of the potential subject as the grounds for the action. One can attempt to evaluate such action by asking what decision any reasonable person would make under these particular circumstances. Most likely, the characteristics of the ideal observer would be helpful in making the decision. Having all the information available, understanding potential consequences, coupled with the ability to visualize the experience as if it were happening to the observer, but also having the ability to be impartial, this observer ideally can make the best morally based decision. This observer, however, represents an ideal, and not necessarily a reality, in any given individual.

Some doubts can be raised about the moral motivation of some parents in giving consent for their retarded institutionalized child to be part of a research study. This does not mean that all such parents are morally suspect, but a possible conflict of interest does exist in the situation. The child may possibly have been institutionalized because the parents rejected the child. In such a case, potential conflict of interest looms larger than in a situation where the child has been placed in an institution because he or she cannot be physically managed at home or elsewhere. The staff members who conduct research with the mentally retarded in such an institution may have more of a conflict than some other researchers.

Some of the same issues come into play in research with minors.[74–76] One of the most serious questions with any group—and especially vulnerable ones, including well children—involves research that is nontherapeutic or nonbeneficial to the subject. On what ethical grounds should research be conducted using either well children or mentally ill or retarded children where risks must be weighed against benefits? For normal children, the benefits will be neither direct nor immediate in any tangible way. The questions become: Should physically well, normal children ever be human subjects? If so, on what moral grounds? Should mentally ill or retarded children participate in any research, and, if so, should it only be research that can potentially benefit them directly? If other research is to be permitted, on what moral grounds would these children become human subjects and who will speak for them in the informed consent procedure?

One area that has aroused much debate, that of fetal research, has also raised the issue of possible medical benefits gained as measured against the possible ethical costs of such research to society. Some of this impassioned debate surrounding fetal research is tied to the different moral positions that people have taken on abortion. A federal ban on fetal research initiated in 1988 was recently lifted in response to the arguments that many diseases and possible treatments could be explored through research on fetuses.[77–79] A discussion of the rights of the fetus can be found in Chapter 8.

The elderly, and particularly those in institutions such as nursing homes, represent another vulnerable group in the human subjects controversy. Many of the same issues mentioned above also arise with this group. Because cognitive functioning is frequently impaired, competence is of particular concern.[80] And, as with some of the other groups, we tend to have negative attitudes toward the elderly that may blur some of the ethical considerations.

Because we live in a time of scientific totalitarianism,[81,82] where science and technology are seen as the solution to human problems,[83] the advancement of medical knowledge can become an ideology. The pursuit of medical knowledge can overshadow all other considerations, including the interests of those who serve as research subjects. This is why we had the abuses as revealed by Beecher and not because we had investigators untrained in the finer points of informed consent. With all potential subjects for research projects, and certainly with these special problem groups, many ethical issues emerge. Although some think that the goal of having human subjects spontaneously volunteer rather than being conscripted cannot be achieved, nevertheless, most believe that efforts to promote educated, informed consent are in order. This effort to educate and inform should reach everyone, including these groups and others, such as the poor, who depend more on public facilities, where more training of health care personnel and more research occurs than in the private sector of the health care delivery system. Even more important, however, than the education of potential subjects is the attitude of the researchers themselves. It is imperative that they be committed, in Katz's words, to the *idea* of informed consent.[84] Such a commitment would serve to keep at bay the powerful pull to advance medical knowledge at any cost long enough to look at the interests and hear the voices of those rendering that knowledge.

INFORMED CONSENT AND TREATMENT

The elements of informed consent that operate in research situations are valid in treatment situations as well. Patients should not receive treatment, except in emergencies, until they have given consent that is informed. In treatment we assume that patients benefit directly, whereas in research they may or may not benefit directly in return for participation. Treatment is routine in the sense that a given intervention, which has been demonstrated to be both safe and effective against a specific disease or symptom, is accepted as a standard of practice. On the other hand, it is just this safety and effectiveness that research sets out to determine. And yet, the boundaries between treatment and research are often less distinct, particularly with certain diseases.

The introduction of what has come to be called compassionate use protocols demonstrates this blurring of boundaries. Compassionate use protocols are research protocols designed to test interventions on human subjects that have not been proven but may be helpful in treating a disease. Cancer and AIDS are two cases where they have been used fairly extensively. They have been justified because the known risk (or inevitability) of mortality is seen as sufficient to balance the unknown risks that might be associated with possible benefit. It cannot be assumed that someone with a fatal disease for which there is no cure would automatically desire to participate in a compassionate use protocol. At the same time, it should be noted that patient groups, particularly those with AIDS and breast cancer, have been very active in lobbying for earlier access to potential therapies. In these situations, as in all clinical situations, it is important that patients receive honest and detailed information about the interventions that are available and that may profoundly affect how they will be able to live their lives.

Truth telling is not uncomplicated, however. While it was not always commonplace for physicians to tell patients their diagnosis and other information, the practice has become part of the mainstream culture of American medicine since the changes that occurred from the mid-1940s to the 1970s. Many of these changes emanated from concerns with informed consent. If the patient is a competent adult who is capable of acting autonomously, the decision to withhold information from him or her violates the ethical principle of veracity and renders the patient less than autonomous. The decision to withhold information often is derived from the ethical principle of nonmaleficence, or the obligation to do no harm. The reasoning is as follows: The patient is very ill and is suffering. We should not further burden him or her with knowledge of the seriousness of the diagnosis. Such good intentions in the name of doing no harm result in curtailment of the patient's autonomy and create a deceitful situation for all those around the patient. The truth can be cruel, and the way we inform patients must take this into account. Great sensitivity and adequate emotional support for the patient are required. When this sort of ethical dilemma arises, it needs to be reasoned through and the ethical principles weighed to determine which is to be followed and which is to be violated, since in these situations, both cannot be followed. How this is to be accomplished must then be worked out.

Unique challenges to this view can be presented by persons from differing cultures where decision making is left more explicitly to medical authority or is more communal than we customarily understand it.[85-88] A current research project on ethical decision making regarding end-of-life decisions among Chinese-Americans, Hispanic-Americans, African-Americans, and Anglo-American is showing similar findings.[89-90] Because informed consent exists, in principle, to honor and respect a person's autonomy and should not be a mere routinized procedure, these situations may require additional time and effort to understand the meaning of autonomy to the people involved. In these situations, there is no hard and fast rule but taking the time to listen carefully to patients combined with sound ethical reflection can help clinicians in their commitment to the idea of informed consent.

How information is conveyed is not unrelated to whether informed consent is conceived of as an event or a process. As an event, informed consent is seen as occurring in a single time period whereas, as a process, informed consent takes place over time.[91] In the complex reality of practice, it is not likely that these are mutually exclusive although the social context of the particular situation contributes to which view is predominate. For example, one author points out that informed consent in the context of an emergency in an intensive care unit where physician and patient are strangers will look very different from informed consent in a primary care setting where physician and patient have known each other over an extended time.[92] Regardless of how physicians envision their duty regarding informed consent, it is important to keep in mind that patients may change their minds at any time during a research project or a treatment regimen.

Another contemporary issue regarding informed consent and treatment concerns managed care and the disclosure of treatment availability. In the move to managed care, insurance companies increasingly dictate what treatments will and will not be paid for. These policies, however, are not routinely made available to patients and this raises questions as to the ethical obligation that these institutions have to those for whom they are responsible for the provision of care. Several works are addressing these issues and others related to managed care.[93–99]

A major criticism of informed consent is that patients cannot understand the complex information they need to be able to give informed consent. Poor distribution of power and information exists. Informed consent is not a perfect tool, but with more attention to the ethics underlying it and a focus on the pragmatic aspects of the process, the patient should be better able to participate in the decision making involved in his or her treatment and care.

INFORMED CONSENT AND NURSING

Over the past 30 years, the discipline of nursing has continued to address the ethical issues as related to nursing practice and research. The following is a brief overview of selected aspects of informed consent in research and treatment and the nurse's obligations as presented in those writings. Abdellah, in a paper based on a presentation at the 1967 National League for Nursing Convention, noted that as nursing research focuses more on clinical problems, the legal and ethical aspects will become more apparent. Although clinical nursing research may differ from medical research in the extent and kind of risk to patients, in both disciplines many similar problems exist regarding the conduct of research. Nonetheless, there are a number of ethical issues, including the right to privacy or to withhold information.[100]

In the mid-1960s, nurse investigators were just beginning to make inroads in biological research. At that time, the nature of consent to participate in research as a human subject could be implicit, explicit, or in the form of a written statement and, for example, the fact that a patient was admitted to a hospital implied a certain degree of implicit consent. Recall that Beecher's paper chronicling abuses was published in 1966.[101] With the advent of governmental guidelines for the use of human subjects and the establishment of peer review committees to assist in safeguarding the rights of human subjects through a formal informed consent procedure, the informal and blanket mechanisms, which could be too easily abused, became ancient history.

In 1969, Berthold wrote a detailed paper based on a review of the literature and focused on the larger topic of maintaining human rights and values amidst a scientific–technological revolution and the concomitant social revolution. She developed the idea that the right of the individual in American society to dignity, self-respect, and freedom of self-determination has been in conflict with the rights and long-range interests of society on many occasions and on various issues. Berthold went on to say that these conflicts have generally been characterized as involving humanitarian, libertarian, and scientific values. Humanitarian values have to do with respect for the sanctity of human life and the safeguards needed to protect the subject from physical or emotional harm. Libertarian values have to do with the individual's political, civil, and individual rights to self-respect, dignity, freedom of thought and action, and the safeguards needed to protect the individual from invasion of privacy without his or her knowledge for the sake of knowledge. Scientific values concern the safeguards needed to protect the right to know anything that may be known or discovered about any part of the universe. In specific situations these different values lead to competing moral claims that must be balanced against one another within the process of moral reasoning.[102]

Today we might wonder if this value of the right to know anything has contributed to the scientific totalitarianism mentioned earlier.[103,104] Might not this cultural value be responsible at least in part for some of the abuses committed in the name of the advancement of medical knowledge? Evidence of this is given in the argument published in 1977 by a nurse and physician working in a burn center.[105] They argued that in burn cases where survival is unprecedented, the person should be allowed to die. The answer by the NIH consensus conference on the treatment of burns was that people must always be treated because to do otherwise would impede research.[106] Informed consent would be irrelevant in such a situation—the patient would not have to consent because he or she could not refuse.

Scientific inquiry can involve several specific ethical issues, all of which should be considered by the nurse investigator when designing the research as well as by the potential human subject giving informed consent. These issues include: (1) loss of dignity and autonomy, (2) invasion of privacy, (3) time and energy requirements, (4) mental and physical discomfort or pain, and (5) risk of physical or emotional injury. These issues must be weighed against potential benefits for the subject himself, for people like him (e.g., diabetics), and for the general good of all people. Although respect for autonomy has been increasingly questioned as a basis for practice, it is essential if the demand for the advancement of medical knowledge is not to trump individual wishes to the contrary. ✺

In 1970, Batey raised the question as to when and to what extent the issue of the rights of human subjects becomes a methodological issue in nursing research. She also asked whether there is a metaprofessional ethic or a set of values guiding nurse researchers who are both researchers and clinicians. In addition, she asked whether nurse researchers share a set of values directed toward optimizing the conditions needed for fulfillment of the aims of science.[107]

The American Nurses Association (ANA) has been active in developing guidelines on ethical values for the nurse in research. In 1968, the Committee on Research and Studies said that nursing was committed to the identification and elaboration of a body of scientific knowledge that guides nursing practice for the provision of optimal nursing services to society. The ANA reaffirmed its belief in the rights and the responsibilities of members of the profession to conduct research and to meet its obligations to those members by establishing guidelines on ethical values. In discussing these ethical dimensions within the framework of protecting human rights, the ANA elaborated on the rights to privacy, to self-determination, to conservation of personal resources, to freedom from arbitrary hurt, and to freedom from intrinsic risk of injury. The rights of minors and incompetent persons, such as young children or unconscious patients, and the informed consent process were also discussed. Essentially, the ANA's position rests on the idea that the relationship of trust between subject and investigator requires that the subject be assured that he or she will be treated fairly and that no discomfort, risk, or inconvenience, beyond that initially stated in obtaining informed consent, will be imposed without further permission being obtained from the subject.[108]

The nurse who conducts research does not differ from her colleagues in other disciplines. Her research protocol and activities must ensure that the human subject will be informed in understandable language and will in no way be coerced to participate or continue in the study but will be free to exercise his or her freedom of self-determination. As stated previously, the integrity and ethics of the investigator are essential to preserve the safety and the rights of the human subject. Nursing must continue their discussions within the profession of the issues involved in research with human subjects, informed consent, and the conflicting moral claims that create ethical dilemmas for the nurse researcher who is the principle investigator and for the nurse in the clinical setting who assists in another's research.

The ethical issues that might arise for nurses who assist in another's research received official attention in the 1975 ANA position paper on human rights developed by the Commission on Nursing Research. One very important aspect of this document is its statement on human rights for the nurse.[109]

> Implementation of this guideline implies the need for written statements about conditions of employment and any special expectations about work performance above and beyond that usually expected of a person occupying the position of nurse. In advance of such employment, nurses need to know if they will be expected to provide medicine, treatment, and other procedures as part of double-blind investigations. They need to know in advance if the work requires them to function as data collectors for research in addition to their role as nurses engaged in the delivery of patient care services. Conditions of employment must also provide for the option of not participating in clinical research if these work expectations are not spelled out in advance of employment.*

Little is known about the ethical experiences of nurses who participate in the research of others. Nurses, however, bear an instrumental relationship to the ends of medicine, that is, in carrying out orders they become the means to the therapeutic ends set by others, usually physicians.[110,111] Although not specifically looking at nurses conducting research, in a study examining the ethical concerns of nurses, Liaschenko showed that nurses are harmed when they must carry out treatment which they consider destructive.[112] They are harmed because they experience moral distress[113] and they are harmed because the integrity of their practice is violated.

Another important group about which we know little are the nurses who run clinical trials. So far we have been talking about nurses conducting nursing research. Yet it is nurses who largely run the clinical trials of medical research. These nurses are paid by research money, hired by physicians, and responsible to them. From informal talking with some of these nurses, we have learned that serious concerns about informed consent are not uncommon. These nurses potentially face very difficult ethical dilemmas around issues of responsibility and conflict of loyalty. The world of practice is not neat and tidy and living by one's commitments can be difficult, rarely done in a pure way. As Aristotle acknowledged, ethics is a practical matter because it deals with the contingencies of human existence.[114] Most of us make compromises and indeed, doing so wisely can be a matter of ethical

---

*Reprinted with permission of the American Nurses Association.

behavior.[115] What we compromise and to what end is a matter of our integrity and integrity is shaped by ethical reflection.

The most recent work identifies nine principles essential to the ethical conduct of research. These include:

1. Respect for the autonomous person to consent
2. The prevention of harm and the promotion of good
3. Respect for personhood and the valuation of diversity
4. Respect of benefits and burdens of research in terms of the selection of subjects
5. Protection of privacy
6. Maintenance of the integrity of the researcher
7. Reporting of scientific misconduct
8. Maintenance of the investigator's competence
9. A concern for animal welfare, if they must be used[116]

These principles and the commentary that accompanies them provide a framework for critical ethical reflection in nursing research.[117]

Informed consent was explored in detail in the first book on ethics and nursing research, *Patients, Nurses, Ethics*, by Davis and Krueger.[118] As we have seen, it continues to figure centrally in the literature on nursing ethics whether in relation to research or treatment.[119–136] Although most of this recent work is not data based, it does support earlier studies showing the concerns of nursing in informed consent.[137–139] For example, one of these studies identified five roles in which nurses have assumed active involvement in informed consent. These roles are:

1. Watchdog to monitor informed consent situations
2. Advocate to mediate on behalf of patients
3. Resource person to provide information on alternatives
4. Coordinator to preserve an open, friendly atmosphere for discussion
5. Facilitator to clarify differences between involved parties

Such studies raise the larger issue of disclosure of information in informed consent. Questions arise about what information should be disclosed, how much, and by whom. One study on the attitudes of nurses and medical students toward nurses disclosing information to patients pointed to areas of possible conflict. Generally, this conflict can be seen as one between a strong view of patients' rights and the need of hospital bureaucracies to maintain orderly channels of communication.[140]

The nurse's ethical obligation in informed consent is to ascertain whether the patient understands what he or she has been told and what has been consented to. Informed consent is an imperfect tool and patients may have questions about the research or treatment they have agreed to. Even if the patients do not initiate this subject, the nurse needs to find out if they actually do understand the nature of the treatment regimen. This is an ethical matter for nurses not just because they work in in-between positions[141-143] but also because they act directly for patients physically, psychologically, and in ways that help them preserve the integrity of who they are as a person.[144]

Once the nurse has discovered that the patient does not understand aspects of the treatment, his or her ethical obligation is to report this to the physician so that he or she can meet the ethical obligation to inform. Usually physicians follow through and speak further with patients regarding their treatment. If a physician decides not to provide additional information, however, or not to clarify what has already been said, the question arises as to the nurse's obligation in the situation. Has the nurse met his or her professional obligation by telling the physician that the patient needs additional input about treatment, or does he or she need to do something more when the physician does not follow through? The nurse must ethically reason through to some conclusion, and on that basis he or she will decide the ethical thing to do. It is important to remember that ethical dilemmas may not have been solved merely by replacing the physician's values with the nurse's. The central question is what does the patient want, or if the patient cannot make his or her position known because of a compromised physical or mental status, then, who is to speak in his or her best interest?

■ CASE STUDY I.

Marjorie is a spry and independent woman. She is very strong minded and practical. At 87, she is diagnosed with pancreatic cancer and a Whipple operation is offered as a potential cure. Her surgeon carefully explains to her the risks of the procedure, which, given her age, include the real possibility of death. As she understands the situation, she will either die a lingering death from cancer, she will be cured by the surgery, or she will die "under the knife." She consents to the surgery. She gets her affairs in order and appoints a conservator to manage her financial affairs.

Marjorie does not die on the table but she lingers for seven months in the intensive care unit as a result of successive complications. She is conscious, but unable to communicate. As is typical in these complex medical situations, each physiological problem is addressed individually. Therefore, each of Marjorie's complications was considered "potentially treatable" since her cancer was gone.

The nurses were disturbed by Marjorie's prolonged suffering as were her friends. They questioned if she really understood the potential consequences of such a radical surgery. Their concerns were discussed with her physicians who justified the continued aggressive treatment on the grounds that she must want this since she had agreed to such radical treatment in the first place.

Suggested Questions for Discussion

1. How do you understand what the patient is consenting to and what difference does this make?

2. Was her consent informed?

3. Do physicians and nurses understand informed consent differently? If so, why?

■ CASE STUDY II.

Ms. Y is a 34-year-old woman who has been under medical care for a severe seizure disorder. During one of her medical visits, her physician discusses advance directives with her. He advises her to obtain one because her seizures are likely to worsen and leave her incapacitated in the future. She does so and appoints her mother Mrs. X, who has a fifth grade education, as durable power of attorney for health care.

One month later, she has a devastating seizure. Her mother is present in the emergency room where the physicians repeatedly seek her consent to provide emergency care, including placing her on a ventilator and other forms of life support. Mrs. X asks if the ventilator is life support saying "That ain't life support is it? She doesn't want life support." She is told it is not life support, it is just to make her comfortable. Ms. Y stays in a coma for two months from which she emerges totally incapacitated; she must be fed, bathed, and diapered. She can speak only a few words such as "water" and "bury me," must be tied to the bed because she thrashes around violently, and screams for many hours each day.

Suggested Questions for Discussion

1. When is consent informed?

2. What are the assumptions we make regarding the average person's understanding of the practice of medicine and how hospitals work? How does this affect the process of informed consent?

3. What other factors influence the process of informed consent? Do you think Mrs. X's educational level was a factor here?

4. Should health care providers even attempt to engage in the process of informed consent in emergency situations?

REFERENCES

1. Miller B: Autonomy and the refusal of lifesaving treatment. *Hastings Cent Rep* 11(4):22–28, 1981.
2. Kant I: *Groundwork of the Metaphysics of Morals.* New York: Harper Torchbooks; 1964.
3. Capron A: Informed consent in catastrophic disease and treatment. *University of Pennsylvania Law Rev* 123:364–376, 1974.

4. Beecher H: Ethics and clinical research. *N Engl J Med* 274(24):1354–1360, 1966.

5. Rothman D: *Strangers at the Bedside: A History of How Law and Bioethics Transformed Medical Decision Making*. New York: Basic Books; 1991.

6. Cunningham S, Mitchell P: The use of animals in nursing research. *Adv Nur Sci* 4(4):72–84, 1982.

7. Crowley M, Connors D: Critique of "The use of animals in research." *Adv Nur Sci* 7(4):23–31, 1985.

8. Donovan J: Animal rights and feminist theory. *Signs* 15(2):350–375, 1990.

9. Slicer D: Your daughter or your dog? *Hypatia* 6(1):108–124, 1991.

10. Midgley M: Is the biosphere a luxury? *Hastings Cent Rep* 22(2):7–12, 1992.

11. Nelson JL: Transplantation through a glass darkly. *Hastings Cent Rep* 22(5):6–8, 1992.

12. Donnelley S: Bioethical troubles: Animal individuals and human organisms. *Hastings Cent Rep* 25(7):21–29, 1995.

13. Liaschenko J: The moral geography of home care. *Adv Nurs Sci* 17(2):16–26, 1994.

14. Liaschenko J: Artificial personhood: Nursing ethics in a medical world. *Nurs Ethics* 2(3):185–196, 1995.

15. McGrath P: It's ok to say no! A discussion of ethical issues arising from informed consent to chemotherapy. *Cancer Nurs* 18(2):97–103, 1995.

16. Holmes H, Purdy, L: *Feminist Perspectives in Medical Ethics*. Bloomington, IN: Indiana University Press; 1992.

17. Sherwin S: *No Longer Patient: Feminist Ethics and Health Care*. Philadelphia: Temple University Press; 1992.

18. Ehrenreich B, Ehrenreich J: The system behind the chaos. In McKenzie N (ed): *The Crisis in Health Care: Ethical Issues* New York: Meridian; 1990, pp 50–69.

19. McKenzie N: The new ethical demand in the crisis of primary care medicine. In McKenzie N (ed): *The Crisis in Health Care: Ethical Issues*. New York: Meridian; 1990, pp 113–126.

20. Callahan D: Bioethics: Private choice and common good. *Hastings Cent Rep* 24(3):28–31, 1994.

21. Katz J: Ethics in clinical research revisited. *Hastings Cent Rep* 23(5):31–39, 1993.

22. Brody H: The best system in the world. *Hastings Cent Rep* 25(6 suppl):S18–S21, 1995.

23. Fox R, Swazey J: Leaving the Field. *Hastings Cent Rep* 22(5):9–15, 1992.

24. Ehrenreich B, Ehrenreich J: *op. cit.*

25. Bernard C: *An Introduction to the Study of Experimental Medicine*. New York: Macmillan; 1927.

26. *Fortner v Koch*. 272 Mich 273, 282, 261, NW (Mich 1935).

27. Lifton RJ: *The Nazi Doctors: Medical Killing and the Psychology of Genocide*. New York: Basic Books; 1986.

28. Proctor R: *Racial Hygiene: Medicine Under the Nazis*. Cambridge, MA: Harvard University Press; 1988.

29. Steppe H: Nursing in the Third Reich. *Hist Nurs J* 3(4):21–37, 1991.

30. Steppe H: Nursing in Nazi Germany. *West J Nurs Res* 14(6):744–753, 1992.
31. Davis A: *Nursing's Role in Creating the Ideal Society*. Presented at the conference, The Value of the Human Being: Medicine Under the Nazis; August 22, 1992; San Francisco, CA.
32. Faden RR, Beauchamp, J: *A History and Theory of Informed Consent*. New York: Oxford University Press; 1986.
33. *Grants Administration Manual*. United States Department of Health, Education and Welfare; 1971.
34. Beecher H: *op. cit.*
35. *Final Report of the Tuskegee Syphilis Study Ad Hoc Advisory Panel*. United States Public Health Service; 1973.
36. Jones JH: *Bad Blood: The Tuskegee Syphilis Experiment*. New York: Free Press; 1981.
37. Caplan AL: Twenty years after: The legacy of the Tuskegee Syphilis Study. When evil intrudes. *Hastings Cent Rep* 22(6):29–32, 1992.
38. Edgar H: Twenty years after: The legacy of the Tuskegee Syphilis Study. Outside the community. *Ibid.*, pp 32–35.
39. King PA: Twenty years after: The legacy of the Tuskegee Syphilis Study. The danger of difference. *Ibid.*, pp 35–38.
40. Alderson P: Consent and the social context. *Nurs Ethics* 2(4):347–350, 1995.
41. Katz J: *op. cit.*, p 38.
42. Presidents Commission for the Study of Ethical Problems in Medicine and Biomedical and Behavioral Research: *Making Health Care Decisions*. Washington, DC: United States Government Printing Office; 1982.
43. Katz J: *op. cit.*
44. *Ibid.*, p 37.
45. Beecher H: *op. cit.*
46. Sheldon M, Whitely WP: Commentary—Case studies-Nazi data: Dissociation from evil. *Hastings Cent Rep* 19(4):16–17, 1989.
47. Folker B, Hafner AW: Commentary. *Ibid.*, pp 17–18.
48. Gaylin W: Commentary. *Ibid.*, p 18.
49. Caplan AL: In brief—The Meaning of the Holocaust for Bioethics. *Hastings Cent Rep* 19(4):2–3, 1989.
50. Seidelman W: In memoriam: Medicine's confrontation with evil. *Hastings Cent Rep* 19(6):5–6, 1989.
51. Barber B: The ethics of experimentation with human subjects. *Sci Am* 234:25–31, 1976.
52. Katz J: *op. cit.*
53. Gray BH: *Human Subjects in Medical Experimentation*. New York: Wiley; 1975.
54. McMullen P, Philipsen N: Informed consent: It's more than just a signature on paper. *Nurs Connections* 9(2):41–43, 1993.
55. Curtin L: Informed consent: Cautious, calculated candor. *Nurs Management* 24(4):18–20, 1993, p 18.
56. Jonas H: Philosophical reflections on experimenting with human subjects. In Freund PA (ed): *Experimentation with Human Subjects*. New York: Braziller; 1969, pp 1–31.

57. Katz J: *op. cit.*
58. Tesch R: *Qualitative Research: Analysis Types and Software Tools.* New York: Falmer Press; 1990.
59. Holloway I, Wheeler S: Ethical issues in qualitative health research. *Nurs Ethics* 2(3):223–232, 1995.
60. Parsons T: *The Social System.* Glencoe, IL: Free Press; 1951.
61. Brody H: *The Healer's Power.* New Haven, CT: Yale University Press; 1992.
62. Baumrind D: Principles of ethical conduct in the treatment of subjects. *Am Psychol* 27:1083, 1973.
63. Milgram S: Some conditions of obedience and disobedience to authority. *Hum Relations* 18:57–75; 1965.
64. Hofling C, Brotzman E, Dalrymple S, et al: An experimental study in nurse-patient relationships. *J Nerv Ment Dis* 143:171–180, 1966.
65. Humphreys L: *Tearoom Trade: Impersonal Sex in Public Places.* Chicago: Aldine; 1970.
66. Rosenhan DL: On being sane in insane places. *Science* 167:250–258, 1973.
67. Teasdale K, Kent G: The use of deception in nursing. *J Med Ethics* 21(2):77–81, 1995.
68. Appelbaum PS, Grisso T: Assessing patients' capacities to consent to treatment. *N Engl J Med* 319:1635–1638, 1988.
69. Erlen J: Informed consent: The information component. *Orthopaedic Nurs* 13(2): 75–78, 1994.
70. Erlen J: Informed consent: The consent component. *Orthopaedic Nurs* 13(4): 65–67, 1994.
71. Erlen J: When the patient lacks decision-making capacity. *Orthopaedic Nurs* 14(4):51–54, 1995.
72. Silva MC: Competency, comprehension, and the ethics of informed consent. *Nurs Connections* 6(3):47–51, 1993.
73. White BC: *Competence to Consent.* Washington, DC: Georgetown University Press; 1994.
74. Fowler M: Pediatric informed consent. *Heart Lung* 17:584–585, 1988.
75. Broome M, Stieglitz K: The consent process and children. *Res Nurs Health* 15(2):147–152, 1992.
76. Thurber F, Deatrick J, Grey M: Children's participation in research: Their right to consent. *J Ped Nurs* 7(3):165–170, 1992.
77. Markowitz MS: Human fetal tissue: Ethical implications for use in research and therapy. *AWHONNS Clin Issues Perinatal Womens Health Nurs* 4(4):578–588, 1993.
78. Sanders LM, Giudice L, Raffin T: Ethics of fetal tissue transplantation. *West J Med* 159(3):400–407, 1993.
79. Shorr AS: Abortion and fetal research: Some ethical concerns. *Fetal Diag Therapy* 9(3):196–203, 1994.
80. Alt-White A: Obtaining "informed" consent from the elderly. *West J Nurs Res* 17(6):700–705; 1995.
81. Liaschenko J: *op. cit.*, 1994.

82. Liaschenko J: *op. cit.*, 1995.

83. Drought TS, Liaschenko J: Ethical practice in a technologic age. *Crit Care Nurs Clin N Amer* 7(2):297–304, 1995.

84. Katz J: *op. cit.*

85. Orona CJ, Koenig BA, Davis AJ: Cultural issues in nondisclosure. *Cambridge Quart Healthcare Ethics* 3(3):338–346, 1994.

86. Carrese JA, Rhodes LA: Western bioethics on the Navajo reservation: Benefit or harm? *JAMA* 274(10):826–829, 1995.

87. Blackhall LJ, Murphy ST, Frank G, Michel V, Azen S: Ethnicity and attitudes toward patient autonomy. *JAMA* 274(10):820–825, 1995.

88. Marshall PA, Koenig BA: Bioethics in anthropology: Perspectives on culture, medicine, and morality. In Sargent CF, Johnson TM, (eds): *Medical Anthropology: Contemporary Theory and Method* (rev ed). Westport, CT: Praeger; 1996.

89. Davis AJ, Koenig BA: A question of policy: Bioethics in a multicultural society. *Nurs Policy Forum* 2(1):6–11, 1996.

90. Koenig BA, Marshall P: Bioethics and the politics of race and ethnicity: Respecting (or constructing) Difference? Paper presented at "Cultural Diversity and Bioethics," American Anthropological Association Annual Meeting: December 2, 1994, Atlanta, GA.

91. Wear S: *Informed Consent: Patient Autonomy and Physician Benefience Within Clinical Medicine.* Dordrecht: Kluwer Academic Publishers; 1993.

92. Brody H: *Stories of Sickness.* New Haven, CT: Yale University Press; 1987.

93. Menzel P: *Strong Medicine: The Ethical Rationing of Health Care.* New York: Oxford University Press; 1990.

94. Rodwin MA: *Medicine, Money, and Morals: Physicians' Conflicts of Interest.* New York: Oxford University Press; 1993.

95. Reiser SJ: The ethical life of health care organizations. *Hastings Cent Rep* 24(6): 28–35, 1994.

96. Council on Ethical and Judicial Affairs, American Medical Association: Ethical issues in managed care. *JAMA* 273(4):330–335, 1995.

97. Rodwin MA: Conflicts in managed care. *N Engl J Med* 332(9):604–607, 1995.

98. Morreim EH: *Balancing Acts: The New Medical Ethics of Medicine's New Economics.* Washington, DC: Georgetown University Press; 1995.

99. Morreim EH: The ethics of incentives in managed care. *Trends Health Care Law Ethics* 10(1–2):57–62, 1995.

100. Abdellah FG: Approaches to protecting the rights of human subjects. *Nurs Res* 16(4):316–320, 1967.

101. Beecher H: *op. cit.*

102. Berthold JS: Advancement of science and technology while maintaining human rights and values. *Nurs Res* 18:514–522, 1969.

103. Liaschenko J: *op. cit.*, 1994.

104. Liaschenko J: *op. cit.*, 1995.

105. Imbus S, Zawacki B: Autonomy for burned patients when survival is unprecedented. *N Engl J Med* 297(6):308–311, 1977.

106. Schwartz SI: Consensus summary on fluid resuscitation. *J Trauma* 19(suppl): 876–877, 1979.

107. Batey MV: Some methodological issues in research. *Nurs Res* 19:511–516, 1970.

108. American Nurses Association Committee on Research and Studies: The nurse in research: ANA guidelines on ethical values. *Nurs Res* 17:104–107, 1968.

109. American Nurses Association Commission on Nursing Research: *Human Rights Guidelines for Nurses in Clinical and Other Research.* Kansas City, MO: American Nurses Association; 1975.

110. Liaschenko J: *op. cit.,* 1994.

111. Liaschenko J: *op. cit.,* 1995.

112. Liaschenko J: *Ibid.*

113. Wilkinson J: Moral distress in nursing practice: Experience and effect. *Nurs Forum* 23(1):16–29, 1987–1988.

114. Aristotle: *The Nichomachean Ethics.* Trans. by D. Ross. New York: Oxford University Press; 1989.

115. Winslow B, Winslow G: Integrity and compromise in nursing ethics. *J Med Phil* 16:307–323, 1991.

116. Silva MC: *Ethical Guidelines in the Conduct, Dissemination, and Implementation of Nursing Research.* Washington, DC: American Nurses Association Publishing, 1995.

117. Silva MC: *Annotated Bibliography for Ethical Guidelines.* Washington, DC: American Nurses Association Publishing; 1995.

118. Davis AJ, Krueger JC: *Patients, Nurses, Ethics.* New York: American Journal of Nursing Company; 1980.

119. Alderson P: *op. cit.*

120. McMullen P, Philipsen N: *op. cit.*

121. Curtin L: *op. cit.,* 1993

122. Holloway I, Wheeler S: *op. cit.*

123. Erlen J: Informed consent: The information component. *op. cit.*

124. Erlen J: Informed consent: The consent component. *op. cit.*

125. Erlen J: *op. cit.,* 1995.

126. Silva MC: *op. cit.,* 1993.

127. Fowler M: *op. cit.*

128. Broome M, Stieglitz K: *op. cit.*

129. Thurber F, Deatrick J, Grey, M: *op. cit.*

130. Alt-White A: *op. cit.*

131. Pieranunzi VR, Freitas LS: Informed consent with children and adolescents. *J Child Adol Psych Mental Health Nurs* 5(2):21–27, 1992.

132. Hooker E: Informed Consent. *Sci Nurs* 9(3):86–91, 1992.

133. Farkas M: Use of informed consent with therapeutic paradox. *Issues in Mental Health Nurs* 13(3):161–176, 1992.

134. Gift AG: Informed consent and vulnerable subjects. *Clin Nurs Specialist* 7(4): 183, 1993.

135. Harrison L: Issues related to the protection of human research participants. *J Neuroscience Nurs* 25(3):187–193, 1993.

136. Summers S: The research process: Informed consent. *J Post Anesthesia Nurs* 8(6):406–409, 1993.

137. Davis AJ: The clinical nurse's role in informed consent. *J Prof Nurs* 4:88–91, 1988.

138. Davis AJ: Informed consent process in research protocols: Dilemmas for clinical nurses. *West J Nurs Res* 11:448–457, 1989.

139. Davis AJ: Clinical nurses ethical decision making in situations of informed consent. *Adv Nurs Sci* 11(3):63–69, 1989.

140. Davis AJ, Jameton A: Nursing and medical student attitudes toward nursing disclosure of information to patients: A pilot study. *J Adv Nurs* 12(6):691–698, 1987.

141. MacIntyre A: To whom is the nurse responsible? In Murphy C, Hunter H (eds): *Ethical Problems in the Nurse-Patient Relationship.* Newtown, MA: Allyn & Bacon; 1983, pp 78–83.

142. Englehardt HT: Physicians, patients, health care institutions—and the people in between: Nurses. In Bishop A, Scudder J (eds): *Caring, Curing, Coping.* Tuscaloosa, AL: University of Alabama Press; 1985, pp 62–79.

143. Bishop A, Scudder J: Nursing ethics in an age of controversy. *Adv Nurs Sci* 9(3):34–43, 1987.

144. Liaschenko J: Ethics in the work of acting for patients. *Adv Nurs Sci* 18(2):1–12, 1995.

8

Abortion

The field of reproductive technology has exploded over the past several years. Neonatal intensive care is a dramatic example of high-technology medicine and nursing. Embryo freezing as an adjunct to in vitro fertilization (IVF) is another technique in the treatment of infertility and control of human reproduction. Technologies such as artificial insemination, IVF, surrogate motherhood, and ovum transfer raise numerous ethical issues. Fetal research as one part of these developments has received much attention as an ethical concern in public policy. The experimental drug RU486 and other chemicals such as methotrexate used to terminate early pregnancy, raises again the question about the status of the early embryo. And yet, with all these scientific developments and the attending ethical dilemmas raised by them, it is the ancient act of abortion that holds center stage in the debates.

Abortion, the expulsion or removal of the products of conception from the uterus, generally occurs before the 28th week of pregnancy. Spontaneous abortion occurs as a result of a variety of endogenous and exogenous causes, excluding intentional human interference. Such human interference, called induced abortion, to deliberately terminate a pregnancy, performed either legally or illegally, relies on a number of different methods. The method used depends, in part, on timing, or how long the pregnancy has existed. Medically speaking, abortion during the first trimester is easiest to perform and safest for the woman involved. However, women do undergo abortion during the second trimester and even up to the point the fetus becomes viable. Viability of the fetus means that it has the potential ability to live outside the uterus, albeit with artificial means, if necessary. Traditionally, viability was thought to occur around 28 weeks, but developments in technology have begun to move the time to an earlier date in the pregnancy. In the last trimester, abortion presents increased dangers to the woman, and the likelihood of delivering a live fetus also increases. However, third trimester abortion is sometimes considered in cases of severe fetal abnormality.

Abortion is an ancient form of birth control and has been used in all parts of the world for centuries. The argument can be made, however, that other effective methods of contraception have been developed that could replace abortion as a means of birth control in most cases. Furthermore, these alternatives to abortion have the potential of presenting fewer ethical dilemmas for those who use them. Several factors must be taken into account before pursuing this line of argument very far, however. First, not all people receive sound knowledge about sex and reproduction, and in many places people still continue to do battle over sex education in the schools. Second, research findings have begun to throw into question the safety of the most effective birth control device, the pill, for many individuals. And finally, the fact remains that people do not necessarily act on information and knowledge they have, even when the results of their actions may prove detrimental to their health or lives. For example, behaviors such as smoking, driving while intoxicated, unprotected sex in the era of AIDS, and having sexual intercourse without using some form of contraception when the couple does not want a pregnancy, all support this fact. Contraceptive devices succeed in preventing unwanted pregnancies only if used consistently. The nature of human sexuality and the complex motivations that people bring to their sexual experiences favor mishaps. For these and other reasons not discussed here, abortion as a form of birth control remains with us.

Few other recent topics have caused so much outcry and activity, although assisted suicide may do so in the near future. One side of the debate has been called *The Right to Life,* while the other side has come to be known as *The Right to Choice.* Many people take a position somewhere between these two stances but are not so visible or vocal in their stance. The ethical dilemmas in abortion are complex and require that we examine them carefully. It seems reasonable to assume that such an examination will need to take into account the social and religious diversity in the United States and to recall that a major philosophical basis here is the separation of church and state.

A great many factors intersect in any discussion of abortion: medical, sociological, psychological, technological, and the attitudes grounded in philosophical and moral concerns that the public has developed. This background information, along with the overview of the historical and social context of abortion to follow, will help us to understand more fully the ethical dilemmas surrounding abortion.

THE RELIGIOUS AND HISTORICAL CONTEXT

At the time of the Persian Empire, abortifacients were accessible, though individuals who performed criminal abortions received severe punishment. In ancient Greece and during the Roman era, people resorted to abortion without scruple.[1] Plato in *The Republic* and Aristotle in *Politics* described abortion as a means of preventing excess population. Neither Greek nor Roman law afforded protection to the unborn fetus. Furthermore, the religions practiced in these cultures did not bar abortion; however, philosophers, religious teachers, and physicians debated the morality of performing abortions. In this climate, the Hippocratic Oath developed and took a position against abortion. One theory explains this radical departure from the prevailing practice of the time in light of Pythagorean dogma.[2] Most Greek thinkers, except for the Pythagorean school, commended abortion, at least prior to viability. For the Pythagoreans, the embryo became animated or infused with a soul from the moment of conception, so that abortion meant destroying a living being. The abortion clause in the Hippocratic Oath reflects Pythagorean doctrine, a small segment of Greek opinion at the time. However, medical writings down to Galen's time (AD 130 to 200) provided evidence of violation of almost every injunction of the oath. For example, Soranos (AD 98 to 138), a Greek from Ephesus, became Rome's leading gynecologist, and in his writings he lists the reasons for abortion and the means to achieve it.[3] Only at the end of antiquity, with the emerging teachings of Christianity, which agreed with the Pythagorean ethic, did the oath become the nucleus of all medical ethics and become regarded as the embodiment of truth. For some, this historical context explains what appears to them as the rigidity of the Hippocratic Oath.

The Greco-Roman world, distinguished by its indifference to fetal life, also saw the development of Christianity, which gave rise to values in opposition to and in conflict with the generally held popular beliefs. Early Christian teachings on sexuality and abortion developed as a means of resistance to the political influence of the Roman Empire. To adopt different attitudes toward sexuality and abortion was a means of repudiating Roman power.[4,5] The specific Christian teaching on abortion was grounded in the Old Testament command to love your neighbor as yourself (Leviticus 19:18). The basis for fulfillment of this commandment, found in the New Testament, emphasized the sacrifice of a man's life for another (John 15:13). From this commandment of love, the Christian valuation of life evolved.[6]

Abortion, as a subject of concern to secular humanists and theologians, has a long history. At the heart of this complex discourse lies the question of how one determines the humanity of a being. The Roman Catholic position on abortion has been clearly stated since the late 1880s and has been reaffirmed by recent popes. Roman Catholics, as well as some other religious leaders, believe the embryo becomes a human being with a soul from the moment of conception. Some of the early teachers of the Church, however, including St. Thomas Aquinas, did not consider it possible for an unformed embryo to have a soul and placed ensoulment at about three months after conception, when the fetus had developed a recognizable human shape. Along with this concept of ensoulment at conception, Roman Catholics reject abortion on the grounds that unborn children need baptism.

Although not as strongly upheld in the Church today, this doctrine of baptizing the endangered fetus still holds. The current official position of Catholic leaders accepts the concept of ensoulment that defines the fetus as a human being from conception. This position can be characterized as a refusal to discriminate among human beings on the basis of their varying potentialities.

Protestant views vary according to the numerous sects and groups involved. Although many Protestants do not agree with the Roman Catholic Church on ensoulment, they do regard abortion as undesirable, though not a mortal sin, since the embryo as an entity should be preserved from unnecessary destruction. Generally, for Protestants, the concept of the sacredness of life has served as an obstacle to the wanton and thoughtless performance of abortion. In attempting to determine when human life begins, most Protestant leaders agree that by the time of quickening, or the first recognizable movements of the fetus in utero, one can define the fetus as a human being.

One Protestant writer outlined pertinent principles that can be stipulated for reflection and reduced them to the following simplified scheme. First, life must be preserved rather than destroyed; second, protection must be provided, especially to those who cannot assert their own right to life; and third, exceptions to these rules exist, such as (1) medical indications that make therapeutic abortion morally tolerable, (2) pregnancy resulting from a sexual crime, (3) social and emotional conditions that do not appear beneficial for the well-being of the mother and child.[7] This writer replaced the determination of an action as right or wrong according to its conformity to a rule and its application with stressing the primacy of the person and human relationships along with the concreteness of the choice within limited possibilities. In the case of abortion, he maintained that no guarantee of an objectively right action can be given, since several values, all objectively important, exist. Furthermore, these values do not resolve themselves into a harmonious relationship to each other. Since there is no single overriding determination of what constitutes a right action, there can be no unambiguously right act.[8]

Ancient Jewish writings consider the fetus a living being when it detaches itself from the mother. According to the Talmud, this occurs when the head has emerged from the birth canal. In more modern times, Orthodox Jewish leaders maintain that abortion is morally wrong at any time, except when the mother's life becomes seriously threatened. Reform Jews accept more reasons for abortion. For all practical purposes, the relatively permissive attitudes of Conservative and Reform Judaism can be equated with those of a growing number of Protestant sects on the topic of abortion.[9]

To briefly summarize the attitudes of the other great religions, Buddhists condemn killing but define commencement of life rather loosely, whereas the Shinto religion recognizes the infant as a living being after birth. The Islamic religion takes the stance that abortion is permissible until the embryo develops into the human shape, or for 120 days after conception.[10]

THE LEGAL AND POLITICAL CONTEXT

The legal aspects of abortion have been influenced by religious developments and definitions. In the fourth century AD, the Roman Empire developed the first laws against abortion in a time when Christian influence began to be felt. However, in the common law, abortion performed prior to quickening, at 16 to 18 weeks, was not an indictable offense.[11] This lack of criminality in common law for abortion occurring before quickening seems to have been influenced by theological concepts, civil and canonical law concepts, and philosophical concepts of the beginning of life—of when the embryo becomes infused with a soul. Christian theology and canon law fixed the point of animation at 40 days for a male and 80 days for a female, a view that persisted until the 19th century. General agreement developed that prior to animation, the fetus was part of the mother and therefore its destruction was not homicide. However, because of the uncertainty as to the exact time of animation and perhaps, influenced by Aquinas' definition of movement in utero as one criterion of life, Bracton wrote in 1640 in the first references to abortion in English criminal law, that to abort a woman is homicide if the embryo is formed and especially if it is animated.[12] Other English legal scholars, such as Edward Coke, Matthew Hale, and William Russell, used the concept of quickening to develop the common-law precedents regarding abortion. In 1803, England's first criminal abortion statute made the abortion of a quick fetus a capital crime. This law also provided lesser penalties for the felony of abortion that occurred before quickening. In 1967, the British Parliament enacted a new, liberal abortion law.

In the United States, generally speaking, the law in effect until the middle of the 19th century was the pre-existing English common law. In 1800, abortions were not prohibited in American jurisdictions but this progressively changed over the next century with the first anti-abortion laws being introduced between 1821 and 1841.[13] During the middle and late 19th century, the quickening distinction disappeared from the statutory law in most states and the penalties for performing an abortion increased.[14] For approximately 100 years, the United States outlawed virtually all abortions. Yet demand for abortion again changed this policy so that by the early 1970s only the three states of Louisiana, New Hampshire, and Pennsylvania prohibited abortion for any reason. This is in contrast to the following state laws: Alaska, Hawaii, New York, Washington, and the District of Columbia permitted it for any reason; 13 states allowed abortion to protect the physical and mental health of the mother; one state permitted abortion only on the grounds of saving the woman's life and in cases of rape; and 29 states sanctioned it only to save the woman's life.[15] Colorado pioneered this liberalizing trend in abortion laws in 1967 and rather than creating an abortion-mill situation, as feared by its critics, this statute resulted in caution on the part of physicians and hospitals.[16]

Texas was the residence of Jane Roe, a pseudonym for Norma McCorvey, and became the proving ground for abortion rights in this country. Roe could not obtain an abortion because her pregnancy was not life threatening, a criteria for abortion in Texas. She sued the state of Texas, filing a class action suit. This suit, *Roe v Wade* was appealed to the highest court of the land.

The United States Supreme Court decision, delivered on January 22, 1973,[17] declared both an original statute (Texas, *Roe v Wade*) and a reform statute (Georgia, *Doe v Bolton*) unconstitutional. The decision by the majority of seven to two of the Supreme Court justices asserted that the constitutional right to privacy, provided for by the 14th Amendment, is broad enough to encompass a woman's decision whether or not to terminate her pregnancy. Furthermore, a state cannot interfere in the abortion decision between a woman and her physician during the first trimester. In the second trimester, when abortion becomes more hazardous, the state's interest in the woman's health permits the enactment of regulation to protect maternal health. Beyond these procedural requirements, the abortion decision still rests with the woman and her physician. After the fetus reaches viability, approximately in the last trimester, the state can exercise its interest in promoting potential human life. At this stage, the state can prohibit abortion except when the necessity arises to preserve the life or health of the mother. The Court did not support the position that a woman has an absolute right to abortion regardless of circumstances; however, the position it took did make legal abortion potentially more available than at any time in the United States during the 20th century.

What was the effect of this judicial decision? Statistical data on legal or illegal abortions performed in the past cannot be stated with certainty. One study of legal abortion covering the years 1957 through 1962, when there were far more restrictions than after 1973, indicated that the women questioned had 1,039 abortions as compared with 522,600 live births. This means there existed a ratio of about two abortions to every 1,000 live births. Using this ratio and extrapolating it to about 4,000,000 deliveries yearly in this country, we could make an educated guess, that, for the years of the study, approximately 8,000 legal abortions were performed annually.[18]

We have, for obvious reasons, even fewer facts about illegal abortions. However, some observations have been made that suggest certain patterns and concerns. In the United States before the 1973 Supreme Court decision, abortion was largely performed clandestinely by physicians, especially for the financially well off. The poor were more likely to abort themselves or to resort to nonmedical amateurs. As well as we can determine, the majority of those fetuses aborted were from married women with several children. Death and invalidism have not been insignificant as an aftermath of illegal abortion. In the 1960s, almost 50 percent of deaths in New York City associated with pregnancy and birth resulted from illegal abortions.[19] Immediately following *Roe v Wade*, there was a significant decrease in abortion-related deaths.[20] *Roe v Wade* did not, however, increase abortion rates. While the overall rates of abortion pre- and post-*Roe v Wade* remained essentially stable, what did change was the geographical distribution of abortions across states.[21]

Pro-abortionists continue to fight to remove the remaining restrictions in abortion law, while anti-abortionists strive for a Constitutional amendment that would recognize a fetus's right to life. Efforts to overturn the 1973 *Roe v Wade* decision by constitutional amendments have failed, but another strategy, the passage of state abortion statutes that are as restrictive as possible within the *Roe v Wade* framework, aim to see the Supreme Court ultimately modify or abandon *Roe* altogether. Such challenges have gone to the Supreme Court nearly every year. For the court to permit states to outlaw abortion—the most frequently performed medical procedure in the United States—seems unlikely but a narrowing of *Roe* seems inevitable. Other strategies have included congressional measures to limit abortions. For example, in the late 1970s Congress prohibited the use of Medicaid funds for abortions, except when the woman's life is endangered, thus limiting access for poor women. More recent attempts to limit *Roe v Wade* concern restrictions to minors seeking abortions and attempts to confine abortions to earlier points in pregnancy.[22] In light of its long history and the great passions generated by the abortion issue, continuation of this controversy can be expected in and out of legislatures and courts.

The battle over abortion, sometimes called the battle of life versus choice, has become one of the most emotional issues of politics and morality facing the United States today. The language used in this debate is so passionate and polemical, and the conflicting and seemingly irreconcilable values so deeply felt, that this issue could well test the very foundations of a pluralistic system of government that was designed to accommodate deep-rooted moral and ethical differences. This is made dramatically clear with the recent murders of physicians and staff at family planning clinics in different parts of the country. It is possible that nothing since the issue of slavery has the potential of dividing us in our quest for a democratic society as much as abortion.

Some believe that abortion is murder of the unborn person and therefore should be outlawed by constitutional amendment. Others argue that abortion is a right that women must have legally because they must be free to control their bodies and their lives. Along with the ethical dilemma of abortion itself, another issue, that of the government's role, has become paramount. Should abortion be legal or illegal? If legal, should government funds be available to cover the cost of abortion for the poor? The abortion issue continues to be a major political battle of the late 1990s. Indeed, the 1996 primary elections demonstrated that abortion is a central concern in American life.

THE MEDICAL AND SCIENTIFIC CONTEXT

"Medicine stands between biology and social policy, between the 'mysterious' world of the laboratory and every day life." [23] From this position institutionalized medicine has tremendous influence on the control of reproduction in general and abortion in particular. It is not surprising to learn that historically medicine has been extremely conservative.

The medical profession shared the anti-abortion mood prevalent in the United States during the latter part of the 19th century and may have influenced the enactment of stringent criminal abortion legislation. In 1857, the American Medical Association (AMA) appointed a Committee on Criminal Abortion to investigate criminal abortion with a view to its general suppression. In 1859, this committee proposed, and the AMA adopted, a resolution against unwarrantable destruction of human life. They called upon state legislatures to revise their abortion laws and requested the cooperation of state medical societies in pressing the subject. The committee, in 1871, again proposed resolutions that the AMA adopted. This time one recommendation read that it "be unlawful and unprofessional for any physician to induce abortion or premature labor without the concurrent opinion of at least one respectable consulting physician, and then always with a view to the safety of the child—if that be possible." They also recommended calling "the attention of the clergy of all denominations to the perverted views of morality entertained by a large class of females—aye, and men also, on this important question." [24]

Except for occasional condemnation of criminal abortionists, the AMA took no further formal action on abortion until 1967, when the Committee on Human Reproduction urged adoption of a policy in which the Association would oppose induced abortion except where (1) documented medical evidence showed a threat to the health or life of the mother, (2) the child may be born with incapacitating physical deformity or mental deficiency, or (3) a pregnancy resulting from legally established statutory or forcible rape or incest may constitute a threat to the physical or mental health of the patient. In addition, the committee proposed that two other physicians with recognized professional competency examine the patient and concur in writing as to the need for the abortion and that the physician perform the abortion in a hospital accredited by the joint Commission on Accreditation of Hospitals. The AMA House of Delegates adopted this policy.[25] In 1970, the resolutions before the House of Delegates did not differ from the policy adopted in 1967 with the exception of the statement that "no party to the procedure should be requested to violate personally held moral principles." [26]

The reason for the change in the medical profession's stance is unclear. One possible explanation for this change is the increasing development of scientific knowledge as a basis for medicine in the 20th century.[27] Traditional notions of ensoulment and personhood are seen as lying outside the province of science. Questions of viability, however, are thought to fall within the domain of scientific knowledge. However, this too proves problematic.

Science, like religion, finds it difficult to establish the moment when life begins. One embryologist could define the unfertilized egg as a living entity but another embryologist could indicate great limitations in that definition because the unfertilized egg cannot continue to live more than a few days, has only half the chromosome supply that other body cells have, and therefore cannot develop without the addition of the sperm. This situation changes the moment an egg becomes impregnated by a male sperm, and this change results in a complete chromosome supply. The process of division begins and growth occurs rapidly; however, up to the sixth week of the embryo's existence, only an expert embryologist can tell whether the embryo is human or not. At the seventh week, human characteristics begin appearing, and by the 15th or 16th week the mother can feel the movements of the fetus—what has been called quickening.

All along the way of this remarkable process the embryo has what some call the marvelous gift of life, but others would argue that this is true only in the same sense that an animal or plant has life. The question remains as to when during this process this entity develops human life. No clear biological definition has been developed as to the beginning of human life. A larger philosophical question is whether physical life and personhood are the same things. Is it possible to have physical life and not have personhood?

Since the 1973 decision, advances in neonatal care have made 25 weeks the generally accepted time of viability. With this scientific change, the utility of the concept of viability for drawing legal and policy lines for abortion has been called into question.[28,29] The development of neonatal medicine, whose expenditures run in the billions of dollars, allows for the treatment of imperiled or premature newborns who would have died only a few years ago. Some of these neonates scarcely bear a physical resemblance to a baby. This technological capacity raises the question for the abortion debate of how we can ethically justify attempting to save imperiled 22 to 25 week-old neonates while accepting the abortion of perfectly healthy fetuses of the same gestational age.[30] The difference hangs on the notion of whether or not children are wanted. In the one case we speak of a cherished baby and in the other, a product of conception. Some public and health care professionals have difficulties with these distinctions.[31]

THE ETHICAL DILEMMA OF ABORTION

Since the 1973 Supreme Court decision, some believed that further ethical debate would only be academic in the most pejorative sense of that word. Others, however, believed that moral distinctions can be made within the framework of the reformed law and that these distinctions can assist the individual in developing or maintaining a moral position on abortion. The ethical dilemma involved can be limited to three of its dimensions for the purpose of discussion: (1) the rights of the fetus, (2) the rights and obligations of the mother, and (3) the rights and obligations of society.

RIGHTS OF THE FETUS

In presenting *Roe v Wade* before the Supreme Court, the lawyer argued that the Constitution does not define "person" in so many words. Although the 14th Amendment contains three references to "person," there can be no assurance that they have any prenatal application. The lawyer concluded that under the law, the unborn fetus is not a person. One important dimension of this ethical dilemma, however, asks for a definition of human life and some determination of when we can recognize its presence, so that we can then place a value on it and weigh it against other values. In the present state of biological ignorance on the matter and philosophical pluralism, the premise that the fetus is a person can be neither proved nor disproved to the satisfaction of all. Therefore, no one can assert superior moral sensitivity over opponents, and neither moral claim can rightfully eliminate the other from the political arena.[32]

Those concerned with what they consider a helpless minority, the unborn fetuses, judge the direct, intentional taking of innocent human life as unacceptable. Some of the arguments supporting the personhood of the fetus are as follows: The Protestant theologian Paul Ramsey found support in genetic research for the position that we should impute full human dignity to the nonviable fetus. Ramsey argues that genetics tells us that we are what we become in every cell and attribute. Genetic data therefore provide us with a scientific approximation to the religious belief of ensoulment from conception.[33] Schwarz contends that the zygote is not a *potential* person but an *actual* person in a nonfunctioning state. He maintains that fetal life is simply the first phase of the continuum of human life and so any distinction is arbitrary.[34]

If we grant that from conception a fetus possesses humanity, we must then accord it all human rights, including the most basic one, the right to life. To kill that which possesses humanity is murder, except, arguably, in the cases of war, self-defense, and capital punishment. Dealing with this, Bok's moral reasoning raises the larger question of whether the life of the

POTENTIALITY

fetus should receive the same protection as other lives. Basically, she asks the question: Is killing the fetus, by whatever means, and for whatever reasons, to be thought of as killing a human being? By drawing the line between abortions performed early in pregnancy and those done later, she develops the moral position that early abortions do not violate the principle of protection of life.[35] Brody presents an argument allowing abortion prior to six weeks gestation. His argument focuses on the development of brain activity as the indicator of human essence constituting humanity. Once this activity is established abortion would be morally wrong.[36]

One basic moral principle that has received much attention in recent years, that of informed consent, must be addressed in this dilemma. If one defines the fetus as possessing humanity at any point along the developmental continuum prior to birth, then the question must be asked: Who speaks for this human, using what criteria, and who guards his or her rights in this matter so vital to existence? One argument, especially for the severely deformed fetus, says that if the fetus could speak under these circumstances, he or she would consent to abortion. This argument can also be used to support abortions for the unwanted child without deformity. If the parent(s) does not want the child, what quality of life can the child expect to have? Will this child more likely become a victim of the increasing social problem, child abuse? The central question in this quality-of-life argument turns on the location of the line to be drawn. The extreme of this line of argumentation can be found in the phenomenon of wrongful life suits—suits brought on behalf of the severely disabled child for suffering and damages attendant to being born. The premise of these suits is that the disability was known prior to birth and the child's suffering would have been prevented by abortion.[37,38]

RIGHTS AND OBLIGATIONS OF THE PREGNANT WOMAN

The moral principle of autonomy leads to the position that a woman has the right to her own body and the right to determine her own fertility. The dilemma arises out of the fact that the situation involves two lives. According to some, no one has an absolute, clear-cut right to control his or her fate where others share it. The Court took this consideration into account in its debate before changing the abortion law and when it made distinctions between what is allowed during the three trimesters as the embryo develops into a viable fetus.

The question has been raised as to whether anyone, before or after birth, child or adult, has the right to continued dependence upon the bodily processes of another against that person's will.[39,40] Some argue that a woman, pregnant as a result of rape, incest, or in spite of every precaution, has no obligation to continue the pregnancy. In this case abortion is equated with cessation of continued support and not with unjust killing. An involuntarily pregnant woman can cease her support of life to the fetus without moral infringement of its right to life. Even those who support this argument under the circumstances specified might have difficulty using it in the situation of pregnancies entered into voluntarily. In this latter situation, the obligation of the pregnant woman to the fetus could be defined differently and abortion might be considered a less responsible moral choice.

Some take the position that pregnant women, no matter what the circumstances of conception, have obligations toward the life and well-being of the fetus that overshadow any discussion of the woman's rights. In fact, in some discussions in certain political arenas, the woman as a variable is not considered. The variables discussed are the father, the fetus, and the society. So we have a moral argument, where the stakes are high, in which some people support abortion on demand based on the woman's autonomy. At the same time we have people who oppose abortion except perhaps to save the life of the mother, based on the sanctity of life principle and the personhood of the fetus. To think in a simple way about this ethical dilemma, on the one hand the fetus is viewed as an object or thing while on the other, the woman is viewed as an object or thing. The political novel *The Handmaid's Tale* takes this woman-as-object idea and stretches it to a chilling conclusion.[41] In doing so, the darker interconnections between politics and sex are illuminated.

Throughout the history of the world, reproduction has been tied to the passage of property.[42–44] In fact, what we would recognize as modern marriage in the Western world had its origins in the 11th century as a means to determine and assure inheritance.[45] State control of reproduction has an equally long history. Control of reproduction and therefore of sexuality has been imposed on women to these ends. Rossi believes that buried deeply beneath the abortion discussion one finds unresolved attitudes toward sex in this country.[46] This analysis continues in contemporary feminist thought. Any ethical system, including contemporary ones, presupposes a cosmology or a social order. Feminist scholarship has shown that many of the current arguments surrounding abortion and reproductive issues have underlying assumptions about the place of women in the world.[47–49] One can only wonder what role this politicization of reproduction plays in the very conservative stances of some religious groups who are not only opposed to abortion but also to birth control. Prior to her appointment as Supreme Court Justice, Ruth Bader Ginsburg presented an interesting argument criticizing the reasoning behind *Roe v Wade*. Rather than the right to privacy as the basis for the decision, she argued that an appeal to the equal protection clause of the Constitution would have been more appropriate. Men have a distinct advantage over women in social and political advancement due to the unique ability of women to be burdened by pregnancy. This line of argument would have made a clear stand for gender equity based upon the Constitutional right to equal protection under the law.[50]

Thompson drew attention to the fact that the major focus in writings on abortion has been on what a third party, such as a physician, may or may not do when a woman requests an abortion. What the pregnant woman may do legally and morally was deduced from what third parties may do in the situation. Treating the matter of what the pregnant woman may do in such a fashion does not grant her the status of person that others insist on so firmly for the fetus.[51] The pregnant woman and the fetus were considered as a unity until the development of technology enabled the conceptualization and ultimate visualization of the fetus as a separate entity.[52] This has led some to view the woman as merely a fetal container.[53] Witness the recent cases in which brain-dead pregnant women (cadaveric pregnancies) were kept as physiological incubators until the living fetus could be delivered.

Traditionally, little attention has been given to the role, rights, and obligations of the father in the abortion decision. This reflects the law's concern with the individual, in this case the pregnant woman. Recent attention, however, has been focused on the rights of biological unwed fathers in cases of adoption[54] and increasingly in abortion.

RIGHTS AND OBLIGATIONS OF SOCIETY

One of the factors for any society in balancing values is the question of where to draw the line. In this case, that means under what conditions and considering the importance of what variables will society determine its abortion policy? If society develops a fairly restrictive policy, the argument could be made that some women would be threatened by the continuation of pregnancy, the new child would place great economic and psychological burdens on the family, the mode of existence and the career of some women would be seriously disrupted, and physically or mentally damaged infants would be born. On the other hand, if the policy permits women to obtain abortion with no restrictions or at least very limited restrictions, the "slippery slope" argument can be brought into the discussion. This argument says that there may be good reasons adduced for doing or not doing something because of what may possibly or predictably follow: What will come to be the case if our society does "X"? Will this social practice have consequences on other practices? Applied to the abortion situation, the questions develop as follows: If social policy makes abortion available, will this lead society to diminish its reverence for life and possibly to a lessening of its collective instinct for protecting the helpless? Would one such policy lead to other policies affecting the elderly, the mentally ill, and the mentally retarded? Could such policies push a society into disregarding the life of others who may not be productive or who may be a burden on society, such as the chronically ill or the chronically unemployed? As mentioned earlier,

Roe v Wade did not increase abortion rates in this country, likewise, data from other countries with liberal abortion practices, such as Sweden and Japan, do not support the slippery slope argument.

In a world as interrelated as our own, some have taken the position that population control has become an overriding problem affecting every society and have suggested abortion as one method of dealing with this problem. Using demographic, economic, sociological, and psychological data, population experts have argued for and against abortion as an important means of birth control. One such expert has argued the issue from a moral perspective and on that basis has decided against abortion as a permissible means of population control.[55] The problem of population control can be approached from another perspective. In this view, while it is acknowledged that the need for population control is an issue, it is not specific techniques that are the solution. Rather, it has been shown that improving the economic conditions and overall lives of women reduces birth rates, thus reducing or eliminating the need for abortion.

The crux of the question of abortion and the rights and obligations of society can be summarized in two questions. First, does society derive some benefits in legally and socially restricting abortion that override the benefits to the pregnant woman of being able to make her own decisions? This question points out the need to balance the rights and obligations of society as a whole against the rights and obligations of the individual member of that society. Second, what ideals will inform our abortion policy? Will it turn on the definition of what constitutes human life or on the meanings we attach to the conditions—psychological, social, and economic—that are necessary for human life? Is agreement possible?

The moral positions in any pluralistic society tend to reflect many diverse values, which can lead to intolerance of other viewpoints. The most difficult challenge for society and its members is the incommensurability of the positions and the moral passion each side brings to the debate on abortion. There is not a shared language or understanding of the issues and there is no common point from which to begin dialogue. Militant stances result and we have passed into the realm of violence. The question of how we live with each other and each other's different values raises a central ethical dilemma.

Abortion is a societal issue that will not go away and, indeed, some argue that it should not go away. The central moral problems in the debate have remained remarkably stable over the years. The personhood argument says that either (1) the fetus lacks personhood and therefore is not entitled to protection against being killed, or (2) the fetus is a person and has this entitlement. The bodily support argument says that even if the personhood of the fetus were established, the choice of continuing the pregnancy belongs to the woman whose body is involved in that pregnancy. In the final analysis, how we understand ourselves as a people and how we define membership in this community is the larger concern for society.[56]

ABORTION AND NURSING

In 1967, the *American Journal of Nursing (AJN)* published a paper on abortion that pointed out that as society's views change, the law changes.[57] This reflected the ferment going on in the years just before the Supreme Court decision. At the American Nurses Association (ANA) 1968 convention, the Division of Maternal and Child Health Nursing Practice presented a Statement to Study State Abortion Legislation. The delegates approved this statement with some discussion on whether the organization should take a stand on such a controversial issue that might be misunderstood. They expressed concern over the loose application of abortion laws that could result in serious risks to women and their families and expressed support of movements to examine and modify existing abortion laws.[58] At about the same time, an essay on nurses' attitudes and abortion addressed the issue of personal moral positions and professional obligations.[59] During the late 1960s and early 1970s, the *AJN* kept its readers abreast of the changes occurring in the state abortion laws in this country and of the changes and nurses' reactions to them in the United Kingdom. In addition, it reported the proceedings of an interdisciplinary panel on abortion.[60] Throughout the early 1970s, the *AJN* reported activities and experiences of individuals and groups concerned with abortion.[61–65] Occasionally, a paper presenting some aspect of nursing care and abortion appeared.[66,67] In January 1972, the *Journal* editor, Thelma Schorr, said in an editorial on abortion that "the search for moral values is part of what makes one human. Respecting the rights of others in their search also makes one humane." [68]

During this time, the research on nursing and abortion focused, in the main, on attitudes. One study reported that in a sample of 500 nurses, 23 percent favored unrestricted abortion. Half or more favored abortion in cases of rape, defective fetus, physical or mental impairment of the woman, and grave economic hardship. Of the total, 75 percent stated that they would treat the abortion patient with as much understanding as any other patient.[69] Another study found older nurses and those at community hospitals less likely to condone abortion than their younger, university hospital counterparts.[70] A survey found that the kind and quality of involvement each health worker had had in dilemmas of unwanted pregnancy were important determinants of attitudes toward abortion. The organization and administration of abortion services and the social environment, including the attitude toward abortion in the general community and among professional peers, also affected the attitudes of health workers.[71] One year before the Court decision, research involving 50 nurses indicated that 22 did not favor a change in the law for religious, ethical-professional, and social reasons.[72] A report sampling doctors and nurses who had actually participated in large numbers of abortions said that the doctors' involvement was perfunctory. Nursing personnel experienced considerable stress attempting to resolve their ambivalence about their participation in these procedures and reported some feelings of anxiety, depression, and anger toward patients for their sexual acting out.[73] When researchers compared the attitudes of social workers and nurses, they found that social workers evidenced more favorable attitudes toward abortion and explained the difference by the social structure of the two professions.[74] And finally, another study reported that significantly more nursing students and their faculty members opposed abortion on demand than did other health professionals and the general population with comparable education. Fewer nursing students and faculty members voiced willingness to help a client obtain an abortion than did other health professionals.[75]

While the ANA stance has not changed,[76] recent nursing literature is again taking up the abortion debate, although division within the profession, reflecting the division in the greater society, is in evidence. Primarily editorials and letters, the titles reflect the level of concern of nurses: "Gag rule: Gag ME," [77] "Pro-life nurses uniting for service," [78] "Abortion: Clinics prepare for autumn protests," [79] "A closet pro-lifer turns activist," [80] "Us against 'them': Bush's cynical manipulation of the real issues," [81] "Readers advocate Pro-Conscience not Pro-Choice," [82] and, perhaps most telling, "It's the 103rd Congress: Do you know how your members of Congress are going to vote?" [83] There is ongoing research on nurses' attitudes about abortion,[84] how best to meet the needs of women seeking abortion[85,86] and the role of RU486.[87] There is occasional continued discussion of the philosophical issues[88-90] and updates on the legal issues.[91] A new important area of concern for nurses is the role of advance practice nurses, particularly certified nurse midwives (CNMs), in abortion. There is support for expanding the role of the CNM to include the provision of abortion services.[92] A national survey showed that 79 percent of the CNMs opposed governmental efforts to decrease access to abortion services and almost 25 percent willing to include the provision of abortion services within their personal practice.[93] Summers provides a history of the position of American College of Nurse Midwives.[94]

In a philosophical analysis of ethical issues in refusing to provide patient care, the authors concluded that nurses may morally refuse a patient care assignment if, and only if, certain conditions are met. One such condition was refusal on religico-moral grounds when those objections have been made known in advance. No emergency can exist nor can the patient be placed in jeopardy by the refusal.[95] This condition would cover refusal to participate in the act of abortion itself. Whether it covers a refusal to care for the patient before or after the abortion is problematic in light of the ANA Code for Nurses, which states that nurses care for patients regardless of the patient's values and life style.

If the nurse finds that because of her values she cannot condone abortion on any grounds, then the likelihood of her being able to care for an abortion patient without exhibiting unkind or even punitive behavior seems greatly diminished. Laws have been enacted in most states that protect the individual who refuses to perform or participate in an abortion because this procedure is contrary to his or her conscience or religious beliefs. Such laws make the violation of this provision by an employer a misdemeanor. Furthermore, these laws indicate that no civil action for negligence or malpractice shall be maintained against a person refusing to perform or participate in an abortion. Every nurse confronted with this situation has both the right and the obligation to obtain information regarding state laws and institution policies on this matter.

A slightly more complicated situation may arise when a nurse approves of abortion for certain reasons but not for others, or when she believes abortion should be limited to the first trimester. Some nurses can work with patients admitted for a dilation and curettage procedure, since these abortions occur early in their pregnancies, while these same nurses find it difficult, if not impossible, to work with patients aborted by the saline method, since the fetuses will be further along in development. If the type of patients admitted match the nurse's category of permissible abortion, she should have no real ethical problems in providing nursing care; however, if they do not, she will need to work out a solution to her ethical dilemma in which her personal value system and her professional obligations conflict. A head nurse or nursing supervisor can play an important role here by discussing the issues with the staff nurse, provided his or her awareness of the ethical dilemma includes the balancing of the rights of the nurse-as-person with the obligations of the nurse-as-professional.

Perhaps the most worrisome type of situation arises with nurses who either have given little thought to their moral position on abortion or in order to maintain their jobs deny to themselves that they harbor resentment toward abortion patients. One can only hope that each nurse will seriously think about his or her beliefs on the sanctity of life. It is important for the nurse to know where he or she morally draws the line for what he or she thinks is right or wrong, have some understanding of how he or she reached that conclusion, and realize how it will affect the provision of nursing care.

In the last analysis, the nurse must arrive at a balance between his or her own values and the professional obligations to the patient. In the process of reasoning through the ethical dilemmas involved in abortion, the least that can be hoped is that the patient not be abandoned. The most that can be hoped is that each nurse regard the rights of others as precious, as he or she would want his or her own regarded. Within this complex context the nurse must engage in critical ethical reflection on the obligations to self, to the patient, to the nursing profession, and to his or her place of employment.

■ CASE STUDY I.

Julie is a 17-year-old pregnant teenager who is receiving prenatal care at a nurse-run pre-natal clinic. She had a baby last year that she decided to keep with the help of her family, with whom she lives. She has been attending high school and had hoped to graduate next year. However, she dropped out of school recently as she had not been feeling "up to par" with this pregnancy. She works part time as a cashier at a local coffee shop.

You are the nurse practitioner caring for Julie, who told you on her first visit that she had been exposed to rubella 3 weeks earlier when her little brother and several of his classmates had "the measles." She is just entering the second trimester. You have explained to Julie and her mother the risks to the fetus from this exposure. Her mother wants her to have an abortion as she already provides most of the care for Julie's child. Julie, however, refuses to have an abortion saying that she loves this baby and is praying the baby will not be damaged.

Suggested Questions for Discussion

1. What are the ethical issues or concerns in this situation?

2. What is the unit of ethical analysis: the fetus, the mother, the grandmother, the family, society?

3. What are the nurse's obligations, to whom, and why?

■ CASE STUDY II.

Ms. B. recently graduated *magna cum laude* from a very prominent law school. She is married to a very successful architect, Mr. C., and they currently live on the West Coast. They have been waiting to start a family until she completed law school, and she quickly became pregnant after graduation. She is somewhat ambivalent about the pregnancy, but her husband is anxious to start a family.

Ms. B. is offered the very prestigious honor of clerking for a Supreme Court Justice just as she enters her eighth week of pregnancy. This is a life long dream come true and she wants very much to accept this position. However, she realizes it would be impossible to care for a child in the way she and her husband value while carrying out the demanding work of a Supreme Court Clerk. She now views this pregnancy as a hindrance and wants to obtain an abortion. Her husband would like to have the child. She decides to have an abortion.

Suggested Questions for Discussion

1. What constitutes a legitimate reason for an abortion? Is having a legitimate reason necessary?

2. What are Ms. B.'s rights and Mr. C.'s rights in this situation?

3. What are your moral judgments in this case and how would they affect your care of Ms. B.?

REFERENCES

1. Castiglioni A: *A History of Medicine*. New York: Aronson; 1973.
2. Edlestein L: *The Hippocratic Oath: Text, Translation, and Interpretation*. Baltimore: Johns Hopkins University Press; 1967.
3. Noonan JT: An almost absolute value in history. In Noonan JT (ed): *The Morality of Abortion*. Cambridge, MA: Harvard University Press; 1970, p 4.
4. Brown P: *The Body and Society: Men, Women, and Sexual Renunciation in Early Christianity*. New York: Columbia University Press; 1988.
5. Pagels E: *Adam, Eve, and the Serpent*. New York: Random House; 1988.
6. Noonan JT: *op. cit.*, p 7.
7. Gustafson JM: A protestant ethical approach. In Noonan JT (ed): *Ibid.*, p 116.
8. *Ibid.*, p 119.

9. Margolies IR: A Reform rabbi's view. In Hall RE (ed): *Abortion in a Changing World*. New York: Columbia University Press; 1970, pp 30–33.

10. Nazer IR: Abortion in the Near East. In Hall RE (ed): *Ibid.,* p 268.

11. Stern L: Abortion: Reform and the law. *J Crim Law*, 59:84, 1968.

12. Louisell DW, Noonan JT: Constitutional balance. In Noonan JT (ed): *op. cit.*, p 223.

13. Callahan JC: *Reproduction, Ethics, and the Law*. Bloomington: Indiana University Press; 1995.

14. Saltman J, Zimering S: *Abortion Today*. Springfield, IL: Thomas; 1973.

15. Wetstein ME: *Abortion Rates in the United States*. New York: SUNY; 1996.

16. Heller A, Whittington HG: The Colorado Story: Denver General Hospital experience with the change in the law on therapeutic abortion. *Am J Psychiatry* 125: 809–816, 1968.

17. *Roe v Wade*, 410 US 113 (1973).

18. Cook RE, Hellegers AE, Hoyt RG, et al (eds): *Terrible Choice: The Abortion Dilemma*. New York: Bantam; 1968, pp 40–41.

19. Guttmacher AF: Abortion—Yesterday, today, and tomorrow. In Guttmacher AF (ed): *The Case for Legalized Abortion Now*. Berkeley, CA: Diablo; 1967, pp 8–9.

20. Legge JS: *Abortion Policy: An Evaluation of the Consequences for Maternal and Infant Health*. New York: SUNY Press; 1985.

21. Wetstein ME: *op. cit.*

22. *Ibid.*

23. Ehrenreich B, English D: *Complaints and Disorders: The Sexual Politics of Sickness*. New York: Glass Mountain Pamphlet No. 2/The Feminist Press; 1973, p 5.

24. American Medical Association: *22 Transcript* 258, 1871.

25. American Medical Association: *Proceedings of the House of Delegates*, June 1967, pp 40–51.

26. American Medical Association: *Proceedings of the House of Delegates*, June 1970, p 221.

27. Starr P: *The Social Transformation of American Medicine: The Rise of a Sovereign Profession and the Making of a Vast Industry*. New York: Basic Books; 1982.

28. Fost N, Chudwin D, Wilker D, et al: The limited moral significance of fetal viability. *Hastings Cent Rep* 10(6):10–13, 1980.

29. Dunn PM, Stirrat GM: Capable of being born alive. *Lancet* 8376:553–554, 1984.

30. Perinatal care at the threshold of viability. American Academy of Pediatrics, Committee on Fetus and Newborn. American College of Obstetrics and Gynecology, Committee on Obstetric Practice. *Pediatrics* 96(5):974–976, 1995.

31. Callahan D: How technology is reframing the abortion debate. *Hastings Cent Rep* 16:33–42, 1986.

32. Cook RE, Hellegers AE, Hoyt RG, et al: *op. cit.*, p 82.

33. Ramsey P: Points in deciding about abortion. In Noonan JT (ed): *op. cit.*, p 67.

34. Schwarz S: *The Moral Question of Abortion*. Chicago: Loyola University Press; 1990.

35. Bok S: Ethical problems of abortion. *Hastings Cent Rep* 4:33–52, 1974.

36. Brody B: On the humanity of the fetus. In Goodman MF (ed): *What is a Person?* Clifton, NJ: Humana Press; 1988, pp 229–250.

37. Steinbock B, McClamrock R: When is birth unfair to the child? *Hastings Cent Rep* 24(6):15–21, 1994.
38. Botkin JR, Mehlman MJ: Wrongful birth: Medical, legal, and philosophical issues. *J Law Med Ethics* 22(1):21–28, 1994.
39. Thomson JJ: A defense of abortion. *Phil Pub Affairs* 1:47–56, 1971.
40. Bok S: *op. cit.*
41. Atwood M: *The Handmaid's Tale.* New York: Ballantine Books; 1987.
42. Westoff LA, Westoff CF: *From Now to Zero.* Boston: Little, Brown; 1971.
43. Staples R: The sexuality of black women. *Sex Behav* 2:4–15, 1972.
44. Strathairn M: *After Nature: A History of English Kinship.* London: Routledge; 1992.
45. Duby G: *The Knight, the Priest, and the Lady: The Making of Modern Marriage in Medieval France.* New York: Pantheon Books; 1983.
46. Rossi AS: Public views on abortion. In Guttmacher AF (ed): *op. cit.*, pp 31–33.
47. Holmes HB, Purdy L: *Feminist Perspectives in Medical Ethics.* Bloomington: Indiana University Press; 1992.
48. Sherwin S: *No Longer Patient: Feminist Ethics and Health Care.* Philadelphia: Temple University Press; 1992.
49. Callahan JC: *op. cit.*
50. Ginsburg RB: Some thoughts on autonomy and equality in relation to *Roe v Wade*. In Pojman LP, Beckwith FJ (eds): *The Abortion Controversy.* Boston: Jones and Bartlett; 1994, pp 119–128.
51. Thompson J: *op. cit.*, pp 47–66.
52. Mattingly SS: The maternal-fetal dyad: Exploring the two-patient obstetric model. *Hastings Cent Rep* 22(1):13–18, 1992.
53. Purdy L: Are pregnant women fetal containers? *Bioethics* 4:273–291, 1990.
54. Shanley ML: Fathers' rights, mothers' wrongs? Reflections on unwed fathers' rights, patriarchy and sex equality. In Callahan JC (ed): *op. cit.*, pp 219–248.
55. Dyck AJ: Is abortion necessary to solve population problems? In Hilgers TW, Horan DJ (eds): *Abortion and Social Justice.* New York: Sheed and Ward; 1972, pp 159–176.
56. Meilaender G: Abortion: The right to an argument. *Hastings Cent Rep* 19(6): 13–16, 1989.
57. Hershey N: As society's views change, laws change. *Am J Nurs* 67:2310–2312, 1967.
58. ANA convention: A week of "firsts." *Am J Nurs* 68:1258–1277, 1968.
59. Fonseca JD: Induced abortion: Nursing attitudes and actions. *Am J Nurs* 68: 1022–1027, 1968.
60. Abortion. *Am J Nurs* 70:1919–1925, 1970.
61. Nurses' feelings a problem under new abortion law. *Am J Nurs* 71:350, 1971.
62. Catholic nurse-legislator files for abortion reform. *Am J Nurs* 71:459, 1971.
63. Personal experience at a legal abortion center. *Am J Nurs* 72:110–112, 1972.
64. Abortion yes or no; nurses organize both ways. *Am J Nurs* 72:416–418, 1972.
65. Nurses' Association of American College of Obstetricians and Gynecologists: Principles and guidelines on abortion. *Am J Nurs* 72:1311, 1972.

66. Cronenwett LR, Choyce JM: Saline abortion. *Am J Nurs* 71(9):1754–1757, 1971.

67. Ketter C, Copeland P: Counseling the abortion patient is more than talk. *Am J Nurs* 72:102–106, 1972.

68. Schorr TM: Issues of conscience. *Am J Nurs* 72:61, 1972.

69. The RN panel of 500 tells what nurses think about abortion. *RN* 33(6):40–43, 1970.

70. Brown NK, Thompson DJ, Bulger RJ, et al: How do nurses feel about euthanasia and abortion? *Am J Nurs* 71:1413–1416, 1971.

71. Survey finds determinants of attitudes toward abortion. *Am J Nurs* 71:1900, 1971.

72. Branson H: Nurses talk about abortion. *Am J Nurs* 72:106–109, 1972.

73. Kane FJ, Feldman M, Jain S, et al: Emotional reactions in abortion service personnel. *Arch Gen Psychiatry* 28:409–411, 1973.

74. Hendershot GE, Grimm JW: Abortion attitudes among nurses and social workers. *Am J Public Health* 64:438–441, 1974.

75. Rosen RAH, Werley HH, Ager JW, et al: Some organizational correlates to nursing students' attitudes toward abortion. *Nurs Res* 23:253–259, 1974.

76. deVries CM: ANA opposes Bush gag rule memo. *Am Nurse* 24(5):3, 1992.

77. Billingsley M: The gag rule: Gag ME. *Nurs Connections* 5(2):10–11, 1992.

78. Sutherland K: Pro-life nurses uniting for services. *J Christian Nurs* 11(3):28–29,45, 1994.

79. Eaton L: Abortion: Clinics prepare for autumn protests. *Health Visitor* 66(2):309, 1993.

80. Schoonover-Shoffner K: A closet pro-lifer turns activist. *J Christian Nurs* 9(2): 40,26, 1992.

81. Rait C: Us against "them": Bush's cynical manipulation of the real issues. *Neonatal Network* 11(7):5–6; 1992.

82. Goller PL, Burchfield H, Wilson R, Glenn MH, Schlais LK: Readers advocate Pro-conscience and Pro-choice. *Nurse Prac* 17(10):8–9, 1992.

83. Havens DH: Its the 103rd Congress: Do you know how your members of Congress are going to vote? *J Ped Health Care* 7(1):43–45, 1993.

84. Marshall SL, Gould T, Roberts J: Nurses attitudes toward termination of pregnancy. *J Adv Nurs* 20(3):567–576; 1994.

85. Wells N: Reducing distress during abortion: A test of sensory information. *J Adv Nurs* 17(9):1050–1056; 1992.

86. Frye BS: Abortion. *AWHONNS Clinical Issues in Perinatal and Women's Health Nurs* 4(2):265–271, 1993.

87. DiPierri D: RU486 mifepristone: A review of a controversial drug. *Nurse Prac* 19(6):59–61, 1994.

88. Griffin KL: Abortion issue is more complex than many realize. *Nurse Prac* 18(3):15–16, 1993.

89. White VM: The moral status of the fetus. *Midwives* 107(1281):375–379, 1994.

90. Curtin LL: Abortion: The limits of moral repugnance. *Nurs Management* 25(10): 22,24, 1994.

91. Horsley J: Abortion and nursing: A legal update. *RN* 55(12):57–58, 1992.

92. Hord CE, Delano GE: The midwife's role in abortion care. *Midwifery* 10(3): 131–141, 1994.

93. McKee K, Adams E: Nurse midwives attitudes toward abortion performance and related procedures. *J Nurse Midwifery* 39(5):300–311, 1994.

94. Summers L: The genesis of the American College of Nurse Mid-wives 1971 statement on abortion. *J Nurse Midwifery* 37(3):168–174, 1992.

95. Brown JS, Davis AJ: Ethical issues in refusing to provide patient care. In Chask N (ed): *The Nursing Profession: Turning Points.* St. Louis: CV Mosby; 1990, pp 313–320.

9
Dying and Death

Issues surrounding dying and death raise many ethical concerns and questions for nurses as well as for the nursing profession. Many of these issues evoke our personal feelings of ambiguity about death. Indeed, some forms of dying while under nursing care challenge the medical view that death is the worst thing that can happen to us. Nurses provide care to patients throughout the life span, from before birth to after death. Through the use of sophisticated life-support mechanisms and treatments, the process of dying has often been prolonged in hospitals, nursing homes, or other institutions, where eight out of ten Americans die and where most nurses have been employed. In the face of these facts, it is not always clear that ethical principles such as respect for persons, or the noninfliction of harm have been considered in practice.

Over the last several decades, we have encountered troubling questions about when death actually occurs, the quality of life, the sanctity of life, verbal do-not-resuscitate orders, disclosure of terminal diagnoses to patients, and the individual's right to die with dignity including the right to receive active assistance in dying from health professionals. There are other questions too. How should the interests of the individual patient, the family, health workers, and the community be weighed in making a decision about a congenitally deformed infant who will die without a sequence of surgical interventions and the use of costly medical resources? Who should decide? Does an individual have the right to choose death? Is there a moral difference between letting a person die and taking an action to hasten death? When, if ever, should life-sustaining treatment be withheld from patients who are unable to make this decision themselves? The implications of these questions are far reaching and demand a thoughtful response from health care professionals, patients, families, the community, and society.

When the landmark Quinlan case in New Jersey (1976) was brought to public attention through the mass media, it served to refocus some of these questions for health professionals, for other professions (such as law and theology), and for the entire community.[1] Another case that also resulted in wide-spread ethical reflection involved the death of a newborn with Down's syndrome and duodenal atresia at Johns Hopkins Hospital a few years earlier. The parents refused permission for surgery and the infant was allowed to die by starvation. This was extremely difficult for the nurses giving care to the baby. Many health professionals and students have engaged in hours of agonizing discussion and moral questioning elicited by this case. These and other situations poignantly illustrate the burdens placed on nurses and nursing by decisions made by others in the system, but which nurses, nonetheless, are expected to implement. On the other hand, it is also in the areas of terminal illness and dying that nurses have made a difference in the options available to patients and their families, such as the development of hospice care, and in initiating changes in the decision-making process related to development of guidelines for orders not to resuscitate.

The ethical, legal, medical, social, cultural, psychological, and economic factors to be considered in near-death interventions (or decisions not to intervene) reflect individual, family, community, and professional values and these factors must arbitrate between and among them. The numbers and kinds of factors, including values and clinical facts, intersecting in each situation serve to further muddy the waters. The immediate decision is also often fraught with more distant implications, not the least of which includes social policy. But, before we discuss end-of-life treatment, we would be well advised to reflect on the end of life, *per se.*

DETERMINING WHEN SOMEONE IS DYING OR DEAD

According to *Webster's Third New International Dictionary* (1971), death is "the ending of all vital functions without possibility of recovery: the end of life: the act, process, or fact of dying: the state of being no longer alive: a joyless, dull, tasteless existence: the state of being without full possession of enjoyment of the intellectual or physical faculties." When is an individual *dead*, with this tremendous range of ideas about death? This range implies the social, psychological, and physical dimensions of death. But which is determinative of death in the sense that one can say, "X" is dead? There is similar variability with use of the word "dead." The definition ranges on a continuum from having ended existence as a living or growing thing, to being without power to move, feel, or respond, to being incapable of feeling or of being stirred emotionally or intellectually. Can one then be dead socially but not physically? This is a metaphysical question beyond the scope of this chapter. But both a process and an event are implied in these various notions.

Tolstoy's novel, *The Death of Ivan Ilyich,* offers a telling description of the social, psychological, and physical aspects of death as a process for the individual and family.[2] Again, these varied ideas of "death" and "dead" raise all the questions mentioned previously and increase the complexity for those who make decisions about whether or not respiratory support equipment should be discontinued or extraordinary measures begun for a particular individual.

Traditionally, the physician made decisions concerning the dying patient. Sixty years ago, these decisions involved primarily the provision of comfort and reassurance for the patient and family. With the trend toward "death with dignity," the patient is or should also be involved in the choices of how to live while dying, the use of drugs to relieve pain, and the decision not to use medical measures that do not promote a cure. Recently, three possible areas of decision making for the physician have been identified by Morison. They are as follows:

1. Using all possible means, including "extraordinary" measures to keep the patient alive
2. Discontinuing "extraordinary" measures but continuing "ordinary" means
3. Taking some "positive" steps to hasten the individual's death[3]

In making such decisions, one must take into account such factors as the determination of what is extraordinary or burdensome, versus ordinary or beneficial in the treatment to be used for a particular patient, whether it be experimental drugs, complicated life-maintaining equipment, or even antibiotics. (It must be noted that though they are still commonly used in clinical settings, the terms ordinary and extraordinary have largely fallen into disuse among ethicists.) These decisions also raise moral questions about the factors that *ought* to figure in the decision-making process. For example, patients may be perceived as being more valuable to the living if they can be declared dead so that organs or tissues from their body can be used to benefit others. Some would see this as using one person primarily as a means to prolonging or improving another's life. In addition to factors already mentioned that may or may not enter into a decision of this nature, a basic question one asks is whether one has the right to die and if so, under what circumstances? In the 1976 Quinlan case, Judge Muir declared that physician decisions were overriding in the care of dying patients. The decision still remained primarily with the physician. But the Supreme Court of New Jersey modified the Muir decision to allow for such decisions to be made in consultation with an ethics committee.[4]

While the dictionary definitions of death give us clues about the process of death, they do not help in determining the moment of death. In contemporary health care, that moment is often obscured because of the use of ventilators, balloon pumps, or other life-sustaining technologies. Actually, medical technology can maintain biological life for a very long time. A question that must be factored into these discussions is whether there is more to life than biological life. Obviously, biological life is necessary to life and living but the question remains whether that is the all of life.

Issues concerning the determination of death clearly demonstrate the interaction of ethics and the law. Some states have legislated a definition of death based on ordinary standards of medical practice, including loss of spontaneous brain function. Other states have passed legislation that include brain death criteria. Both the clinical criteria and the statutes provide guidelines and a process for determining that biological death has occurred. The President's Commission for the Study of Ethical Problems in Medicine and Biomedical and Behavioral Research (the President's Commission) developed uniform criteria for brain death to present to the states as a model for possible legislative action.[5]

Questions about attempting to determine a specific time of death have been raised, since life in any organism, including humans, is not a clearly defined entity with sharp beginning and end points. Issues of life are often clouded with those of personhood and humanity.[6] This is particularly evident in discussions of abortion. The human organism can be conceptualized as a complex interaction among individual cells, the totality of the cells, and the environment. The human system does not usually fail as a unit and so we may have to make clinical or ethical judgments about the value and intactness of the complex interactions of the organism; life is a continuous rather than a discontinuous process.

Some would argue from another viewpoint and would say that the organism does die as a whole and there is still validity for the whole-body concept of death as an event and for using "reasonable criteria" for determining that a person has died. These two viewpoints, presented only very briefly, again give the reader some notion of the complex philosophical, biological, and social issues involved in decisions made about death and the dying process.

To some extent the process of dying is partially controlled today by individuals themselves in the choices they make about the use or refusal of available technologies or treatments. With this relative control over the time of death comes the necessity to think very carefully about who should be involved in decisions relating to this control and again what elements are important in the decision-making process.[7]

Death can be delayed or prevented with the use of sophisticated technologies. Should these technologies be used simply because they are available? This raises the ethical issue of what is called the technological imperative. Should elderly comatose patients be taken from a nursing home to a renal dialysis center for thrice-weekly dialysis? A patient-centered ethic requires that the individual patient remain the center of the decisions. All of these issues and questions seem to pivot on questions about the sanctity of life and the quality of life when dying is prolonged through medical and nursing intervention. Discussions of euthanasia nip at the heels of discussions of the quality of life when dying is prolonged through the use of technology.

EUTHANASIA OR THE GOOD DEATH: ALLOWING TO DIE AND HELPING TO DIE

The concept of *euthanasia* comes from the Greek, meaning good or pleasant death. Is death ever preferable to life? Is there a moral difference between letting die and hastening death, in light of the moral law that thou shalt not kill? At present, there are mixed responses on answers to these questions.[8-14] One needs to consider carefully what the best interests are for a particular patient in a specific situation and to distinguish this from the interests of the provider, institution, and society. The following discussion focuses primarily on the dying adult patient and on ethical (as distinct from religious) considerations *per se*.[15,16]

In attempting to provide at least tentative solutions to euthanasia, an examination of the following criteria for decision making serves as a first step.

1. Who decides? The physician, guardian, patient, family member, clergyman, or a committee or some combination of these?
2. For whom does one decide? Oneself, one for whom one is acting as a proxy, or others?
3. What additional criteria are used (e.g., psychological, religious, economic, social) after the medical status of the patient has been established?
4. What degree of consent is required of the patient?

Decision-making should also consider the moral principles involved, such as respect for autonomy, the obligation to do no harm, and the requirement to tell the truth. Are these being affirmed or negated by particular alternatives proposed? Some believe that euthanasia should be considered only in relation to those who can ask to die (what is commonly called voluntary euthanasia). This position eliminates newborns and infants from its consideration. It is also problematic in that it excludes, as well, those individuals kept alive on machines and the severely senile elderly who are unable to participate in decision-making.

Others in health care and bioethics, take another position on decision making in relation to newborns and argue that in certain circumstances, some severely deformed newborns should be allowed to die by withdrawing or withholding treatment. They feel that these decisions should be made by parents with the assistance of professional advisors, usually physicians, since the parents are the most familiar with the human complexities of a given situation. In past years, when parental decisions for nontreatment of infants have been brought to the courts, most court decisions have required that treatment be given. These decisions make it clear that there has been a general legal duty to treat a child. These opposing views again reflect the complexity and conflict that exist when we attempt to answer the questions surrounding dying and death.

To look further at questions related to euthanasia, there is a continuum of intervention for decision makers ranging from an anti-euthanasia absolutist position on the sanctity of life, to an equally absolutist pro-euthanasia view based on some determination of an inadequate quality of life, or on a supposed absolute right to decide. The absolutist anti-euthanasia position commits one to vigorous treatment to preserve life at any or all costs, and is not in accord with a general understanding of the sanctity of life principle. More moderate positions require the use of nonburdensome treatments without necessarily requiring the use of heroic measures. There is difficulty in determining exactly what constitutes (and who decides what constitutes) burdensomeness and heroics. If we follow the general norm that the patient's decisions are determinative about his or her own care, what constitutes burdensomeness becomes particularly difficult when the patient cannot express the degree of burden that he or she feels.

Over 20 years ago, there was a generalized agreement and many defined *ordinary* (or *nonburdensome*) means of preserving life as including all medicines, treatments, and surgical procedures that offer reasonable hope of benefit to a patient and could be obtained and used without excessive pain, expense, or other inconveniences. *Extraordinary* (or *burdensome*) means are those that are very costly, unusual, difficult, or dangerous, or do *not* offer a reasonable hope of benefit to the patient at a given time and place. These determinations may vary in a large teaching hospital from the ones made in a small community hospital, or in the particular setting where the dying individual is placed. What may be considered ordinary or nonburdensome treatment to or for one patient may be considered extraordinary or burdensome to or for another, for example, the use of antibiotics for a patient with pneumonia only as opposed to their use for the patient who has terminal cancer with metastases to the brain and liver who develops pneumonia.

Some regard withdrawal of treatment to let the patient die as a form of passive euthanasia, while others maintain that it is the intent (i.e., that the patient's death is intended) rather than the withdrawal of treatment itself that determines whether or not euthanasia is involved. In letting die, treatment is withheld, or ongoing treatment withdrawn, with or without the consent of the patient. The withdrawal of treatment to allow a patient to die is still a morally controversial topic for some health professionals even though it has received ample attention in the ethical and clinical literature, to the point of being considered a settled question, as we shall see in a moment.[17,18]

Active euthanasia is considered to include such actions as giving patients the means to kill themselves (assisted suicide) or directly bringing about the patient's death with or without consent, for instance through the lethal injection of potassium chloride.

Do patients have the right to control their dying and if so where does this right of patients to control their own dying fit into our consideration of euthanasia? Do individuals have the right to die, or even to kill themselves in a hospital historically committed to preserving life? Can a patient refuse life-saving treatment? Some have said that institutional inhumanity is the enemy, not death *per se.*

There is no provision in the law that compels a competent person to seek medical care, except when the illness is a threat to the public health or safety—for example, with a communicable disease. In several legal cases, the hospital and the attending physician were not required to perform surgery or transfusions against the patient's will. There have been contradictory legal findings in various cases where individuals refused life-saving blood transfusions due to religious beliefs. In 1977, the Massachusetts Supreme Court decided in the famous Saikewicz case that the courts should most appropriately make decisions about nontreatment for those incompetent to make their own decisions. This court also affirmed that all patients have the right to refuse life-sustaining treatment that will not cure or preserve life.

In the landmark Karen Quinlan case, mentioned earlier, Judge Muir said that when an adult is rendered incompetent, society expects that the attending physician's decision will prevail even when there is a conflict with a family decision.[19] The Quinlan decision also supported a role for ethics committees in the decision-making process (though this concept of an ethics committee was what would more commonly be regarded as a prognosis committee). Judge Muir's decision conflicted with that of a national public opinion poll. When asked about a patient dying in the hospital with no hope of cure, over 50 percent of the sample said that is was alright to let the person die and that the decision should be made by family members or by the physician in conjunction with family members. Only 7 percent felt that it was the decision of the patient's physician alone. Physicians seem to agree with the public rather than with Judge Muir. In 1973, the AMA House of Delegates adopted a statement that condemned physicians agreeing to perform mercy killing (active euthanasia), but said that stopping extraordinary means to prolong biological life is the decision of the patient or his immediate family, with freely available advice and the judgment of the physician.[20] A general social consensus was developing that physicians should not be the only individuals to make decisions related to prolonging life or hastening death.

In the early 1980s, the President appointed a commission to investigate several major ethical issues. That commission was formally named the President's Commission for the Study of Ethical Problems in Medicine and Biomedical and Behavioral Research. Of the reports that it issued, the one entitled *Deciding to Forego Life-Sustaining Treatment* is of special importance to the discussion here.[21] In that report, the President's Commission maintained that:

> Nothing in current law precludes ethically sound decision making. Neither criminal nor civil law—if properly interpreted and applied . . . forces patients to undergo procedures that will increase their suffering when they wish to avoid this by foregoing life-sustaining treatment.[22]

The commission further held that:

> The distinction between failing to initiate and stopping therapy—that is, withholding versus withdrawing treatment—is not itself of moral [or legal] importance. A justification that is adequate for not commencing a treatment is also sufficient for ceasing it.[23]

Life-sustaining treatment may be withheld, or may be withdrawn when it is against the patient's wishes, providing that the patient is fully informed and freely consenting; it may be withheld or withdrawn when it will or has begun to harm the patient; or when it is not benefitting the patient or will not.

Thus, for the most part, ethicists have agreed that when life-sustaining treatment will constitute the violation of the patient's dignity, humanity, well-being, or integrity, it need not be given or continued. This has become a settled issue to a very large extent. The one area of concern that has yet to be fully resolved is the administration of food and fluid, particularly by medical means.

The Cruzan case dramatically brought ethical issues surrounding this specific form of treatment into the public arena in the 1980s.[24] Nancy Cruzan, a 32-year-old woman, was tragically rendered in a persistent vegetative state as the result of an auto accident 6 years earlier. Before the accident, Cruzan had made a number of statements that she would never wish to live as a vegetable, and that she did not view death as the worst possible thing that could happen to her. Thus, in accord with what they believed to be her wishes, and on the basis of her former life style and personality, her parents, who were also her legal guardians, sought to have Cruzan's gastrostomy tube removed so that she might be allowed to die.

The Supreme Court of the state of Missouri refused to allow the removal of the gastrostomy tube. This decision flew in the face of the trend in law and ethics and many previous court precedents regarding withdrawal of treatment. The court decision was lengthy and poorly argued, but it essentially held that the state had a compelling interest in preserving life. It did not matter that Cruzan would not emerge from the persistent vegetative state, nor that she had stated to her parents and others that she would never have wanted treatment under the conditions to which she was subject. The court, instead, demanded clear proof of Cruzan's position—such as a written statement to that effect. This case was argued before the Supreme Court of the United States on December 6, 1989.[24] The 1990 decision of the Supreme Court had profound implications for how the issue of nutrition and hydration was to be approached in clinical practice, particularly in terms of whether such treatment may be withdrawn in accord with the patient or family wishes, and patients be allowed to die.[25-30] A constitutional right to refuse life-preserving medical therapy was recognized, while allowing states to develop procedures for determination of patient intent. In addition, artificial nutrition and hydration was deemed a medical treatment.

In using the term *euthanasia,* some authors make a distinction between mercy killing or active euthanasia and allowing people to die or passive euthanasia. They claim that one is an act of commission, the other an act of omission. A further distinction is made between voluntary (with patient permission) and involuntary (without patient permission) euthanasia. Others consider euthanasia to be any act done by another that results in intentionally bringing about death, whether it is an act of omission or commission, and that treatment withdrawal without intent to bring about death does not constitute euthanasia. It has also been argued that there is no moral distinction between active and passive euthanasia because the end result, death of the patient, is the same. Acts of omission are seen as not interfering with the natural process of dying, where euthanasia-as-mercy-killing is seen as inducing death, (as in the AMA House of Delegates' statement). Another distinction is that the right to die is associated only with the individual, while euthanasia demands that someone else, or society, intervene to induce, or to assist in inducing, death. This raises the question as to whether society or any of its members should accept such an obligation.

While in the Netherlands both a social consensus and the law support active euthanasia, in the United States, there have been some serious gaps in the law for dealing with the broad issue of euthanasia.[31] Euthanasia has been regarded as a form of homicide; patient consent or request for euthanasia is not legally acceptable as a defense. The law has taken into account whether the situation involves an act or failure to act. To some extent, the law does make a distinction between active and passive euthanasia. There has been no case in the Anglo-American tradition of law in which a physician has been convicted of murder or manslaughter for having committed a passive act to end the suffering of a patient. This tradition, then, seems to consider intent of the physician.

There are different ethical points of view on euthanasia that are significant to the nurse, other health professionals, and society, seeking to articulate a moral position on euthanasia. One position, sometimes called the new morality, supports a value system that puts humanness, human dignity, and personal integrity above biological life and functions. This position arises from the ancient religious belief that the core of humanness lies in the rational faculty, that is, in one's ability or potential to be rational. What counts as ethically right action is whether or not human needs come first.

The moral defense is that euthanasia reduces suffering and helps the patient die rather than prolonging a slow, ugly, dehumanizing death. This position holds the value that death is not the worst thing that can happen to an individual. Both Eastern and Western religious traditions agree that one is not morally obligated to preserve life in all cases. For example, the Roman Catholic position, as represented in the Pope's position as long ago as 1957, is that it is not necessary to use extraordinary means to prolong life for the terminally ill person.[32]

One objection to the general idea of euthanasia is that the same thing will happen as happened in Nazi Germany; this is a kind of slippery slope or wedge argument. This particular wedge argument claims that if beneficent euthanasia, a kindly act, can be morally justified, then euthanasia for other and possibly unethical purposes may be practiced and justified. This kind of thinking ignores the fact that the Nazis engaged in genocide and killing for experimental purposes, *not* mercy killing in the sense of a merciful act of kindness. On the other hand, one should not ignore the findings of an earlier classic study in which, a sample of university students in the United States was asked a variety of questions related to euthanasia and a final solution to problems of overpopulation and misery. Over half of the respondents said that society should get rid of unfit persons as a final solution.[33]

It is still more difficult to morally justify letting someone die a slow, dehumanized death than not letting him or her do so. The practice of euthanasia-as-merciful-killing implies compassion on the part of the agent and society. Others do not agree, because killing for them always has evil characteristics, even when killing is in self-defense.

In considering whether or not suffering justifies killing, the principle of proportionate good may be used. This is the principle of balancing the benefits and harms of an action for the suffering individual. A reminder of the Rawlsian criterion for moral principles follows, to be used in deciding whether or not one can morally justify the proportionate good principles for any form of euthanasia. A moral principle should be:

1. *General* in the sense that it expresses general properties and relationships and is not specific to individual persons or relationships
2. *Universal* in the sense that it applies to everyone and is chosen with a view of the consequences if everyone complies
3. *Public* in the sense that everyone knows and recognizes the principle as operative in society
4. An *imposition of order* on conflicting claims in terms of using justice and right to make the adjustment rather than the capacity to coerce
5. *Final* in the sense that this is the last court of appeal and overrides law, custom, social rules, and self-interest[34]

One may question whether the proportionate good principle meets all these criteria in relation to the question of active euthanasia. One could say that this principle is in line with a quality of life ethic, which says that some lives are not worth living. In other words, death is not always the worst thing that can happen to a person according to this thinking.

In the face of continuing debate by proponents of active euthanasia and opponents of it, the ethic of obligation suggests the following kinds of care for patients who are considered to be imminently dying:

1. The relief of pain
2. The relief of suffering
3. Respect for the right of an individual to refuse treatment
4. Universal provision of health care in the sense that individuals and families would not have to bear alone the burden of catastrophic medical care

A third position on euthanasia as "mercy killing" states that mercy killing as active euthanasia is never permissible and that respectful treatment of patients as persons is the fundamental principle of health care ethics. This position does make a moral distinction between killing and allowing to die. Disease is accepted as a cause of death, but a human agent should not be the cause of death, according to this position. This seems to actually rule out both active and passive euthanasia. Another distinction that could be made is between not actively fighting death and actively putting an end to life. A further argument is that the starting point for considering the morality of any kind of killing is that evil is always present in the act of killing. However, this idea of killing may be in the process of being changed and redefined as helping to die. With this wording this idea is gaining more acceptance in some quarters.

This third position holds that the physical cannot be separated and excluded from what makes a person a person. A person is not just cerebral function. How does one determine what is a person for decision-making purposes? Some believe that the sanctity of life ethic should not be put aside in favor of a quality of life ethic, as this will weaken our respect for the dying person and will present a dehumanizing ethic to the human community. The basic questions remain: What is best for the individual? What is best for society, now and in the future?

The view above says that there does come a time to cease prolonging life and to concentrate on the needs of the dying person in an attempt to provide a peaceful death for the overall good of the individual patient. Health care providers must be aware that what is considered to be the medical good for the patient is not always what the patient wants. What the patient wants may change over time, making decisions even more difficult. A further complication is that the physician may have developed an ethic, which claims that it is a physician's duty to preserve life as long as possible. Consequences to the patient are not considered as important as the physician's hope to avoid criticism for stopping life-support mechanisms prematurely.

Decisions Not to Resuscitate and Advance Directives

In discussing the decision not to resuscitate, many in the health professions as well as the general public believe that this decision is fully compatible with respect for the intrinsic value of human life. Not to resuscitate under specific circumstances can be seen as a refusal to attempt to control life and death further through the use of technology.[35,36]

Further efforts to clarify the position of individuals and society on the right to die with dignity are seen in the development of advance directives sometimes referred to as a *Living Will* or the *Durable Power of Attorney for Health Care (DPAHC)*. These are documents in which competent adults can indicate their end-of-life wishes and values. People can change their minds at any time and replace an advance directive with a new one. The living will prepared by Concern for Dying (formerly the Euthanasia Educational Council) was used as a model for death with dignity bills introduced into state legislatures in the early stages of this legislation.

The landmark Natural Death Act (1976) in California (its living will legislation) recognized the rights of adults to prepare written instructions authorizing their physicians to withhold or withdraw life-sustaining procedures in specified circumstances of terminal illness.[37] A major purpose of the original bill was to settle a number of legal issues concerned with professional liability and insurance coverage. This Act relieved physicians, health facilities, and other licensed health professionals of civil liability for carrying out directives as defined in the bill. The bill declared that death resulting from carrying out a directive does not constitute suicide, thus resolving this issue in relation to insurance policies, as well. Although this legislation provided answers and guidelines for some problems, it has always been recognized that public policy of this import will raise a host of additional issues in relation to interpretation.

In addition to the living will, a number of states have provisions for designating a durable power of attorney for health care (DPAHC). Though the legislation varies from state to state, the DPAHC allows adults to designate another (and an alternate) as decision maker for health care decisions when the person cannot make his or her own decisions. Such documents allow for the power of attorney to be given to any adult, including a nonfamily member. While the DPAHC is not a living will, some forms allow the person to specify the sorts of treatments that would or would not be acceptable at the end of life. For the person who holds the power of attorney (emphasis is on *power;* the person need not be a lawyer) his or her decisions have the force of the patient's own decisions and cannot be challenged unless they appear to be clearly contrary to the patient's own wishes.[38-42] In 1991, the Patient Self-Determination Act became law.[43] Congress passed this law as the first federal legislation to ensure that hospitals and other health care facilities inform patients regarding their rights under state law. In addition, patients were to be informed about institutional policies to accept or refuse medical treatment and their right to have an advance directive. In some health care institutions, nurses are the ones who discuss these issues with patients and their families.

Previous discussion of the problem of active euthanasia and passive euthanasia focused primarily on adult and elderly patients. These issues were mentioned only briefly in relation to severely deformed newborns and children with terminal illness. Many of the same issues and questions involving adults apply to children and newborns. A basic issue when children and infants are involved concerns who should make what decisions. The physician? The parents? The child? One concern is whether or not a society should even consider the nontreatment option for children. What are the implications for individuals and the human community, again, in terms of the value of life? Some see this as a question of infanticide, others see it as a quality of life issue. There are other special concerns arising in relation to euthanasia and young children—for example, the legal standing of the rights of children, the status of parental rights, and the obligations of adults to prevent suffering in children. All of these concerns are still raised whenever severely deformed infants and terminally ill children receive care. What are ordinary and extraordinary measures in a newborn intensive care unit? Do they depend on the locally available technology? Do health professionals have obligations to always use the technology available without looking at how lives are affected by it now and in the foreseeable future?

In discussions of nontreatment of newborns with birth defects, some have said that the current haphazard, arbitrary patterns of selection for nontreatment will probably continue unless substantive and procedural criteria are developed as guidelines for decision making in this area that is full of stress and pain. It would be possible to develop guidelines that would identify those situations where treatment would invariably be required, such as low-lesion spina bifida; those situations in which treatment could invariably be withheld, such as anencephaly; and those cases in which the situation is less clear and decisions depend on the facts of the individual case.

In summary, this brief overview of some of the issues and complexities of decision making related to euthanasia, death, and dying does not provide us with any ready-made answers. What it does do is give the reader some idea of directions taken by individuals, institutions, and society in seeking ways to make more ethically appropriate decisions in this area.

SUICIDE AND ASSISTED SUICIDE AS AN ETHICAL DILEMMA

Suicide is a major leading cause of death in the United States. Suicide has been seen variously as an affirmation of life, a denial of life, and a questioning of life. The traditional religious teachings of the Western religions have historically condemned all intentional acts of self-destruction. Though it is all too simple a reduction of their position, traditionally Western theologies have regarded life as a gift of God, belonging to God, but given to humankind for its stewardship. Suicide, then, has been seen as a usurpation of God's authority, thus as sin, because it involves the claim that one's life is one's own (and not belonging to God) to do with as one pleases.

According to the philosopher Kant, who was concerned to separate religion and ethics, humans rightfully do not have the power of disposal of their own bodies. One can only treat one's body as one chooses in relation to self-preservation.[44] These traditional religious and philosophical views are being challenged in today's society. Realizing that suicide often occurs when a person is despondent or under duress, and thus less than fully voluntary, the Act of 1961 declared that suicide should not any longer be regarded as a criminal act.

If one believes that there is a right to commit suicide, then it is useful to distinguish between rational and irrational suicide. Rational suicide may be ascribed to those rational persons suffering from a terminal disease and who with understanding of their act, exercise their self-determination. However, the majority of persons who commit suicide are not terminally ill. The majority suffer from clinically recognizable psychiatric illnesses and have sought help from physicians. These are cases of irrational suicide and health providers have an obligation to do good by not allowing patients to harm themselves.

Recently, the debate has focused on assisted suicide, which means that under certain circumstances the group of people who are severely ill, near death, and who wish to commit suicide should receive help to die from their physicians. Laws exist in the Netherlands, Uruguay, Switzerland, Peru, Japan, and Germany, but not the United States, for such assistance by the physician. However, fearful of a slippery slope situation, those who support physician-assisted suicide say that this group of patients must be considered separately from the lonely, the elderly, and the physically handicapped who may also seek to commit suicide and ask another's assistance.

The question of the individual's right to self-determination is a basic consideration in talking about the ethical dimensions of suicide and assisted suicide. There are positions on both ends of the continuum. They range from the position that individuals have the right to self-determination and that they should retain this right even if they are considered by some to be potentially dangerous or suicidal, to the view that the physician has the obligation to support the desire for life that exists even in those who feel that this desire has left them—e.g., individuals with terminal illness. Other major arguments against suicide are that it is a crime against society, a cowardly act, a violation of one's duty to God, unnatural, and an insult to human dignity, and that it is cruel because it inflicts pain upon one's family and friends.

Arguments have been made that suicide may be ethically justifiable under certain conditions. These arguments include the idea that no rational morality would require that certain lives be continued in the face of disastrous accidents of birth or illnesses for which there are no effective remedial measures. Another argument is that no social morality can be equally binding on everyone in society unless there is more equality in distributing the necessities, sometimes called the goods, of life. Here one thinks in terms of justice as fairness, and a more equal distribution of society's benefits and harms. The obligation to provide a just society in which all can live well seems to especially rest with those who say that one should not commit suicide.

In summary, the question of suicide and assisted suicide is still controversial in our society and raises many profound ethical questions for the health professional about the individual's right to self-determination vis-a-vis the right of the human community to preserve itself. Assisted suicide raises profound questions about the aims of the health sciences, the obligations of health professionals to patients, and redefines what historically has been considered as good and harm in the relationship with patients.[45-50]

FURTHER THOUGHTS FOR NURSING PRACTICE

The nursing literature in the recent past has focused primarily on attitudes toward death and dying patients; the depersonalized, institutionalized dying process; and the nurse's personal experiences with dying patients and their families. Now much more is written on the ethical dilemmas faced by nurses in relation to the dying patient, the family, and other health professionals, particularly the physician.

Nurses should examine, individually and collectively, their own values in relation to death, quality of life, the importance of the individual needs of patients, and such moral principles as self-determination for the dying patient, the bases of respect for the person, the obligation to do no harm, distributive justice, and the caring dimensions of the nurse–patient relationship.

The nurse's *legal* responsibility is to respect the medical decision. One issue, however, that arises for nurses is that they do not always have written orders on which to rely. For example, decisions will be made by nurses for specific patients if they have a cardiac arrest and only verbal no code orders exist. It is generally understood that if written orders for no code do not exist and a patient arrests, the nurse must code the patient.

One example of hospital efforts to recognize a patient's right to refuse available medical procedures, in light of the hospital's primary philosophy to preserve life, is the development of guidelines for orders not to resuscitate. According to these guidelines, physicians have the primary obligation to explore the implications of this decision with the patient and family, but the initial judgment should be discussed first with the other physicians, nurses, and any others directly involved with the patient's care. This provides an opportunity for nurses to add their observations and assessment of a patient to those of others in the decision-making process and to carry out the *caring* process for the dying patient. It is the responsibility of the physician not only to actually record the order not to resuscitate but to convey the meaning of this order for a particular patient to medical, nursing, and other appropriate staff members. Nurses are in a key position to notify the physician if the patient's condition changes.

Nurses are involved in the emotional support needed by the patient's family as they are often the most constant resource for families. Nurses can be most helpful to families of dying patients. Some specific needs of spouses of dying patients are to be with the dying person, to be helpful to the dying person, to be assured of the comfort of the dying person, to be informed of the mate's condition, to be informed of impending death, to be able to air emotions, to have the comfort and support of other family members, and to have acceptance, support, and comfort from health professionals. Spouses often note that nurses had been helpful to their dying mates but are perceived as being too busy to help the families. Nurses can be facilitators for meeting most of these needs, even in intensive care settings, by making themselves available to families. This is not without strain and tension for the nurse.

An important question is whether nursing administration has a moral obligation to provide support systems for nursing staff members involved with critically ill and dying patients. Some institutions already provide such support for nurses and physicians. Nurses can also initiate collaborative efforts with others, such as chaplains and social workers, to meet the needs of families of dying patients.

Clinical ethics committees often discuss issues of care for the dying. These discussions can fall into two categories: those with the participant point of view and those with the administrative perspective. Nurses and physicians are usually in the first group—that is, they often identify with the patient and what they assume to be in the best interests of the patient. The second perspective views the dying patient as a managerial problem and is more concerned with such issues as the use of hospital resources. Problems are implicit in these two viewpoints. The participant perspective in advocating death with dignity and the rights of patients to refuse treatment often ignores when and under what conditions patients might choose death. Health professionals must also guard against imposing their own values on patients and families. The administrative viewpoint, frequently a more utilitarian view, is concerned with efficient use of resources and the equality of treatment for all patients, thus ignoring the diversity of individual patient needs. With the development of managed care, these two perspectives, which can conflict, become even more important to examine from an ethical perspective.

Some have taken the position that in disagreements between these viewpoints, questions should be resolved as *patient* policy questions, not as hospital or public policy questions, such as those concerning limited beds or other limited hospital resources.[51] The danger exists that more and more decisions will be based on economic considerations and needs that can be accommodated or on a utilitarian ethic that considers only the common good as the determinant in decision making. In light of this, one needs to refocus on the moral principles of doing no harm, justice as equal treatment, and respect for values of patients and families, with both the common good and individual needs considered.

Nursing emphasizes the importance of *caring* for dying patients when they are beyond the point where life can be preserved. Nurses and other health professionals are healers and menders of patients. However, in caring for patients there are some dimensions of the patient's life that are beyond the professional's appropriate concern. These areas are more appropriate to the concern and attention of the family or the patient's significant others because these persons are most intimately involved with the patient. Concerns about decision making arise when nurses are caring for an individual who does not have family or significant others when particular problems that concern only the patient and the family or significant others arise, and when it is inappropriate for health professionals to intervene. This becomes a particularly sensitive issue when the patient is unable to make these decisions; legal intervention may be necessary to secure a guardian or conservator.

There is a duty never to abandon *care.* In caring for the dying person one may eventually cease doing what was once called for and begin to do what is now required in the individual situation. This does not mean that one is required to assist the dying process, but that one must assure the person that she or he is not alone and that others are aware of this dying and will be there during the dying process. Recall the needs and concerns of family members of dying persons mentioned earlier.

These caring values and practices are clearly demonstrated in the hospice movement. It has been suggested that we could formulate a moral rule that the *only* circumstance in which positive action might be taken to hasten a person's death is if there is the kind of prolonged dying where it is medically impossible to control the individual's pain or other distressing symptoms. Physician-assisted suicide and possibly active euthanasia could result from such a formulation. The nurse, through close contact in caring for the patient and managing control of symptoms, may be the first to see that this situation has been reached by a particular patient. It becomes imperative for the nurse to communicate this to the patient's physician in response to an ethic of caring. The ethic and practice of allowing to die, recognized by most health professionals, still leaves the question as to whether physicians can take positive action to hasten death without weakening medicine's life-saving ethic. It must also be noted that actively helping a patient to die is not an acceptable solution to poor symptom control. It is important to realize that the clinical definition of pain is often limited to concerns for physical pain. But there is also psychological pain which is more akin to suffering. Physical pain can often be controlled while psychological pain in some instances may be beyond the reach of health professionals. In concert with others such as family members or a religious counselor such as the hospital chaplain, health professionals can attempt to help patients ease their suffering.

In 1971, a study of nurses' feelings about euthanasia was done at the University of Washington Hospital and Swedish Hospital Medical Center.[52] Findings indicated that nurses heard requests for positive or direct euthanasia from terminally ill patients and their families more frequently than did physicians. The underlying assumption was that nurses have more interaction with the patient and family than do physicians. More nurses were uncomfortable when physicians did not let patients irretrievably dying die than when the physician did follow this ethic. Nurses generally demonstrated more desire than physicians for social changes, such as legislation, to allow euthanasia. These nurses may hold the value that the patient has a right to maintain control and make decisions about the end of his or her life and way of dying. More nurses than physicians supported the concept of using a committee or board for resolving difficult philosophic decisions about questions of euthanasia.

Nursing, as a profession, may want to articulate an ethic of care for the dying. In the recent past, a moral distinction has been made between acts that *permit* death and acts that cause death. According to this ethic, the compassion and freedom of the nurse are increased as the nurse cares for an irreversibly ill patient who has the freedom to refuse interventions that only prolong the dying process and to make choices such as how to live while dying. This ethic adheres to the commandment "thou shalt not kill" and stands in the deontological ethical tradition of principle-based ethics and notions of obligations. Nurses can help patients and families to look at hospice or hospice-like options for care, such as care at home when appropriate support is available. Nurses need to be particularly sensitive to families when home care is not a viable choice. There have been situations where home care has been imposed on families by well-meaning health professionals. The major focus should be on preserving the life and values of the human community, with mercy and compassion for the individual.

Nurses also work with patients such as the elderly and AIDS patients who are, or are considered to be, suicidal. As discussed earlier, suicide and assisting in suicide have been generally considered to be unjustifiable acts of killing. Suicide, in one view, is considered to be the ultimate way of shutting out all other people from one's life and of saying that life is no longer worthwhile. This position negates the view that our lives are shaped by responses to others and their responses to us. This means we have responsibilities to others as members of groups and families. In this viewpoint, suicide in any form negates this aspect of human community. Key elements of this view follow:

1. The individual's life is not solely at the disposal of that person because he or she is part of a human community.
2. The individual has the freedom to make moral choices.
3. Every individual life has some worth.
4. The supreme value is goodness, in Western religious traditions referred to as God, to which the dying and those who care for the dying are responsible.

Others view suicide as a cry for help by those psychologically disturbed or a rational act of a mentally competent person exercising self-determination. While in this view the community is considered, the major emphasis is on the individual person. So what does mercy and compassion for the individual mean?

A March 7, 1996 lead newspaper article said that the U.S. 9th Circuit Court had struck down a Washington state law barring doctor-assisted suicide, becoming the highest court ever to rule that terminally ill patients have a constitutional right to decide when and how to die. This ban on aiding suicide was seen to violate the due-process rights of those who wish to hasten their death with medications prescribed by doctors. Although states have a strong interest in preserving lives, the court indicated that this interest is outweighed by the right of mentally competent patients to determine the time and manner of their deaths. This case, and one like it in the New York 2nd Circuit Court, was granted cert by the U.S. Supreme Court for a ruling in 1997.[53–55]

Obviously, our society has not yet reached a consensus on this ethical issue. As there may be recognized conflict between the authority and autonomy of the health professionals and that of the patient, patients need someone outside of this conflict who represents their interests. Health professionals have traditionally adhered to the ethic that says one should do everything one can to preserve life. Death is seen as the failure of medical technology and knowledge. Now there is a growing division between those who support the patient's right to die and those who do not see this as a right and who give more weight to the health professional's obligation to treat. With the dying patient, what we mean by treatment needs to be examined and perhaps reconceptualized.

The philosophy of the hospice movement provides a starting point for discussion within and outside the profession by nurses confronted with a patient and family who want a respirator turned off or do not want heroic measures instituted. The Dying Person's Bill of Rights offers another framework for discussions and decision making about ethical issues that arise in the care of the dying person, whether an adult or a child. The Dying Person's Bill of Rights includes such ideas as rights to treatment as a living human being until death, maintenance of a sense of hopefulness, expression of one's own feelings and emotions about approaching death, participation in decisions concerning one's care, freedom from pain, the right not to die alone, the right to have one's questions answered honestly without deception, the right to maintain one's individuality, and the right to be cared for by caring, sensitive, knowledgeable people. These rights parallel many of the needs identified by families of dying patients. The last right (to be cared for by caring, sensitive, knowledgeable people) implies that these people, including nurses, have deliberated and continue to consider the ethical dimensions of questions posed by the availability of technologies that may or may not be used to maintain life.[56]

To focus primarily on a patient-centered ethic, as has been done in this section, is not to ignore the hospital policy and public policy issues that have arisen in connection with society's priorities for health and illness and allocation of finite resources. Chapter 12 focuses on some ways that nursing is and can be actively involved in such areas as legislation, including that legislation where death and dying as ethical dilemmas for health providers, consumers, legislators, and the human community at large is considered.

Advance directives, hospital and nursing home guidelines for orders not to resuscitate, and court and legislative actions are all significant steps in seeking paths to resolving some of the ethical dilemmas that exist today concerning dying and death. Nurses should have opportunities to articulate and think through positions on these dilemmas that confront them as individuals and professions. Ethics rounds, courses in basic nursing education, and continuing education efforts in patient care ethics provide forums for doing this within the nursing community and with other health disciplines. The American Nurses Association Center for Ethics and Human Rights provides consultation and serves as a clearinghouse on ethics materials.

Nursing efforts in truly caring for the terminally ill and dying patient have made positive differences at the individual level of care and at the institutional policy level that are reflections of respect for persons. Concerns focus primarily on *how* to treat the dying patient rather than on whether one should treat or not treat. While futility of treatment has become a major topic in medicine, it is not central to nursing because nurses provide care to patients until they die and even after death.[57,58]

■ CASE STUDY I.

You are a hospice nurse who has been caring of Mr. J. for the past 4 months. He is dying of AIDS. He is a high school English teacher and literature has been the love of his life. He has been doing reasonably well until the last 6 weeks. He now has recurrent cytomegalovirus and is losing his vision. His t-cell count is less than 15.

You have had a very warm relationship and he has freely shared his hopes, fears, and concerns about his illness. On your visit today, he tells you how much he misses being able to read, and how full his life has been, and that he wants to die. You explore with him how you could make him more comfortable and he says "I'm just tired of this disease, I don't want anymore surprises. It's time to see what comes next. I've planned my farewell for Thursday, some friends are coming to read my favorite poetry. I'd really like you to be here."

Suggested Questions for Discussion

1. What will you do? What motivates your decision?

2. How would you articulate your reasoning to your colleagues?

3. What is the nature of your responsibility to Mr. J.; ethically, legally, and personally? What are the origins of these responsibilities? Are there limits to these responsibilities?

■ CASE STUDY II.

You are a new grad of 6 months working the night shift on a small cancer unit. There are two RNs on this unit and you are the most senior. Mr. V. has been in and out of this unit several times over the last few months. He has liver cancer and has gone through several episodes of chemotherapy. His last admission, however, was for an unsuccessful suicide attempt. At the time, you learned that he had made several such attempts in the last few weeks.

Mr. V. recently joined the hospice program. His current admission is for pain control and the orders are to start a morphine drip to be titrated for pain. The only set parameters are to decrease the drip for respirations less than four per minute. Mr. V. requests that the drip be increased several times during your shift. Even though he does not appear to be in any discomfort, you accept his assessment and increase the drip. His wife has been staying with him since his admission. On a routine check, you note that his respirations are now four per minute and he is unarousable. You turn off the drip, telling the wife that you will turn it back on if he arouses at all or shows any signs of being in pain but that his respirations are dangerously low. After about an hour he begins to arouse and you resume the drip at a lower level. After about 10 more minutes, Mr. V. wakes up and is furious with you, accusing you of bringing him back from death. "I have a do-not-resuscitate order, you are supposed to let me die." You reply that you did not bring him back, you stopped pushing him toward death.

Suggested Questions for Discussion

1. How do you ethically define what is happening in this situation?

2. If you had kept the morphine turned on, would you be letting him die or causing him to die? Is there a difference? How do you justify your actions?

3. What is at stake in this situation?

REFERENCES

1. Matter of *Quinlan*, 70 NJ 10(1976), 355 A2d 647 (NJ1976).
2. Tolstoy L: The death of Ivan Ilych. In *Great Short Works of Leo Tolstoy*. New York: Perennial Library—Harper Row: 1967, pp 245–302.
3. Morison RS: Death: Process or event? In Steinfel P, Veatch RM (ed): *Death Inside Out: The Hastings Center Report*. New York: Harper & Row; 1974, p 68.

4. *Quinlan: op. cit.*
5. President's Commission for the Study of Ethical Problems in Medicine and Biomedical and Behavioral Research: *Defining Death.* Washington, DC: United States Government Printing Office; 1981.
6. Jonas H: The burden and blessing of mortality. *Hastings Cent Rep* 22(1):34–40, 1992.
7. Kjervik DK: Legal and ethical issues: The choice to die. *J Prof Nurs* 7(3):151, 1991.
8. Liaschenko J, Drought TS: Euthanasia: Pro or con? *Calif Nurse* 89(1):1,6, 1993.
9. Anderson JG, Caddell DP: Attitudes of medical professionals toward euthanasia. *Soc Sci Med* 37(1):105–114, 1993.
10. Aroskar MA: Nursing and the euthanasia debate. *J Prof Nurs* 10(1):5, 1994.
11. Curtin LL: Euthanasia: A clarification. *Nurs Management* 26(6):64–67. 1995.
12. Davis AJ, Philips L, Drought TS, Sellin S, Ronsman K, Hershberger AK: Nurses' attitudes toward active euthanasia. *Nurs Outlook* 43(4):174–179, 1995.
13. Scherbakova S: Why euthanasia? A reflective inquiry. *Nurs Inquiry* 2(3):184, 1995.
14. Sellman D: Euphemisms for euthanasia. *Nurs Ethics* 2(4):315–319, 1995.
15. Moskowitz EH, Nelson JL: Dying well in the hospital: The lessons of SUPPORT. *Hastings Cent Rep* 25:S35–S36, 1995.
16. Hiltunen EF: The nurse's role in end-of-life treatment discussions: Preliminary report from the SUPPORT project. *J Cardiovascular Nurs* 9(3):68–77, 1995.
17. Reckling JB: Withholding and withdrawing life-sustaining treatment. *Medsurg Nurs* 4(4):327–330, 1995.
18. Valko NG: The ethics of death: Selling euthanasia to nurses and doctors. *Revolution* 5(2):47–49, 1995.
19. *Quinlan: op. cit.*
20. Ramsey P: *The Patient as Person.* New Haven: Yale University Press; 1970.
21. President's Commission for the Study of Ethical Problems in Medicine and Biomedical and Behavioral Research. *Deciding to Forego Life-Sustaining Treatment:* Washington, DC: United States Government Printing Office, 1983.
22. Brody H: *Ethical Decisions in Medicine.* Boston: Little, Brown; 1976.
23. *Ibid.*
24. *Cruzan v. Harmon,* 760 S.W.2d 408 (MO 1988), cert. granted sub nom. Cruzan v. Director of Missouri Department of Health et al, 106 L.Ed.2d 587, 109 S.Ct. 3240, 1989.
25. Fiesta J: The Cruzan case—no right to die. *Nurs Management* 21(9):22, 1990.
26. Musgrave CF: Terminal dehydration: To give or not to give intravenous fluids? *Cancer Nurs* 13(1):62–66, 1990.
27. Banja JD: Nutritional discontinuation: Active or passive euthanasia? *J Neurosci Nurs* 22(2):117–120, 1990.
28. Flarey DL: Ethical decisions: What we learned from Cruzan about the right to die. *Nurs Admin Quart* 15(4):13–21, 1991.
29. de Raeve L: To feed or to nourish? Thoughts on the moral significance of meals in hospital. *Nurs Ethics* 1(4):237–241, 1994.

30. Day L, Drought T, Davis AJ: Principle-based ethics and nurses' attitudes toward artificial feeding. *J Adv Nurs* 21(2):295–298, 1995.
31. van de Bunt CE: Euthanasia in the Netherlands. *International Nurs Rev* 41(2): 63–64, 1994.
32. Fletcher J: Ethics and euthanasia. *Am J Nurs* 73(4):670–675, 1973.
33. Mansson HH: Justifying the final solution. *Omega* 3:79–87, 1972.
34. Rawls J: *A Theory of Justice.* Cambridge, MA: Harvard University Press; 1971.
35. Jacobson BS: Ethical dilemmas of do-not-resuscitate orders in surgery. *AORN J* 60(3):449–452 and 60(4):543, 1994.
36. Berky PS: Do not resuscitate orders: The nurses role. *Maryland Nurse* 14(3):4, 1995.
37. Jonsen AR: Dying right in California—The Natural Death Act. *Clin Toxicology* 13(4):513–522.
38. Crisham P: Living wills—Controversy and certainty. *J Prof Nurs* 6(6):321, 1990.
39. Reigle J: Preserving patient self-determination through advance directives. *Heart Lung* 21(2):196–198, 1992.
40. Catalano JT: Treatments not specifically listed in the living will: The ethical dilemmas. *Dimensions Crit Care Nurs* 13(3):142–150, 1994.
41. Brunt B: Advance directives: Two years later. *Medsurg Nurs* 3(8):408–409, 1994.
42. Campbell ML: Interpretation of an ambiguous advance directive. *Dimensions Crit Care Nurs* 14(5):226–332, 1995.
43. *Omnibus Budget Reconciliation Act of 1990,* Pub L No. 101–508 ** 4206, 4751.
44. Kant I: Duties towards the body in regard to life. In Gorovitz S et al (eds): *Moral Problems in Medicine.* Englewood Cliffs NJ: Prentice-Hall; 1976, pp 376–377.
45. Curtin LL: Nurses take a stand on assisted suicide. *Nurs Management* 26(5):71, 73–74, 76, 1995.
46. Bosek MS, Jezuit D: The nurse's role in assisted suicide. *Medsurg Nurs* 4(5): 373–378, 1995.
47. Scanlon C: What if a patient requests assisted suicide? *Maryland Nurse* 14(6):6, 1995.
48. Murphy PA: Nurses speak out on assisted suicide. *Trends Health Care Law Ethics* 10(1–2)124, 1995.
49. American Nurses Association: Position statement on assisted suicide. *Trends Health Care Law Ethics* 10(1–2):125–127, 1995.
50. Coyle N: The euthanasia and physician-assisted suicide debate: Issues for nursing. *Oncol Nurs Forum* 19(7 suppl):41–46, 1992.
51. Emanuel E, Emanuel L: The economics of dying: The illusion of cost savings at the end of life. *N Engl J Med* 330(8):540–544, 1994.
52. Brown NK, Thompson DJ, Bulger RJ, Laws EH: How do nurses feel about euthanasia and abortion? *Am J Nurs* 71(7):1413–1416, 1971.
53. Holding R: Appeals court declares "Right to die." *San Francisco Chronicle.* March 7, 1996, p 1.
54. Annas GJ: The promised end—Constitutional aspects of physician-assisted suicide. *N Engl J Med* 335(9):683–687, 1996.

55. Orentleicher D: The legalization of physician-assisted suicide. *N Engl J Med* 335(9):663–667, 1996.

56. Love MB: Patient advocacy at the end of life. *Nurs Ethics* 2(1):3–9, 1995.

57. Morreim EH: Profoundly diminished life: The casualties of coercion. *Hastings Cent Rep* 24(1):33–42, 1994.

58. Taylor C: Medical futility and nursing. *Image J Nurs Sch* 27(4):301–306, 1995

10
Behavior Control

The long history of social evolution has engaged the human species in an endless struggle to understand, predict, influence, and control human behavior. The notion of the common good has been invoked in most instances as justification for coercing an individual to conform to social mores. Historically, the tyranny of the majority has had limited results, especially in private life, since the machinery of repression has had no efficient ways to cope with the deviance and nonconformity engaged in within the confines of an individual's own home and in private relationships. Laws developed to deal with this area of life to a large extent functioned more as expressions of public morality than as incursions on private liberty. However, recently developed control methods make it possible now to exact conformity with greater reliability and less potential for resistance than has been the case in the past. Increasingly, we have the technology to effectively engineer consent, which can thereby eliminate personal license and still leave individuals with the feeling that they are free. This situation may appeal as a therapeutic tool to those who work with the "hard-core" criminal or the severely mentally ill; however, such developments in behavior control, with widespread use, can also serve to unhinge the conventional political morality essential to modern democracy. The basic ethical problem of behavior control arises in the dilemma of how to maintain personal liberty in situations where suppression of liberty can be rationalized not only by the needs of the common welfare but also by the individual's happiness.

The potential success of behavior control techniques to change people—prison inmates, substance abusers, mental patients, the entire gamut of people seeking psychiatric help with the goal of self-fulfillment and self-realization, the mentally retarded, and people with dementia—has become a source of controversy within the larger debate as to society's proper response to deviant behavior. The concept of unintended consequences, which maintains that reforms and innovations often carry with them effects of a social nature contrary to the stated purpose of the intended goals, becomes a central concern in developing techniques to control behavior.[1] For example, according to sociologists and social historians, the original intent in establishing asylums for the mentally ill was to provide a protective setting with treatment and humane conditions, but this approach also had the unintentional consequence of turning the asylum into a warehouse for the mentally ill where loss of individuality, depersonalization, and dehumanization resulted.[2-4] The concerns surrounding behavior control and its unintended consequences can be understood in the context of the three social dilemmas that prisons and mental hospitals share:

1. How does the institutional social structure affect attempts at treatment and rehabilitation?
2. How can these institutions meet both the demands of society and the needs of the individuals they serve?
3. What kind of control should be exercised over the development and application of behavior control techniques?

Although the criminal justice system and the mental health system—which is a part of the system of medical knowledge—both use forms of behavior control, for the most part this chapter will focus on the latter.

During the 1950s and 1960s, we came to recognize that prisons and mental hospitals fall far short of meeting the goals set for them by society. Critics, both in and out of the mental health field, traced this failure to a number of variables, including the basic factor that the social structure of these institutions did not always support their stated goals but at times tended to undermine their purpose.[5-8] The recognition of these problems led to three changes that affected the "total institution" nature of the mental hospital. In an attempt to alter the social structure of mental hospitals, Jones developed the therapeutic community concept in the United Kingdom, which became a major reform movement during the 1950s and 1960s.[9,10] The second change, the community mental health movement, arose from an awareness of the negative aspects of maintaining a patient in a total institution over a long period of time. This change resulted in a shift away from almost total reliance on public institutions with their involuntary incarceration and treatment to a more voluntaristic and pluralistic system. This shift has come to be known as deinstitutionalization. An awareness of and concern for the civil rights of the involuntarily committed mentally ill during the 1960s was one aspect of a broader social consciousness concerning the rights of women and non-Whites, particularly African-Americans to be full participants in American life. Economics, however, also played a role in deinstitutionalization in that housing patients in large institutions was expensive. The third change has been the development of behavior control technologies, all of which have become more sophisticated, more effective, and more efficient. While the history of behavioral control technology includes electroshock therapy, psychosurgery, behavior modification, and other psychological techniques, it is psychotropic drugs that has had the most influence in shifting the place of care from large institutions to the community.

The issue of behavioral control, however, did not end with the move to a community locus of care. One area in which the issue of behavioral control can be seen is homelessness. Community care done well, like institutional care done well, is expensive and inadequate funding and housing lead to increasing numbers of the homeless mentally ill. The deinstitutionalization of the 1980s occurred in a political climate that effectively saw a decrease in a tax base for public services and then rationalized the poor services with the damaging view that government cannot do anything. These sentiments continue to the present and the result for mental health services is continued inadequate funding. This is not only a matter of concern for public mental health care, however. Over the past 20 years, private insurers have dramatically limited mental health coverage for policy holders. As mental health services have decreased and state mental health hospitals have closed, the mentally ill have become visible to the society at large and there has been increasing demand to control this deviancy. In the absence of services, jails have become an option for the seriously mentally ill.[11] As we stated, the focus of this chapter will be on the mental health system but we want to make a few points about the prison system. First, the jail and prison populations have swelled over the past 20 years largely with nonviolent offenders as a result of the war on drugs. This should lead us to question the wisdom of the policy. Second, in this era of general resistance to taxes, jail construction and operations is one area that has received fairly widespread social endorsement. Finally, it is clear that the mentally ill are increasingly incarcerated in jails and the health care providers who work with them interface with both systems of social control.

Regardless of setting, developments in the technology of behavioral control have raised basic legal and ethical questions regarding the rights of patients and the role of staff members in a situation where some view psychiatric personnel as double agents—that is, as regulatory agents for the state and as therapeutic agents for the patient. This can, and does, create a conflict-of-interest problem.[12,13]

Before proceeding to a more detailed discussion of specific forms of behavior control, it will be helpful to define the term itself and to consider the fundamental problems of deviancy and coercion. London defined behavior control as getting people to do someone else's bidding, as has been depicted in several classic fictional and nonfiction accounts.[14–19] In the broadest sense, behavior control can be understood as a special form of behavioral change. For example, in a psychiatric setting, treatment offered to or imposed on a patient may, to a large extent, be designed to satisfy the wishes of others. Behavioral change that satisfies others—the community or society, for example—may or may not satisfy the patient's wishes to change. The use of behavior control with the mentally ill has been questioned on the grounds that such treatment deprives patients of the fundamental right to choose their course of action. As behavior control technology develops and becomes more available, and as the psychiatric categories seem to expand to include more attitudes and behaviors defined as deviant, numerous ethical questions arise. Preventive psychiatry continues to define more and more problems of human behavior as falling within its jurisdiction, yet the critics maintain that its practitioners are unable to cope with its present scope. This inability to deliver the goods, so to speak, may be considered as both an ethical problem and a safeguard against unchecked power. With recent research probing the biological base of major mental illnesses, some of the ethical questions for the future will be different from those that are central in behavior control today.

DEVIANCY AND MENTAL ILLNESS

Every society has its rules and social norms. It is generally expected in a given society that a majority of the people will conform to these rules and norms most of the time. In addition, every society has its nonconformists, for example artists with a bohemian life style, which most communities within society will tolerate without attempting to control as long as such a life style does not deviate too much from the established norm. The nonconformists considered as deviants and as creating social problems in our society do not constitute a homogeneous group, and the characteristics that bring them societal attention do not lend themselves to easy classification. Generally speaking, the most obvious groups considered deviant in our own society fall into the following nonexclusive categories:

- Medical (the mentally ill)
- Intellectual (the mentally retarded)
- Chronological (the senile)
- Social (the alcoholic)
- Economic (other drug abusers)
- Sexual (the homosexual)
- Doctrinal nonconformity (the sociopolitical radical)

These groups share two things in common. First, their behavior is proscribed or controlled by law, and second, society increasingly seeks them out for "treatment" instead of "punishment."[20] It is of importance to note that social norms change and therefore influence the definition of what is deviant. For example, homosexuals have been eliminated from the category of psychopathology by a vote of psychiatrists. Such action shows the fluidity of the boundaries between normal and abnormal behavior.

The idea of deviancy is rooted in sociological labeling theory.[21,22] Basically, social groups create deviance when they make rules whose infraction constitutes deviance and when they apply those rules to particular individuals and label them as outsiders. It follows, then, that deviance is not solely a quality of the act the person commits, but rather a consequence of the application by others of rules and sanctions to a so-called offender. The deviant person is one to whom that label has successfully been applied and deviant behavior is behavior that people so labeled engage in, according to a classic study on this topic.[23]

Those persons whom we call mentally ill tend to be at variance with the mores and conventions of society. The fact that this condition usually has behavioral rather than physiological symptoms alone casts those so labeled into the role of the social deviant. Mental illness is not easy to define or to determine, and this situation becomes compounded by the fact that different societies may have different tolerance levels for the sort of deviation that becomes labeled as mental illness.

The concept *dangerousness* is the paramount consideration in the legal commitment procedure within our mental health system.[24] This was not always the case, however. Prior to the late 1960s, the major consideration was the idea of *in need of treatment*. The Lanterman/Petris/Short Act of California was highly influential in shifting the criteria for involuntary commitment from the need for treatment to that of dangerousness. Although some states allow involuntary commitments on the grounds of being *gravely disabled*, which means the inability to find food and shelter, the risk of dangerousness remains the standard in contemporary mental health law.[25,26] This means that for the mentally ill deviant, the justification for civil commitment is thought to be a provable likelihood of dangerous acts toward the self or toward others. Despite the fact that the mental health field does not possess the tools to determine, with any degree of precision, those who will be dangerous, the prediction of dangerousness remains a key issue.[27] Three explanations have been offered by noted authorities. First, the courts continue to demand that mental health providers make these assessments. Second, it is a very practical concern because the mentally ill who are violent increasingly comprise the inpatient population—a result of the overall decrease in beds combined with the restriction of admission to that of danger to self or others. Finally, the mentally ill can no longer be committed for indeterminate lengths of stay. This means that commitment is no longer a single solution with the result that the management of the dangerous mentally ill in the community, difficult in its own right, creates anxiety for the community.[28] Dangerousness, like any number of other things, including beauty, is, to some extent, in the eye of the beholder.[29,30] For example, one study conducted by a nurse explored the notion that the concept of dangerousness is a social construction. The study focus was an examination of how nursing personnel on locked inpatient psychiatric units define patients as dangerous to others.[31] While the general public has tended to associate dangerousness with mental illness, numerous experts have pointed to the inadequacy of the criteria for predicting who will commit a dangerous act.[32,33] Although the vast majority of the seriously mentally ill are no more dangerous than the general population, there is a subset who are.[34,35] Among this subset, substance-abuse, noncompliance with medication, and a history of violent behavior are important predictors.

Some critiques of the idea that violence can be predicted emphasize that violent behavior is not only a function of personality but also a function of social context.[36,37] The theory of social context provides one explanation as to why the traditional psychiatric approach, which emphasizes personality, would have limited predictive value.[38–40] The above comments are not intended to imply that no traditional psychiatric clues are valid, only that such validity has yet to be established. The difficulty involved in predicting dangerousness increases when the patient has never actually performed an assaultive act. This problem becomes particularly relevant to involuntary hospitalization situations. Some believe that mental health professionals, since they have no reliable criteria, tend to overpredict dangerousness. In such instances, so the argument goes, these professionals have stereotyped ideas of the personality attributes of dangerous individuals that have no valid relationship to the occurrence of dangerous acts. Rather, they commit themselves to these stereotypes because of theoretical constructs that cause them to attend selectively to certain data. In addition to the problems of identification and prediction of dangerous behavior, some maintain that neither mental hospitals nor prisons are now capable of treating persons labeled as dangerous. It must be seen as a bizarre system of criminal justice that confines mostly those who cannot be identified as dangerous, and equally bizarre a mental health system that commits mostly those who cannot be treated.[41]

Most research on the management of violent behavior is based on inpatient settings.[42–47] The knowledge contributed by such work is important but it is no longer sufficient as the dangerous mentally ill are being discharged rapidly to the community from inpatient settings or they are not being admitted in the first place. While some work on the community management of violent behavior has been done, the complexity of the issues warrants more study.[48]

COERCION AND FREEDOM

The following comments come from an essay by Willard Gaylin, a psychoanalyst who has been for many years the president of the Hastings Center, one of the think tanks in bioethics in the United States. He points out that in the United States, freedom constitutes a dominant value; however, the structure of organized society depends on defined limits of freedom. The legal system supplies the definitions of permissible behavior and also establishes the coercive force that society may use to ensure compliance. Therefore, coercion may not necessarily always be an evil. The basis of civilization depends to a great extent on the right of the state to coerce its citizens. These statements lead to the realization that we must weigh society's right to coerce against the individual's right to freedom. Furthermore, one needs to think through what constitutes a coerced, as distinguished from a free, act. Freedom, a principle to which psychiatry aspires rather than a concept that it often employs, has not been incorporated to any extent into a theory of behavior, since psychiatry has difficulty fitting freedom with theory that tends toward a deterministic view.[49]

Since people's beliefs and experiences form the basis of future behavior, the perception of danger becomes the crucial issue in understanding coercion. If you feel threatened, it is easier to justify coercion on the basis of that perception. To understand coercion one must understand that which threatens man. The problem is not so much the coercion involved in physical force and threatening survival itself, but threats to survival equivalents, such as threat of isolation, loss of love, social humiliation, and so on.

As stated earlier, the social order relies to some extent on the right to coercion. Along with the legal dimensions of coercion, society has given a moral privilege to coercion when such action is done in the individual's best interest. For example, certain parental behavior coerces children, but society permits this because of the assumption that parents have the child's best interest at heart. Also, in the field of health, coercion has a traditional respectability and legal sanction, and psychiatry, as a branch of medicine, has engaged in coercion. Indeed, one might correctly say that, in the recent past, the abrogation of the legal rights of the mentally ill, the denial of due process, and the confinement beyond the limits the law tolerates for criminals represent a gross example of coercion.

Sophisticated and morally reflective nurses know that they bear an instrumental relationship to institutionalized medicine, which is to say that nursing can become the means for ends or goals set by medical knowledge.[50,51] They also know that because they occupy a key place in powerful institutions, they have a great capacity to coerce patients. In one study that examined the ethical concerns of psychiatric and home care nurses, one nurse aptly expressed this reality in stating: "I am the enforcement tool of a large university hospital."[52] In an excellent history of the use of restraints, the authors note that a "reduction of mechanical restraint never became a compelling professional ideal in the United States and, further, that a therapeutic philosophy of control characterizes most health care institutions. Physical restraint and locked seclusion remain a reality in the management of many troublesome patients."[53] Those nurses who recognize the places they occupy in complex positions are particularly sensitive to the potential for coercion and loss of patient autonomy.[54] Other nurse researchers studying the ethical dimensions of psychiatric nursing practice have repeatedly documented that direct–care nurses experience the balancing of patient agency against social control as a central moral concern.[55–61]

Behavior control represents a broad spectrum of activities, including psychiatric therapy, political propaganda, commercial advertising, religious and moral education, and rehabilitation of deviant persons. The major categories of behavior control in the mental health field that will be discussed in this chapter are psychotherapy, psychosurgery, and psychopharmacology. Practitioners in the field readily accept the fact that patients should be protected from outright coercion, and this belief has been formalized in statutes and regulations. The idea that the patient should also be protected from more subtle pressures is not only more difficult for many mental health professionals to accept, but makes the problems of such regulation more difficult as well.

PSYCHOTHERAPY

The history of psychotherapy reveals three developmental stages during the 20th century. Each of these stages has been in response to the psychosocial motif dominating the society at that time. Stage one came into being with the development of psychoanalysis. This occurred around the beginning of this century, when Freud and Breuer first published their works and formed the Psychoanalytic Society in 1902. The psychoanalytic approach to treatment was to uncover and expose unconscious material that had been repressed. It came to be known as the talking cure. The patients, mostly middle class women, lived in the Victorian era of Vienna, known for its standards of proper behavior and repression of sexuality. Psychoanalysis was seen as offering a viable explanation of the human mind and its desires in conflict with a repressing, controlling society. While psychoanalysis is still practiced, it remains limited to the affluent and even its more commonly utilized descendent, psychodynamic psychotherapy, is increasingly rare. One problem identified with all psychotherapeutic approaches requiring long-term therapy has been the lack of evidence to prove its effectiveness for patients. Traditional psychodynamic therapies have not produced empirical validation of the treatment efficacy. Two problems arise with attempts to research this area. The first problem is defining what is to be measured, which rests on the larger problem of the definition of normal or healthy. The second problem concerns methodology, or ways of evaluating possible long-range effects of psychotherapy on both individuals and society as a whole. While these are legitimate issues, it is important to note that these criticisms arose within a context of complex social factors that have changed the focus of treatment from predominately psychological to predominately biological approaches. This shift is not a novel phenomenon; it is another phase in the swinging pendulum that has occurred throughout the 20th century between these two competing systems seeking to explain and control human behavior.[62]

Psychotherapy most frequently occurs between a middle class patient and therapist who share more or less similar attitudes and values, and this process may be a voluntary activity chosen by the patient. However, it can also occur as an involuntary activity when the patient, who may or may not share values and attitudes with the therapist, becomes legally committed. Therapy has been viewed as a political act in either case, in that the therapist can encourage patients to either adjust to or rebel against their environment. However, the potential for using psychotherapy as a coercive tool of social control increases in the situation of involuntary commitment. Psychotherapy can be based on the social and economic biases of the therapist rather than the patient's behavior, and as such can become a coercive tool operating mainly on those very groups that are least able to change the social context in which their problems arise.

Stage two occurred during the 1950s and 1960s with the development of psychotherapy based on principles of conditioning. The generalized term, behavior modification, became the generic name for those methods emphasizing a behavioristic orientation. Another activist treatment, crisis intervention, led to the establishment of crisis intervention centers where clients could come in or telephone at any time in an attempt to deal with their problems. These two approaches shared several things: direct attack on the symptoms presented, without going into the underlying cause; short duration of therapy; and the possibility of a more technological basis for therapy than had been available in previous therapeutic approaches. Stage two represents a shift away from treating causes to an era of treatment geared toward symptom relief.

Stage three grew out of the affluence and leisure that the large middle class had achieved in the late 1960s and the early 1970s, when society passed from the age of anxiety to the age of ennui. The overriding preoccupation for many became the achievement of value and meaning in life. Psychotherapy shifted away from a focus on the relief of discomfort and pain to meeting the demands of the populace who sought a richer life with deeper experiences and relationships. As indicated for stage one, the developments in stages two and three, separately or in combination, can also serve as coercive tools of social control. Developments from all three stages continue to function to meet the different needs of some individuals with a great variety of reasons for seeking help or having it imposed on them. But as stated above, psychotherapy has fallen out of social favor. One reason for this that has not been mentioned is the economics of this care—psychotherapy is expensive in time and money. It is difficult to know exactly how economics figured in the present shift to the primacy of biology but it is certain to have played a significant role. In spite of its markedly reduced status, psychotherapy still has its adherents among both practitioners and those who seek it.

In addition to the problems in each stage of the development of psychotherapy, there are present problems, clinical, social, and ethical. Among these are the homeless mentally ill and the large numbers of the young, chronically mentally ill who often have dual diagnoses as a result of their mental illness and drug taking. These populations represent a failure in the social movement of deinstitutionalization, the goal of which was to empty the mental hospitals and have the mentally ill enter into society.

Substance abuse is an acute social problem and society has declared war on drugs. The fact that great numbers of people are addicted to drugs of all types and that newborn babies begin their lives addicted has grave potential consequences for society and certainly raises numerous ethical issues. For example, should drugs be legalized? Should abusers who are apprehended by the police be forced to enter treatment programs, and who will pay for such programs? Should bus drivers, truck drivers, and others whose jobs may do harm to others if performed under the influence of drugs, undergo drug testing in order to retain those jobs? Should pregnant women who are on drugs either have an abortion or be placed in a treatment program? What obligations does society have to these babies, to these mothers? These problems do not easily fall into a stage, perhaps because we are too close to them and do not have the benefit of a longer view. However, taken together they demonstrate the dynamic interaction among the concepts of democracy, social definitions and issues, behavior control questions, and ethical dilemmas.

Behavior control, as a potential ethical dilemma, varies with the different methods of treatment used. Psychotherapy has been widely accepted and practiced as the major means therapists have to deal with psychological disorders. It has been less recognized or discussed as a means of controlling people. Long-term insight therapy can be utilized systematically to influence attitudes and values, if not overt behavior, toward conventional norms of conduct. One could however, make the argument, that because this therapy method is slow, technologically benign, and limited to a relatively small target population, the risks incurred, as far as behavior control goes, are few. As behavior changes occur, the patient develops an accompanying increase in awareness, enabling the patient to monitor his or her own behavior changes to some extent. Furthermore, to a large degree, clients participating in insight therapy remain outside the large mental hospitals, so that the factors of institutional social structure do not affect the attempt at treatment and rehabilitation.

The second stage of psychotherapy, with its principles of conditioning, deserves more attention since such treatment techniques have been rigorously criticized as being repressive and dehumanizing. Our fascination with technology leads us to overrate the promise as well as the threat of these new techniques. Such techniques received attention in the controversial film of Anthony Burgess' novel, *Clockwork Orange*.[63] Generally speaking, the type of behavior control referred to as behavior therapy or behavior modification is one in which the therapist manipulates the environment and the consequences of a person's behavior in order to change that behavior, otherwise called operant conditioning. The therapist reinforces desired behavior whereas the behavior not wanted receives an adverse response or, at a minimum, receives no reward. A classic report of Ivar Lovaas's work with autistic children who had not been reached by normal methods of love, compassion, and punishment provides us with an example of behavior modification. The therapist placed barefoot autistic children in a room with a metal grid in the floor. The children periodically received an electric shock that they could avoid only by throwing themselves into the arms of an adult. After a time, these children began to seek out adults on their own without the shock.

Success using this type of therapy has been rather limited because of the major difficulty in retaining changed behavior over time. The major question that arises has to do with the possible gains as against the possible losses. Considerable evidence that people's behavior can be programmed fairly easily now exists. Behavior modification has been greatly influenced by Skinnerian behaviorism with its emphasis on environmental control and shaping of behavior.[64,65] The antibehaviorism viewpoint, developed early as a reaction to behavior modification and expressed in the writings of Carl Rogers and others contends that while the so-called behavioristic approach to psychiatry acknowledges an individual's susceptibility to manipulation by another, it also ignores the possible deleterious impact of this manipulation on the whole person and, in addition, on the manipulator himself.[66,67] They believe that the essential factor in the psychotherapeutic encounter is an honest, loving, spontaneous relationship between the therapist and patient.[68-70] A behaviorist might make the argument that apparent spontaneity on the therapist's part can well be the most effective means of manipulating the patient's behavior. The therapist has been programmed by his training into a fairly effective behavior control machine of sorts, and most likely this machine is most effective when it appears least like a machine. The side we take in this debate may not be the result of some appeal to an objective truth but reflect a view of how we want to think of ourselves.

PSYCHOSURGERY

Psychosurgery, or surgery to alter behavior, has virtually disappeared from the realm of treatment options since the 1970s but the continued popularity of such films as *Frances* and *One Flew Over the Cuckoo's Nest* have insured that psychosurgery stays in the public consciousness. It is important to examine this topic from a more historical view to understand the ethical issues involved, including the ways in which certain treatments come to hold center stage in medical practice. This discussion can do no more than highlight a few aspects; for a highly readable but indepth history of psychosurgery, the reader is referred to Elliot Valenstein's book, *Great and Desperate Cures*.[71] The present discussion draws largely on that account.

Biological treatments of mental and behavioral disorders are ancient, for example, the prescription for baths in certain springs in Ancient Rome now found to be rich in lithium salts, a contemporary drug used to treat manic depression. Twentieth century biological treatments have included carbon dioxide therapy, insulin coma therapy, malaria fever therapy, electroconvulsive therapy, drug therapy, and psychosurgery. The shock therapies were introduced in the 1930s at a time when psychiatrists and neurologists were bickering over who would treat the mentally ill. While the neurologists accused the psychiatrists of being "metaphysical," the psychiatrists doubted the supposed scientific foundation of the new somatic therapies. As Valenstein demonstrated, much of the dispute centered on the economic advantages to be had.

In 1935, a Portuguese physician, Egas Moniz, introduced psychosurgery for which he won the Nobel Prize in 1949. The American physician, Walter Freeman, was largely responsible for popularizing the practice. According to Valenstein, tens of thousands of patients were treated by psychosurgery during its peak between 1948 and 1952. Other factors providing the social context for the rise of psychosurgery included its promotion by the media, the lack of adequate funding for mental institutions, and, not unimportantly, "pressure from desperate mental patients and their desperate families." [72]

While there were often improvements in patients' symptoms following psychosurgery, these have been attributed largely to a decrease in emotional intensity rather than a change in thinking. As has happened with so many other treatments in medicine, the initial promise of a miracle cure began to give way to a more honest appraisal. Responses to psychosurgery varied and could be related to numerous factors, just as there were numerous reasons for the tide turning against psychosurgery. One reason was that patients who had undergone the procedure developed a dementia that could not be attributed to other causes. Other reasons included: increased questioning of the procedure by the media; disputes between psychiatrists and neurosurgeons over different techniques of lobotomy that were ultimately about control of the surgery and, therefore, economic advantage; the development of chlorpromazine (Thorazine) in the 1950s; and, the growing popularity of psychotherapy and psychoanalysis. By the end of the 1960s, the practice of psychosurgery had been dramatically curtailed but not obliterated. Some surgery was still being done in the very early 1970s. Yet perhaps it was the social climate of the 60s with its challenge to the perceived wisdom of the status quo that was the final demise for psychosurgery. This challenge came in the form of Vietnam War protestors, civil rights advocates, the Black Panthers, women's rights advocates, alternative health care advocates (for example those promoting birthing centers), and advocates for the elderly such as the Gray Panthers. These social movements signalled a distrust of traditional authority and power and their challenge and its response was often violent.

In 1970, neurosurgeon, Vernon Mark, and neuropsychiatrist, Frank Ervin, wrote a book entitled *Violence and the Brain* that detailed the application of neurosurgery techniques to the problems of violent behavior.[73] While there are disorders with demonstrable brain pathology that are characterized by violent behavior and which may be responsive to psychosurgery, the authors seemed to have extended their reach in advocating for the development of a test that would identify those with "a low threshold for impulsive violence." Furthermore, the introduction by a noted neurosurgeon stated that the knowledge gained by those with brain disease could be used on those with a low threshold for violent impulses but no disease. However this was intended, the political ramifications did not go unnoticed. The response to this book vividly underscored the growing concern with the social role of such experts who have within their power, along with the geneticist, the possibility of turning the classic philosophical question, "What is man?" to a very different question, "What kind of man are we going to construct?"

Psychosurgery, like any other technology, can be misused; nevertheless, the basic problem stems from the dichotomy in fundamental approaches to understanding behavior. There are those who view certain behavioral abnormalities, such as aggressive, assaultive behavior or intractable depression, as resulting primarily from unusual or abnormal environmental stress while others maintain that it is primarily brain function or dysfunction that plays the most significant role in abnormal behavior. Obviously, no human behavior, normal or abnormal, can be the consequence of the brain alone without the environment and equally obviously, no behavior, whatever its environmental determinants, occurs without the brain freighting its mechanical impulses with emotion and culture. Nonetheless, the dichotomy remains for complicated reasons and there are consequences to either side.

In reaction to the response, Mark and philosopher Robert Neville offered some reflections on the social issues involved in psychosurgery, making the point that most criticisms either impute to this type of surgery more capability than it can deliver or assume that such surgery would be appropriate to use for control in those instances when no surgeon would agree to such a use.[74] They articulated three defenses of psychosurgical procedures which illustrate their theses regarding the relationship of medicine to the appropriateness of this type of behavior control. Importantly, they reject the first two alternatives. Alternative one states that medical means should be undertaken to improve any behavior, normal or abnormal, whenever possible. Alternative two states that any undesirable, abnormal behavior should be treated by whatever medical means available, including psychosurgery, if it can be shown to be the most efficient method with the least risk. Alternative three, accepted by Mark and Neville, states that drastic procedures such as psychosurgery should be used only when behavior is abnormal and "bad" primarily because of a brain abnormality. As a result, any abnormal behavior not associated with brain disease should be dealt with by political and social means, not medical ones.

PSYCHOPHARMACOLOGY

Between books and the media, every informed person in the United States must know about both the pharmacological developments potentially enabling us to control human emotions and mental functioning and the extent of drug use in this country. At one time, we commonly thought of psychotropic drugs as limited to use by patients diagnosed as psychotic or depressed. More recently it has been documented that relatively normal people increasingly use these agents to cope with the stresses encountered in daily life. Statistics indicate that the production and distribution of psychotropic drugs have become a major component of the drug industry. At one time diazepam or Valium was the most widely prescribed drug in the country, especially for women; this has no doubt been replaced by Prozac. Newspaper articles, even entire books for the general public have been devoted to the virtues of Prozac.

Yet Americans seem to have an ambivalent relationship to drugs. Over our 200-year-old history, Americans have vacillated between acceptance and intolerance of drugs such as opium, cocaine, and marijuana.[75] Presently, ours is a drug culture where many people think a visit to the doctor's office or clinic has been a waste of time unless they come away with some pills and where the medical professional usually reinforces this attitude. We eagerly endorse and demand the latest therapeutic drug for *us* while condemning street drug use by *them*—we declared war on those drugs, appointed a drug czar and, most dramatically, invaded Panama. Indeed, the drug subculture has grown to such an extent that it has become a major social, economic, and mental health problem for the country. The point we wish to make, however, is that this subculture exists as part of a larger culture in which drugs are readily seen as "magic bullets."

Psychopharmacology emerged as a separate branch within pharmacology after World War II, with the discovery of LSD (lysergic diethylamide) in 1943 and chlorpromazine in 1952. During the next few years, and with great rapidity, dozens of new compounds became available. Psychotropic drugs have been divided into three categories, depending on the purpose for which they are used:

1. Drugs used as therapeutic agents for the treatment of psychiatric disorders
2. Drugs used for nontherapeutic purposes, such as recreation or personal enjoyment
3. Drugs used to enhance performance and capabilities

Of all the techniques that modern technology has developed and that can be used for controlling behavior, drugs are certainly among the most widely disseminated and readily available. In each of the above categories, ethical issues arise, including that of coercion, which can be a special problem in category one. There are numerous reasons why the mentally ill or those with behavioral problems may not want to take psychotropic medications. One is that many people may not see themselves as having a problem in need of control. For another, several of these drugs have numerous, severe side effects. It is not at all uncommon for health care providers to fail to listen to patients as they try to explain their concerns regarding medication. In our present emphasis on biological therapeutics for mental illness, we forget that even if research were to find the "magic bullet," the patient would have to take it—unless, of course, we are to have a truly totalitarian state. Currently there is more discussion about the rights of the mentally ill to refuse medication and some state laws ensure those rights.[76,77]

ETHICAL DILEMMAS

The right to receive treatment and the right to refuse treatment in general, and the right to consent to or decline behavior modification techniques in particular, raise a conflict-of-interest question. Does the therapist satisfy his or her own interests or those of the patients or, most likely, some combination of the two? In some situations, the therapist serves a third party, and this can be a problem, especially when the therapist is an employee of an institution whose interests do not necessarily coincide with the interests of the patient. Third parties often apply subtle and sometimes not so subtle pressures that therapists may not be fully aware of or understand. Conflict of interest represents one facet of the wider problem of what values, especially what conflicting values, are served by the mental health field. One major obstacle to a greater awareness of these value conflicts comes from the fact that mental health professionals have a marked tendency to assume that they function in a value-free frame of reference. Keenly aware of the patient's conflicts, they may be less inclined to see the conflicts of their own social role. The fact remains that regardless of theoretical orientation, these professionals are often a party to such conflict.

The larger ethical question involved in behavior control of any type turns on the problem of personal integrity. The essential question then is, does the individual have an inviolable, defensible, absolute right to be himself or herself, whatever or whoever he or she is, the product of whatever heredity and environment is his or her lot, even if deviant or dangerous to self or others? A whole host of questions for consideration in discussing behavior control include:

- If the individual is a danger to self, does society have the right to intervene to stop him or her from hurting or destroying himself or herself?
- Does society have the right or obligation to protect its members from themselves or from others?
- On what moral ground can the limit be determined where individual rights become outweighed by societal rights?
- Who will decide who is dangerous and on the basis of what knowledge?
- How is normalcy to be defined for therapy?
- If a social deviant receives psychiatric treatment, should the aim of that treatment be adjustment or adaptation?
- Are there ethical grounds for rejecting some or all of the more potent behavior control techniques, even if they prove to be quite effective?
- When are possible risks from such procedures justified?
- How is consent obtained and from whom?
- Is experimentation justified outside of the context of a reasonable belief that the procedure will be therapeutic for the individual?
- If therapists increasingly use these techniques, should there be some type of regulatory mechanism over and beyond informed consent?

One way to answer the last question is that any treatment recommendation for civilly committed disturbed patients who have not consented, that involves brain surgery, electric shock therapy, prolonged use of drugs, or behavior therapy, should be reviewed and approved by a monitoring agency. The question remains who will be on this monitoring agency and who will select the members? Other questions are:

- Should such treatment as long-term use of psychotropic drugs or psychosurgery be considered for children?
- If so, which children will be eligible for this treatment and who will decide on what grounds?
- Is it ethical to deny such treatment to adults or children if all other treatment approaches have failed?
- Should such a technique as brain surgery be used as a means to control violent behavior, even if such behavior is of unknown cause?
- How does any one of these behavior control techniques determine the relationship between the patient and doctor, nurse, or family?
- How does the technology affect the distribution of monetary and other resources for medical care?
- Who pays for such treatment?
- What are the possible potential implications of behavior control?

Essentially, the ethical questions boil down to: What kind of behavior should be controlled? Whose behavior is controlled? Who controls? Who decides who controls? How does behavior control affect dignity and freedom? What are the costs of gaining self-control? What social interests justify social control? What instruments of control are warranted to serve the interest of society? All of these questions evolve from several ethical dilemmas involved in behavior control. The dilemma of maintaining personal integrity versus society's obligation to protect its members remains perhaps the most central dilemma. The dilemma of immunity versus forfeiture of rights raises the question of what rights to privacy and inviolability of body and mind a person should lose once he has been diagnosed as mentally ill, especially if he is committed to an institution. The dilemma of procedural rights is concerned with what rights a patient has to the procedural protection from the suspension, waiver, or forfeiture of these basic rights. The dilemma of rights and goods concerns the possible conflict between the person's right to be different and his potential desire to be free from any misery that his deviance causes. The dilemma of informed voluntary consent raises the problems of mental status and legal status as inhibitions to obtaining informed consent. The dilemma of paternalism and authoritarianism raises the questions that John Stuart Mill addressed:[78] What are the limits on the use of coercion, on the kinds of coercion, and on the actions coercively prevented or elicited that one person may use on another in the name of the latter's own good? The fact that those using the techniques of intervention may be doing so with therapeutic intent does not alter either the paternalistic or the authoritarian character of such use under certain circumstances. The dilemma of deceptive labeling concerns the issue of when enforced treatment, especially that involving irreversible effects, becomes primitive control under a false therapeutic label.

In 1971, Kittrie developed a Therapeutic Bill of Rights because he believed that the philosophical origins of therapeutic programs combined humanism, paternalism, and utilitarian determinism in promoting the public's interest in social defense.[79] This document articulates an ethical view relevant to behavior control today. The general principles of the Therapeutic Bill of Rights are stated below.

Therapeutic Bill of Rights

1. No person shall be compelled to undergo treatment except for the defense of society.

2. Man's innate right to remain free of excessive forms of human modification shall be inviolable.

3. No social sanctions may be invoked unless the person subjected to treatment has demonstrated a clear and present danger through truly harmful behavior, which is immediately forthcoming or has already occurred.

4. No person shall be subjected to involuntary incarceration or treatment on the basis of a finding of a general condition or status alone. Nor shall the mere

conviction for a crime or a finding of not guilty by reason of insanity suffice to have a person automatically committed or treated.

5. No social sanctions, whether designated criminal, civil, or therapeutic, may be invoked in the absence of the precious right to a judicial or other independent hearing, appointed counsel, and an opportunity to confront those testifying about one's past conduct or therapeutic needs.

6. Dual interference by both the criminal and the therapeutic process is prohibited.

7. An involuntary patient shall have the right to receive treatment.

8. Any compulsory treatment must be the least required reasonably to protect society.

9. All committed persons should have direct access to appointed counsel and the right, without any interference, to petition the courts for relief.

10. Those submitting to voluntary treatment should be guaranteed that they will not be subsequently transferred to a compulsory program through administrative action.*

IMPLICATIONS FOR NURSING PRACTICE

The nurse's role in psychiatric settings has ranged from custodial keeper of the keys to skilled therapeutic agent. In any of these roles, the nurse has the power to influence and determine, in part, the patient's course of treatment, since she observes and interacts with him. Nurses in all specialties have such influence, to some extent, but in the mental health field it takes on special significance because the illness is tied to behavioral symptoms. The mental health nurse, like all other members of the staff, has his or her own attitudes and value system, which affect his or her definitions of mental illness and mental health. These attitudes and values become a factor in encounters with patients. For example, the field of psychiatry has, on paper, changed its concept of homosexuality. The fact remains, however, that mental health workers in this country are members of the larger society, which for the most part has had and continues to have deeply ingrained negative attitudes toward homosexuality. These negative attitudes extend to some of society's most marginalized people, such as drug abusers, sex of-

---

*Reprinted with permission from Kittrie NN: *The Right to Be Different*. Baltimore: Johns Hopkins University Press; 1971.

fenders, prostitutes, and criminals. Yet these people often find themselves within the mental health system and working with them can pose a moral problem for nurses.[80]

Another ingrained attitude that reflects membership in the culture is the double standard of mental health for men and women, and the differences parallel the treatment of women in our society. For example, in Illinois in the 1800s when this country was beginning to legislate commitment laws, a person was found to be insane by a lay jury. The one exception to this was a married woman who could be committed by a physician and it was not at all uncommon that many women were confined because physicians acted on the say so of their husbands. Take Mrs. Elizabeth Packard, the wife of a theologically rigid Calvinist minister. In 1860, The Rev. Theophilus Packard had his wife committed essentially for disagreeing with his harsh religious view of the world. After some years of confinement, Mrs. Packard was released and she worked tirelessly to change commitment procedures. Our present system owes much to her.[81] The practice of declaring women insane and incarcerating them was not limited to the state of Illinois—all states condoned such behavior. In many states, exercising economic independence was reason enough for being declared insane. For a revealing moral indictment of the treatment of women within the mental health system, an indictment in the words of the women themselves, the reader is referred to *Women of the Asylum*.[82]

Once a person enters the mental health system as a patient, the nurse becomes a major source of information regarding that person's behavior. This is especially so in inpatient settings where longer contacts can occur between nurse and patient and where the nursing staff is the only group to work a 24-hour day. Many decisions regarding treatment occur in team meetings, and the nurse affects the discussion by either providing information or withholding it. If he or she provides information, what is reported and how it is said influences the perceptions of the patient by others. In Rosenhan's classic study, pseudopatients gained admission to mental hospitals by saying they heard voices. Once admitted, they found themselves indelibly labeled with the diagnosis of schizophrenia, in spite of their subsequent normal behavior. They kept field notes for the research project and the nurses charted that these "patients" engaged in "compulsive writing." Only the other patients suspected that these pseudopatients were not mentally ill and were there for other reasons. The staff was unable to acknowledge normal behavior within the hospital milieu. In such a setting, staff members tended to see pathology more than they saw normal behavior.[83]

Another potential problem with ethical dimensions that adds to the larger problem of behavior control has to do with whether nurses take the patient seriously. Does the diagnosis of mental illness affect our attitudes toward this category of persons in ways that do not allow us to take seriously what the patient says or does? Because someone is "crazy," it may be easier to dismiss him or her by not putting any stock in what he or she communicates, since it does not reflect reality. Such an attitude may be supported by the reward system of the institution where the nurse works as an employee. Not being taken seriously also occurs in situations where adults interact with children.

The medical literature discusses the ethical dilemmas arising from a paternalistic attitude that physicians have toward patients. Such an attitude tends to reduce the adult patient to the status of a child and permits the physician to violate the patient's rights, such as the right to participate in the decision-making process that influences his or her own welfare. Paternalism is interference with a person's liberty of action with the exclusive justification that it is for the welfare, good, happiness, needs, interests, or values of the person being coerced. Some think that self-protection or the prevention of harm to others is a sufficient warrant; however, as stated earlier, the mental health field lacks tools for predicting dangerousness. Others think that the individual's own good is never a sufficient warrant for the exercise of compulsion either by the society as a whole or by its individual members. Currently, few theorists are willing to defend the "old" type of paternalism in which health professionals imposed their own values and wills upon patients. Patient autonomy is now thought to be extremely valuable and has been given great moral value. Of concern is that this claim for autonomy is being used to justify a new form of paternalism.[84]

All nurses in all settings can interfere with a patient's liberty of action. Mental health nurses are in a particularly good position to do so, since either the patient has sought help with his or her behavioral problems or the patient has been committed by legal procedures. In the former case, staff may feel they have been given license to make decisions for the patient's own good, in the latter, the staff may interpret that they have both the right and obligation to interfere with the patient's liberty of action.

The ideas discussed above—namely, influencing decision making regarding mental status and treatment, not taking the patient seriously, and paternalism—can play a part in discussions of using techniques of behavior control. Nurses participate in individual and group psychotherapy as well as in behavior modification programs. Nurses also have a great influence on decisions about drugs, such as type, dosage, and frequency. One often finds in the literature, either explicitly or implicitly, the idea that drugs make the patient more amenable to other types of therapy, such as psychotherapy. Drugs also make the patient more manageable from a nursing point of view, and this raises some ethical issues around the problem of the double-agent role. All the ethical dilemmas raised in the preceding section involve and affect the nurse. To the extent that he or she is aware of them, the nurse can examine these situations not only from a clinical perspective but also from an ethical one.

The mental health field sometimes tends to promise more than it can deliver, given the knowledge and technology it has available. This in itself raises ethical problems and dilemmas. The technology that is available has potential for abuse with regard to behavior control. The single most important factor in the intelligent use of such techniques is an ethically grounded clinician, who for moral reasons hesitates in order to think through the clinical and ethical implications of his or her actions. This cannot be overstated. We live in a violent society and we can be impelled to exercise violence even as we attempt the understandable and laudable goal of controlling it. As feminist ethicist, Claudia Card, warns, we must be wary of "becoming what we despise." [85]*

---

*The authors wish to thank Anastasia Fisher, RN, DNSc for her help with this chapter.

■ CASE STUDY I.

Mary Elizabeth is from a large and well-to-do family. She is 24 years old and living on the streets. Her family has paid to have her admitted to many expensive private psychiatric facilities for treatment of her schizophrenia. Mary Elizabeth always signs herself out. Since she is not judged to be dangerous, she cannot be held against her will.

Mary Elizabeth's symptoms can be well controlled with psychotropic medication. However, she does not take the drugs and says she does not like the way she feels when she is on them. She writes beautiful poetry and says she finds "my own reality" much more interesting than the boring and tedious life she experiences when on the medication. She prefers the friends she makes on the street to the dullness of "so-called normal people."

Her sister arranges to have her poetry published and sends the meager proceeds to Mary Elizabeth. She is occasionally picked up for vagrancy, however, and brought in for treatment. Her parents are always contacted. Mary Elizabeth does not maintain contact with them otherwise.

Suggested Questions for Discussion

1. Does Mary Elizabeth have the right to live in her "own reality"? What are society's rights and responsibilities toward "vulnerable" individuals like Mary Elizabeth?

2. Should Mary Elizabeth be required to take her medications? How? Why? By whom?

3. What responsibility do Mary Elizabeth's parents have for her?

■ CASE STUDY II.

Juan is 34 years old, lives with his extended family, and works sporadically on the local farms, especially during the planting and harvest seasons. He is a large man, 6 feet tall and over 250 pounds. Juan says he sometimes hears voices in his head telling him to do "bad things" so he bangs his head until the voices stop. He bangs his head violently to stop the voices, usually until he loses consciousness. He has had at least one subdural bleed in the past. Juan has been hospitalized 10 or 12 times in the last several years for these episodes. He is brought into the county hospital emergency department during these episodes. His family says they can't control him and are afraid he will hurt himself, or one of them.

You are a nurse practitioner in the Emergency Department. You know from previous episodes that Juan can be a very sweet and gentle man, but it can take six staff members to subdue him when he is having one of these episodes. At least one person on the staff has been injured in the past. He usually tests positive for alcohol when he is brought in. The usual approach is to medicate him heavily, check him for injuries, and transfer him to the county mental health facility. They load him up on psychotropic drugs and discharge him home to his family when he is quiet, usually within 24 or 36 hours. Juan quits taking the drugs after a few days, and never makes his follow-up appointments. His family refuses to acknowledge that Juan has any psychiatric problems saying he's just prone to "fits." You know in the Hispanic culture, mental illness is often highly stigmatized.

You are concerned about this "band-aid" approach and feel Juan's problems should be addressed more comprehensively.*

Suggested Questions for Discussion

1. What are the ethical issues in this case?

2. What role should concerns about the personal safety of the emergency department staff have in Juan's treatment plan? Aren't dangerous patients just part of the job?

3. What responsibility does the mental health clinic have for patients who do not follow the prescribed medication regime or come in for follow-up treatment?

---

*Special thanks to Kathleen Dempsey, MSN, RN, NP for this case.

REFERENCES

1. Klerman GL: Behavior control and the limits of reform. *Hastings Cent Rep* 5(4): 40–5, 1975.

2. Goffman E: *Asylums*. New York: Doubleday; 1961.

3. Grob GN: *Mental Institutions in America: Social Policy to 1875*. New York: Free Press; 1973.

4. Rothman DJ: *The Discovery of the Asylum: Social Order and Disorder in the New Republic*. Boston: Little, Brown; 1971.

5. Stanton AH, Schwartz MS: *The Mental Hospital*. New York: Basic Books; 1954.

6. Greenblatt M, Levinson DJ, Williams R: *The Patient and the Mental Hospital*. Glencoe, IL: Free Press; 1958.

7. Caudill WA: *A Psychiatric Hospital as a Small Society*. Cambridge, MA: Harvard University Press; 1958.

8. Greenblatt M, Levinson DJ, Klerman GL: *Mental Patients in Transition*. Springfield, IL: Charles C. Thomas; 1961.

9. Jones M: *The Therapeutic Community*. New York: Basic Books; 1953.

10. Jones M: *Beyond the Therapeutic Community*. New Haven: Yale University Press; 1968.

11. Torrey EF, Steiber J, Ezekiel J, et al: *Criminalizing the seriously mentally ill: The abuse of jails as mental hospitals*. Washington, DC: National Alliance for the Mentally Ill and Public Citizen's Health Research Group; 1992.

12. Szasz TS: *The Myth of Mental Illness*. New York: Harper & Row; 1974.

13. Boyers R, Orrill R: *R.D. Laing and Anti-Psychiatry*. New York: Harper & Row; 1971.

14. London P: *Behavior Control*. New York: Harper & Row; 1970.

15. Orwell G: *1984*. New York: Harcourt, Brace; 1959.

16. Condon R: *The Manchurian Candidate*. New York: McGraw-Hill; 1959.

17. Huxley A: *Brave New World*. New York: Harper & Row; 1932.

18. Koestler A: *Darkness at Noon*. New York: Bantam; 1970.

19. Appel W: *Cults in America: Programmed for Paradise*. New York: Henry Holt; 1985.

20. Kittrie NN: *The Right to Be Different*. Baltimore: Johns Hopkins University Press; 1971.

21. Gibbs JP: The sociology of deviance and social control. In Rosenberg M, Turner MH (eds): *Social Psychology*. New Brunswick, NH: Transaction; 1992.

22. Trexler JC: Reformulation of deviance and labeling theory for nursing. *Image J Nurs Sch* 28(2):131–135, 1996.

23. Becker HS: *Outsiders: Studies in the Sociology of Deviance*. New York: Free Press; 1963.

24. Monahan J, Steadman HJ: Toward a rejuvenation of risk assessment research. In *Violence and Mental Disorder: Developments in Risk Assessment*. Chicago: University of Chicago Press; 1994, pp 1–18.

25. Appelbaum P: The new preventive detention: Psychiatry's problematic responsibility for the control of violence. *Am J Psychiatry* 145(7):779–785, 1988.

26. Monahan J, Shah S: Dangerousness and the commitment of the mentally disordered. *United States Schizophr Bull* 15(4):541–553, 1989.

27. Mulvey EP, Lidz CW: Conditional prediction: A model for research on dangerousness to others in a new era. *Int J Law Psychiatry* 18(2):129–143, 1995.

28. *Ibid.*, p 130.

29. Finnema EJ, Dassen T, Halfens R: Aggression in psychiatry: A qualitative study focusing on the characterization and perception of patient aggression by nurses working on psychiatric wards. *J Adv Nurs* 19(6):1088–1095, 1994.

30. Fisher A: *The Process of Definition and Action: The Case of Dangerousness*, doctoral dissertation. University of California, San Francisco; 1989.

31. *Ibid.*

32. Steadman HJ: The right not to be a false positive: Problems in the application of the dangerousness standard. *Psychiatric Quart* 52(2):84–99, 1980.

33. Steadman HJ, Morrissey JP: The statistical prediction of violent behavior: Measuring the costs of a public protectionist versus a civil libertarian model. *Law Hum Behav* 5:263–264, 1981.

34. Torrey EF: Violent behavior by individuals with serious mental illness. *Hosp Comm Psychiatry* 45(7):653–662, 1994.

35. Mulvey EP: Assessing the evidence of a link between mental illness and violence. *Hosp Comm Psychiatry* 45(7):663–668, 1994.

36. Campbell J, Stefan S, Loder A: Taking issue: Putting violence in context. *Hosp Comm Psychiatry* 45(7):633, 1994.

37. Morrison EF: A coercive interactional style as an antecedent to aggression in psychiatric patients. *Res Nurs Health* 15(6):421–431, 1992.

38. Monahan J: The prediction of violent behavior: Toward a second generation of theory and policy. *Am J Psychiatry* 141(1):10–15, 1984.

39. Steadman HJ: A situational approach to violence. *Int J Law Psychiatry* 5(2): 171–186, 1982.

40. Lidz CW, Mulvey EP, Gardner W: The accuracy of prediction of violence to others. *JAMA* 269(8):1007–1011, 1993.

41. Mulvey EP, Lidz CW: *op. cit.*

42. Davis DL, Boster L: Multifaceted therapeutic interventions with the violent psychiatric inpatient. *Hosp Comm Psychiatry* 39(8):867–869, 1988.

43. Kirkpatrick H: A descriptive study of seclusion: The unit environment, patient behavior, and nursing interventions. *Arch Psych Nurs* 3(1):3–9, 1989.

44. Morrison EF: Violent psychiatric inpatients in a public hospital. *Image J Nurs Sch* 4(1):65–82, 1990.

45. Outlaw FH, Lowery BJ: Seclusion: The nursing challenge. *J Psychosocial Nurs Ment Health Serv* 30(4):13–17, 1992.

46. Corrigan PW, Yudofsky SC, Silver JM: Pharmacological and behavioral treatments for aggressive psychiatric inpatients. *Hosp Comm Psychiatry* 44(2):125–133, 1993.

47. Fisher WA: Restraint and seclusion: A review of the literature. *Am J Psychiatry* 151(11):1584–1591, 1994.

48. Dvoskin JA, Steadman HJ: Using intensive case management to reduce violence

by mentally ill persons in the community. *Hosp Comm Psychiatry* 45(7):679–684, 1994.

49. Gaylin W: On the borders of persuasion: A psychoanalytic look at coercion. *Psychiatry* 37(1):1–9, 1974.

50. Liaschenko J: Artificial personhood: Nursing ethics in a medical world. *Nurs Ethics* 2(3):185–196, 1995.

51. Liaschenko J: The moral geography of home care. *Adv Nurs Sci* 17(2):16–26, 1994.

52. Liaschenko J: *Faithful to the Good: Morality and Philosophy in Nursing Practice*, doctoral dissertation. University of California, San Francisco; 1993.

53. Strumpf NE, Tomes N: Restraining the troublesome patient: A historical perspective on the contemporary debate. *Nurs Hist Rev* 1:3–24, 1993.

54. Liaschenko J: Ethics in the work of acting for patients. *Adv Nurs Sci* 18(2):1–12, 1995.

55. Garritson S: Degrees of restrictiveness in psychosocial nursing. *J Psychosocial Nurs* 21(12):9–16, 1983.

56. Garritson S: Ethical decision making patterns. *J Psychosocial Men Hlth Nurs* 26(4): 22–29, 1988.

57. Forchuk C: Ethical problems encountered by mental health nurses. *Issues Men Hlth Nurs* 12(4):375–383, 1991.

58. Lutzen K, Nordin C: Benevolence, a central moral concept derived from a grounded theory study of nursing decision making in psychiatric settings. *J Adv Nurs* 18(7):1106–1111, 1993.

59. Lutzen K, Nordin C: Modifying autonomy—a concept grounded in nurses experience of moral decision-making in psychiatric practice. *J Med Ethics* 20(2):101–107, 1994.

60. Fisher A: The ethical problems encountered in psychiatric nursing practice with dangerous mentally ill patients. *Sch Inq Nurs Prac* 9(2):193–208, 1995.

61. Mattiasson AC, Andersson L: Nursing home staff attitudes to ethical conflicts with respect to patient autonomy and paternalism. *Nurs Ethics* 2(2):115–130, 1995.

62. Valenstein ES. *Great and Desperate Cures: The Rise and Decline of Psychosurgery and Other Radical Treatments for Mental Illness*. New York: Basic Books; 1986.

63. Burgess A: *Clockwork Orange*. New York: Norton; 1963.

64. Skinner BF: *Walden Two*. New York: Macmillan; 1948.

65. Skinner BF: *Science and Human Behavior*. New York: Macmillan; 1953.

66. Rogers CR: Persons or science: A philosophical question. *Am Psychol* 10:267–278, 1955.

67. Rogers CR: Implications of recent advances in prediction and behavior control. *Teachers Coll Bull* 57:316–322, 1956.

68. Rogers CR, Skinner BF: Some issues concerning the control of human behavior. *Science* 124:1057–1066, 1956.

69. Jourard S: I-Thou relationship versus manipulation in counseling and psychotherapy. *J Indiv Psychol* 15:174–179, 1959.

70. Jourard S: On the problem of reinforcement by the psychotherapist of healthy behavior in the patient. In Shaw FJ (ed): *Behavioristic Approaches to Counseling and Psychotherapy*. University, AL: University of Alabama Press; 1961.

71. Valenstein E: *op. cit.*
72. Valenstein E: *op. cit.*, p 5.
73. Mark VH, Ervin FR: *Violence and the Brain.* New York: Harper & Row; 1970.
74. Mark VH, Neville R: Brain surgery in aggressive epileptics: Social and ethical implications. *JAMA* 226(7):765–772, 1973.
75. Musto DF: Opium, cocaine, and marijuana in American History. *Sci Am* 265(1): 40–47, 1991.
76. Clayton EW: From Rogers to Rivers: The rights of the mentally ill to refuse medication. *Am J Law Med* 13(1):7–52, 1987.
77. Brushwood DB, Fink JL. Right to refuse treatment with psychotropic medication. *Am J Hosp Pharm* 42(12):2709–2714, 1985.
78. Mill JS: *On Liberty.* Indianapolis, IN: Hackett Publishing; 1978.
79. Kittrie NN: *op. cit.*, pp 400–408.
80. Liaschenko J: Making a bridge: The moral work with patients we do not like. *J Palliative Care* 10(3):83–89, 1994.
81. Lombardo PA: Mrs. Packard's revenge. *Bio Law* 11:S791–S797, 1992.
82. Geller JA, Harris M: *Women of the Asylum: Voices from Behind the Walls,* 1840–1945. New York: Anchor Books; 1994.
83. Rosenhan DL: On being sane in insane places. *Science* 179(70):250–258, 1973.
84. Strasser M: The new paternalism. *Bioethics* 2:103–117, 1988.
85. Card C: *Feminist Ethics.* Lawrence, KS: University Press of Kansas; 1991, p 26.

11

Mental Retardation

ETHICAL DILEMMAS

Any discussion of ethical dilemmas and the mentally retarded must take into account the concept of respect for persons. Private morality concerns itself with respecting the distinctive human endowment as we find it in ourselves, whereas public morality is concerned with respecting the distinctive human endowment as we find it in others. Private and public morality therefore represent two aspects of a single, fundamental moral principle.[1-2] We feel brotherly love, *agape*, respect toward those regarded as persons. This notion, however, leaves open the possibility of debate as to who or what properly and truly constitutes a person we are to regard with respect. The concept of *person* has a long and complex history within philosophy. Teichmann made note of the many senses of the word person as given in the Oxford English Dictionary; these include, dramaturgical, legal, moral, theological, grammatical, and zoological.[3] Trendelenberg traced the etymology of the word person from its earliest use until the late 19th century.[4] The meaning of the word person underwent several shifts beginning with the use of the word in Greek theater. Interestingly, from its earliest beginnings, the word person was associated with the power of speech. The "persona" or mask of the Greek theater served to concentrate and focus the voice, thus enabling clearer and more forceful speech. Three characteristics emerged through the evolution of the meaning in Greek thought. First, the word person came to be associated with roles, that is, with the holding of rights and responsibilities within the polis. Thus, persons were distinct from slaves who did not have rights within and responsibilities to the polis or community. In another sense of the word, persons came to mean beings with self-consciousness as distinct from the inanimate class of objects referred to as things. Third, persons came to be seen as beings in themselves and not merely instrumental to the ends of others.

The latter became particularly important to Immanuel Kant, a supreme representative of the Age of Enlightenment. He argued that the distinctive endowment of a human being is his ability to reason. For Kant, the possession of a rational will is the quality that gives a human being absolute worth because it is through willingness to do one's duty that one becomes a member of the moral universe.[5] In this way, the word person comes to mean more than a certain kind of being, in this case a human being, as contrasted with another kind of being, for example a dog or a bird. Rather, for Kant, the term person conveyed a certain moral status and for that reason, a person cannot be used as a means to another's end. It should be noted that throughout the history of Western thought, the ability to reason has been associated with language and the capacity to manipulate symbols. Kant's thesis has profoundly influenced directly or indirectly our attitudes toward a number of groups, including the mentally retarded.

The concept of a *person* is an evaluative concept with something of the force of "that which makes a human being valuable" implied in it. But the questions remain: Why do we respect or value a person? What makes a human being a person?[6] In the field of developmental disability, as we move along the continuum from severely to borderline retarded, do we perceive each individual as a person or do we draw the line based on moral reasoning ability and think only of some on the continuum as persons we respect? If personhood is *not* dependent on moral reasoning ability, what is it that indicates that someone is a person and what is it about persons that requires our respect?

The term *person* seems to refer to a cluster of features including *biological factors* (descended from humans; having a certain genetic make-up; having a head, hands, arms, eyes; capable of locomotion, breathing, eating, and sleeping); *psychological factors* (having a concept of self and of one's interests and desires; the ability to use language or symbol systems); *rationality factors* (the ability to reason and draw conclusions; the ability to learn from past experiences); *social factors* (the ability to work in groups; the ability to recognize and consider the interests of others; the abilities to love and sympathize); and *legal factors* (the ability to own property and inherit goods; subject to the law and protected by it; citizenship).[7-8] This is not a list of necessary and sufficient conditions for personhood but simply features that are more or less typical of those who are referred to as "persons."

If individuals lack some of the above mentioned biological, psychological, and rationality factors, are they less qualified as persons? Is respect for them as persons dependent on which factors are present and which are lacking? Or do individuals merely need to be members of the human community to be counted as persons? Respect for them is then dependent on whether or not the community values them and accords them full rights and responsibilities as members of the community. These questions point to the complexity of the concept. This confusion may result from the fact that the same word, person, is used in two senses: as a kind of ontological being and as a being in the moral or evaluative sense, that is, as a being who is held accountable for his or her actions.[9-10] Some authors find the term so confusing as to advocate for its removal from the discourse of health care ethics, arguing that the work of health care concerns human beings.[11] We have some sympathy with this view and would reframe the issue from a concern over personhood to one of respect for human beings.

Respect can mean several things.[12] In one author's analysis, respect is used in four senses: as esteem for some particular talent or capacity; as regard for agency which refers to the capacity of someone to manage their own affairs; as a recognition of limitations; and as regard for class membership, in this case, the class of human beings.[13] Kopelman argues that respect in terms of esteem can apply to all of us in some degree but few of us attain the esteem of a Michelangelo. On the other hand, all of us respect in the sense of limitations; for instance, we respect the power of nature displayed in earthquakes and hurricanes. Respect in the sense of regard for agency reflects the issues of autonomy, such as the capacity for voluntary action and the capacity to give reasons for those actions. According to Kopelman, most mentally retarded people can do these things to varying degrees. Yet when someone is profoundly retarded and cannot, she believes that the individual is still owed respect on the grounds that they are a human being. We are in agreement.

Human beings are a class of beings that have a certain embodiment and the capacity for consciousness and/or social interaction. For that reason they have rights and responsibilities that may vary according to a variety of factors, and they have a moral claim on other members of the community. As Kopelman states, "we depend on each other for support and protection in a way that makes or should make the interests of all human beings of special importance to us." [14] In our view, the advantage of the term human being circumvents the major difficulty associated with the concept of person in philosophy, which is its focus on rationality. This is particularly important when addressing those individuals whose capacity for rationality is, in some way, compromised. Our position is that mentally retarded and physically disabled individuals are worthy of our respect simply because they are human beings.

The ethical dilemmas discussed with regard to the mentally retarded can be listed as concerning the concept of *person*; how we define mental retardation and the consequences this definition has; problems encountered by the mentally retarded in institutions and in the community regarding their rights; and the moral reasoning that society uses in balancing its resources and values to determine the risks and benefits for the individual and for society itself. Consider, for example, the ethical issues that arise around respect for the autonomy of mentally retarded people. If we believe that support for the enactment of autonomy is central to the ethical treatment of each other, we must ask what autonomy might mean in the case of those individuals who are mentally retarded. The same question has been raised by those concerned with the elderly in long-term care with the answer that it is not enough to offer choices but that choices must be meaningful.[15] This is significant because it is through our identification with meaningful choices that we define who we are. A recent court decision in New Jersey recognized the right of a mentally retarded woman to choose whether to live with her mother or father.[16] Practitioners who work with the mentally retarded within the theoretical framework of behaviorism might take issue with the notion of meaningfulness but they, nonetheless, stress the complexity of the notion of choice and the ethical obligation to avoid coercion.[17] This is particularly important because the act of choosing, which involves an evaluation of consequences, is a difficult task for those with limited verbal or symbolic capacities.

The focus of concern is thus how society fulfills its duties and obligations to safeguard the basic rights of the mentally retarded and physically disabled individuals when they cannot, by virtue of their retardation or disabilities, completely do so themselves. Crocker and Cushna, for example, outline the "normal rights" of the mentally retarded that must be defended as including the right to family living, educational opportunities, treatment and habilitation services, employment, support in the development of contracts, and confidentiality in personal records. They also outline "special rights" as including qualified advocacy and guardianship capacity; protection against use of drugs and behavior modification techniques, including experimental procedures; counseling and safeguards regarding reproduction; and intelligent exposure to life situations involving risk.[18]

Friedman, on the other hand, outlines the rights of mentally retarded persons according to whether they reside in an institution or in the community. Mentally retarded persons in institutions should be recognized as having the right to habilitation and the right to protection from harm; freedom from hazardous, intrusive, and experimental procedures; the right to sexual expression; the right to fair compensation for institutional labor; the right to a humane physical and psychological environment; the right to dignity and privacy, religious freedom, behavioral and leisure time activities; and prompt and appropriate medical treatment consistent with the accepted standards of medical practice in the community.[19] Mentally retarded persons in the community should be recognized as having the right to education; the right to reside in the community; sexual and marital rights; the right to a barrier-free environment; employment rights; the right to be free from discrimination in voting, driving, and other rights of citizenship; the right to medical care; and the right to participate in federal financial assistance and other benefit programs.[20]

DEFINITION AND LABELING

It is not uncommon for people, including some health care providers to speak of mental retardation as if it referred to a single capacity, most commonly construed as IQ, or intelligence quotient, rather than a range of abilities across a variety of domains. However, mental retardation is a "state of impairment" rather than a single entity and can have multiple causes.[21] Yet precisely because it is fluid, the definition of mental retardation has been fraught with difficulties and is frequently unsatisfactory. As early as the first century, the words imbecile, idiot, and witless were in use although only the latter referred to mental retardation. It was not until several centuries later that imbecile, which designated any type of debility, and idiot, which originally meant a private person, also came to categorize mentally retarded people. We want to move ahead to modern times but the reader is referred to Scheerenberger's *History of Mental Retardation* for a review of this history.[22]

Contemporary ideas of mental retardation are associated with IQ, which had its origins in the 1800s. By that time mental retardation, or idiocy as it was called, had been differentiated and was no longer viewed as a single entity. As a result, classification issues focused on concerns with performance and its measurement. Although work on intelligence testing had been common during the end of the 19th century, it was Alfred Binet and Theodore Simon who left the most prominent legacy. The Binet–Simon intelligence test was intended to assure that mentally retarded children received necessary educational help.[23] IQ testing figured prominently in classifying the mentally retarded. For instance, in 1969, the eighth publication of the World Health Organization's *Manual of the International Statistical Classification of Diseases, Injuries and Causes of Death* listed the following criteria for mental retardation: borderline, 68 to 85; mild, 52 to 67; moderate, 36 to 51; severe 20 to 35; and profound under 20.[24] IQ as a measure of mental retardation has had its proponents and detractors. A balanced position seems to hold that it is quite useful when not the exclusive measure.

The American Association on Mental Deficiency holds the following definition: "Mental retardation refers to significantly subaverage general intellectual functioning existing concurrently with deficits in adaptive behavior and manifested during the developmental period." In this definition, significantly subaverage means an IQ of 70 or below.[25]

Mental retardation, ultimately a social attribute, comprises at least three components: organic, functional, and social. The organic component we refer to as impairment, the functional component as disability, and the social component as handicap. Epidemiological understanding of any disorder will differ depending on which of the three components is counted. In mild mental retardation, the rule is the absence of recognized impairment but the presence of functional disability measured in terms of an IQ below a given point. The extent of social handicap varies with age and social setting. Unfortunately, occasionally the social role of mental handicap has been conferred on a person with neither brain impairment nor functional disability. In this country and in England, there have been reported cases of individuals with IQs within the normal range being placed in institutions for the retarded and so acquiring the social role of mental retardation.[26]

It has been suggested that the human propensity to classify is a basic aspect of our cognitive faculties.[27] Through classification, we impose a certain order on the world.[28] We classify phenomena for a variety of reasons, one of which is to determine etiology. The etiological classification of mental retardation can be divided into two overall categories, genetic and acquired. The genetic category contains such examples as Down's syndrome, a chromosomal abnormality; phenylketonuria (PKU), a disorder of amino acid metabolism; and Tay–Sachs, a disorder of lipid metabolism, to mention only a few conditions. Examples of acquired mental retardation can be further categorized into (1) prenatal, when infection such as rubella, toxin effects, and placental insufficiency occur; (2) perinatal, when prematurity, anoxia, or cerebral damage occur; (3) postnatal, when brain injury, infection such as meningitis, anoxia, effects of poison, and sociocultural factors such as deprivation and child abuse occur. The examples given here do not exhaust the possibilities but serve to give some idea of the complexities of mental retardation. We believe that these distinctions are sometimes conflated but that they are quite important in this era of genetic hyperbole. The exact cause of mental retardation in many cases can be most difficult to elucidate and the difficulty becomes compounded by genetic and environmental interaction, prematurity, low birth weight, and perinatal complications. The causes of mental retardation and other developmental disabilities overlap and are inextricably related in complex ways.

Another reason for classification is that it allows access to certain societal resources. For example, in 1970 Congress enacted Public Law 91-517, which defined developmental disability as:

> . . . a disability attributable to mental retardation, cerebral palsy, epilepsy, or another neurological condition of an individual found by the Secretary to be closely related to mental retardation or to require treatment similar to that required for mentally retarded individuals, which disability originates before such individual attains age 18, which has continued or can be expected to continue indefinitely, and which constitutes a substantial handicap to such individual.

The concept of developmental disability recognizes mental retardation, regardless of cause, as a facet within a spectrum of possible abnormalities.[29] Not as specific as it might be, this definition does, however, recognize disorders of adjustment, communication, locomotion, and intellectual function and emphasizes the generally nonprogressive nature and irreversibility of these disabilities.

The Developmentally Disabled Assistance and Bill of Rights Act, Public Law 94-103, which became law in October of 1975, broadened the definition of developmental problems and the strategies for strengthening services and safeguarding individual rights. This act authorized grants for the purpose of developing services and training personnel and established a National Advisory Council on Services and Facilities for the Developmentally Disabled.

Most recently is the American with Disabilities Act (ADA) of 1990 that became effective in 1992. The goals of this legislation are to fight discrimination, protect access to goods and services, and promote equality of opportunity for people with disabilities. Here disability is defined very broadly and encompasses a variety of physical, mental, and developmental disorders.[30]

While the purpose of these laws is to offer protection and resources to those so delineated, the process of classification is not without risk of harm. Classification is not a neutral practice in that actions are taken on behalf of the classifications we make. Some authors point out that most commonly, it is some administrative action. There is an interesting historical example dating from the reign of Edward I (1272 to 1307) during which the first recorded distinction is made between a fool and a lunatic. In the reign of Edward II, the distinction is made between the born fool and the person who is, at times, clearheaded. This was not just a point of interest because if you were declared a born fool, the Crown could take your property. If, on the other hand, you had periods of lucidity, the Crown could lay claim to your property only during the periods of insanity.[31]

In addition to the administrative, the other purpose of classification is scientific, which includes diagnosis, prognosis, and research. Classification systems are designed primarily to provide statistical data about groups of similar individuals or cases, furnish the basis for measuring incidence, prevalence, characteristics, and other information, including the success of programs established to prevent or ameliorate the condition.[32] Such a procedure as classification has many problems. The most basic problem stems from the difficulty of any effort to categorize the totality and complexity of a human being. No matter how multidimensional the classification methods, their imperfections and inadequacies will soon become apparent. An interesting paradox that compounds this serious problem in classifying any group can be noted—the more knowledge science develops about a given entity, in this case mental retardation, the more difficult classification becomes because of the additional dimensions and complexities. The classification system presents special problems in dealing with individuals in the mild or moderate categories. Frequent discrepancies occur between adaptive behavior and measured intelligence, making it difficult to determine who should be classified in which category.

These problems may be further compounded by the sociopolitical processes at play in the society at any given time. For example, as we mentioned above, IQ has a controversial history. In recent years, questions have been raised about the use of IQ testing as a basis for classifying and placing individuals in programs. The limitations of IQ tests and the possible errors in using them point to their disadvantage as the only source of information used to classify people. Other problems with IQ testing are the presumed-cultural-bias controversy and the difficulty in assessing social competence. The IQ and social competence tests must be supplemented by life history data, biomedical information, and clinical judgment.

Classification would not be possible without the labeling process. The label of mental retardation, like all such labels, serves as a shorthand way of saying a number of things about an individual or group. Although labels may be necessary to facilitate communication, they do tend to conjure up stereotypes, especially socially defined pejorative ones of the labeled person. For example, people hold an image of the alcoholic as a skid-row bum and not as a business executive, although in this latter group alcoholism constitutes a problem of some magnitude. Labels are not inherently bad, although they can be, and sometimes are abused. With the mental retardation label, one abuse derives from overlooking the vast range of individual differences found in the people so labeled. This abuse can lead us to interact with all mentally retarded persons as if no differences existed. All of us, including the mentally retarded, gain and maintain our concept of self from interaction with others. If we constantly respond to a retarded individual in stereotyped ways, he or she continually receives feedback that may be based more on our preconceptions and stereotypes than on the individual himself or herself. This could lead to a self-fulfilling prophecy, in that the mentally retarded person begins to respond to us on the basis of our notion of him or her. For example, if we view the retarded individual as dependent and unable to do for himself or herself, then he or she may behave to fit this view. Labeling can function in two ways. In one way, it stigmatizes people thereby excluding them from participation in the larger society. If the reader wishes to pursue the important topic of stigma, they are referred to the classic works of Goffman and Edgerton.[33,34] On the other hand, labeling does provide access to beneficial services. One scholar has described this beautifully as a world gained and a world lost. Gained is the world of special services but lost is "the world of the rest of us who are, as it were, 'normal'."[35] Ethically speaking, perhaps the most important thing we can do for the mentally retarded, as nurses and as citizens, is to work to see that the doors to both worlds are kept open and freely traveled.

SOCIAL TREATMENT

In the United States before 1810, the majority of the mentally ill and retarded lived in homes with their families or friends or, if without a social network, they could be found in poorhouses and jails. The era of the Industrial Revolution, which brought with it waves of immigrants and a beginning shift from a rural society to an urban one, defined deviant behavior as a product of the social, political, and economic environment of the time. Social reformers viewed this environment as chaotic, disordered, and lacking stability. The traditional social procedures and institutions were breaking down and in some cases dissolving. This situation, in turn, created great societal stresses and strains.[36] From Europe at about this time, news came of cures for insanity and deviant behavior, with emphasis on humane care in special residential institutions. This "moral treatment" developed along with the increasing belief in the physical base of certain deviant behaviors. Within this context, individuals exhibiting these behaviors became the legitimate concern of physiology and medicine.[37] By 1860, 28 of the then 33 states had built public institutions to house and care for this segment of the population. This growth in institutional care, occurring mostly between the 1830s and the 1850s, was due to its new status as the most proper treatment method.[38]

This era, which emphasized the social origins of disease, also defined idiocy and feeblemindedness as social problems. Major reformers of the day had their ideas applied to a large extent because they fitted the pervading assumptions about the therapeutic effects of institutionalization. And so the transformation of these institutions from residential schools to custodial asylums had support from the society at large, as well as from the professionals who ran them. One writer maintains that these professionals did not necessarily invent the concept of the "menace of the feebleminded," but they did support its propagation, benefited from it, and until the 1920s opposed alternatives to residential segregation.[39] Essentially, the patterns of development in the institutions for the mentally retarded paralleled those used in the treatment of other forms of dependency and deviancy.

These larger social changes also had an impact on the educational system of the country. Society increasingly called on schools to train for economic, social, and civic roles, and in assuming these functions the school became the primary defender of the social order. By the 1920s, the experts and the general public assumed that by making an educational problem out of any social problem it could be effectively treated.[40] Other changes in the educational system affecting the mentally retarded also occurred during these years. The adoption of a corporate-industrial model of educational organization—in which the administration became managers, teachers the workers, the curriculum the technology, and the students the raw material for processing,[41]—combined with a rise in vocationalism that led to a definition of equality of educational opportunity.[42] This and the development of intelligence testing affected the role of the school vis-a-vis the mentally retarded. These changes, occurring in the first three decades of this century, combined to provide a major impetus to the emergence of special education for the mentally handicapped.[43]

The special education movement, although gathering support from various groups, never achieved the full public acceptance enjoyed by the earlier asylum movement.[44] A variety of reasons accounted for the lack of acceptance, one of which was parental hostility that was kept in play by the school's failure to distinguish among the different categories of children— that is, the mentally retarded, the behaviorally disruptive, the physically handicapped, and the truant children. In short, these special classes became the custodial places for children whom, because it lacked ways of accommodating them, the educational system could not tolerate.[45] By the second half of this century, however, special education experienced a substantial growth, due largely to President Kennedy's interest and support. In October of 1961, he established a Presidential Panel on Mental Retardation, which articulated four principles to be used in program development for services. These principles were normalization, the developmental model, the least restrictive alternative, and mainstreaming.[46] The principle of normalization originated in Denmark, the idea being to make available to mentally retarded people, as much as possible, the patterns of life that exist for society in general. The developmental model was very significant because it challenged the notion of irreversibility, replacing it with the idea that mentally retarded people are capable of growth and learning. The least restrictive alternative had its roots in legal doctrine and basically means that if the state must interfere with someone's freedom, they must do so in the least restrictive way possible. Finally, mainstreaming refers to the placement of mentally retarded children in regular classroom situations. These principles continue to exert influence on services for the mentally retarded.

The enactment of the Education for All Handicapped Children Act of 1975 (PL 94-142) attempted to make many of these principles a reality in that a variety of special services such as speech therapy, psychological services, and even transportation were mandated. In one authority's view, this act changed the very idea of what constitutes special education.[47] The idea of mainstreaming is about inclusion, about who can and cannot participate in the routine life of a community and that makes it an ethical issue. It is a matter of how we as a society want to live, of who counts as one of us. Such an articulation of ideals is critically important because it motivates us, calls us to account for our actions, and provides reasons for the justification of our actions. But ideals, if they are to be more than words, must be enacted in the complex world of day to day life and it is here that we, as individuals and collectively as a society, face some of our most difficult ethical dilemmas. Resources, neither human nor monetary, are not infinite. Suppose, for example, that a special needs child is placed in a regular classroom but requires an educational aid in continuous attendance as well as speech therapy four times a week. The school, however, has the resources for only half of these services. Obtaining everything the child needs could be done only at the cost of decreasing other services, perhaps physical education or art. What should be done? Human life seems to have embedded within it a tension in the relationship between the individual and the group and there are no pat answers. Treating the mentally retarded as persons demands that we address the issues of the provision of services in general,[48] as well as regular school inclusion,[49,50] the nature of medical decision making for the retarded individual,[51-55] the degree to which we submit parents to scrutiny,[56,57] capital punishment and incompetent offenders,[58] sexual abuse,[59] and the morality of such treatment interventions as aversive therapy.[60-65] Ethical reflection is imperative if we are to continue to strive for an ethical world in which the virtues of justice and compassion flourish.

LAW, ETHICS, AND SOCIAL POLICY

Earlier in the chapter we stated that the ethical dilemmas discussed with regard to the mentally retarded can be listed as concerning the concept of *person*; how we define mental retardation and the consequences this definition has for the person so labeled; problems encountered by the mentally retarded in institutions and in the community regarding their rights; and the moral reasoning that society uses in balancing its resources and values to determine the risks and benefits for the individual and for society itself. While law and ethics are not equivalent, they stand in important relationship to each other. Laws have significant ethical implications because they structure a society, thereby setting up minimal standards of expectation. Rights, when codified legally, incur binding obligations. The relationship between the law and issues of mental retardation is complex and fluid reflecting many social factors and influencing public policy. One social factor of profound importance was the interest and leadership of President Kennedy who influenced every aspect related to our social policy for mental retardation. As a result of the work of the entire Kennedy family, social consciousness was awakened, concrete services improved, and legal rights procured; in short, social policy was altered. Social policy is a form of collective action and in terms of mental retardation four perspectives have been identified: protecting society; protecting the mentally retarded individual; helping society to accommodate the person; and assisting the individual to participate fully in social life.[66] In the first section we listed some of the rights claimed for retarded citizens over the past several decades and our purpose is not to repeat them here. Rather, we want to discuss three items that well illustrate the intersection of law, ethics, and public policy. These are sterilization, confinement, and the Americans with Disabilities Act.

   Although sterilization is no longer a widespread practice for the mentally ill and mentally retarded, we believe that its lessons are instructive for many reasons. Most importantly, it shows how specific procedures can become enactments of ideas whose purpose is to justify excluding others from participation in the goods of social life. Large scale immigration during the second half of the 19th century, social Darwinism, beliefs in heredity over social conditions as the cause of behavior that violates social norms, and the means to measure IQ were factors that converged and fueled the social movement of eugenics.[67] New immigrants were tested at Ellis Island with the Binet–Simon IQ test and when this finding was coupled with the contemporary evolutionary theories, the *perceived* inferior status of the immigrants was quickly labeled as genetic.[68] Another mass screening of IQ was conducted on United States Army recruits during the first World War. Within these two groups, lower scores were most often found among African-Americans, Jews, or those from Central or Southern Europe or of that descent. This supposed genetic inferiority was used as evidence to support a certain moral order, that is, a certain view of the world and who is entitled to full membership in it.[69]

From beliefs in the hereditary cause of social problems, combined with "scientific evidence" and powerful theories, it was a small leap to sterilization laws and practices. This century witnessed laws prohibiting marriage involving the mentally retarded and laws mandating compulsory sterilization.[70] It is estimated that in the first six decades of this century, 60,000 mentally retarded or mentally ill people were sterilized.[71] The most famous U.S. Supreme Court case (*Buck v Bell* 1927) regarding sterilization concerned a Virginia woman named Carrie Buck. As reported by Bourguignon, there was no evidence that Carrie was "feebleminded . . . but she did have an illegitimate daughter who was slow and this apparently satisfied the broad statutory requirement for sterilization." [72]

On the face of it, sterilization might readily be seen as the solution to a legitimate concern for the well-being of children born to certain people. But too often such "solutions" are unreflective and morally suspect. In our view, there are at least four ethical problems with sterilization. The first, the relation between sterilization and eugenics, was discussed above. Second, the focus on sterilization can obscure the important underlying issue of what good parenting does involve and who is capable of enacting it. In 1949, the renowned child psychiatrist, Leo Kanner stated:

> In my 20 years of psychiatric work with thousands of children and their parents, I have seen percentually at least as many 'intelligent' adults unfit to rear their offspring as I have seen such 'feeble-minded' adults. I have . . . and many others have . . . come to the conclusion that to a large extent independent of the IQ, fitness for parenthood is determined by emotional involvements and relationships.[73]

Third, sterilization of the mentally retarded is a power-sanctioned procedure by which we mean that the state in conjunction with medical authority dictates what kind of life is possible for these individuals. Such decisions can too easily be made without understanding the perspectives of those who will be affected and failing to do so is a moral wrong. Research done in the early 1960s documented the effect of sterilization on the ability of mentally retarded people to live happy, meaningful lives. The following is a woman interviewed by the researchers, Sabagh and Edgerton:

> I was all engaged to marry a man that I really loved. He loved me too, but one day we were sitting and talking with his mother and father and they were saying how happy they would be when we were married and had children. When I heard this, I said, "No, I don't never want to get married." I almost told her (the mother) why but I just couldn't bear to tell her.[74]

We want to make an important point about the power of the state, especially since government bashing is currently in vogue. In a representative democracy, we, as individuals bear a great deal of responsibility for the policies of our goverment because we vote for people who will take action in one way or another. To put it somewhat differently, the state is not just *them*—it is *us.*

Finally, the usual social response to correcting the abuses of something such as sterilization is to prohibit the practice and to see the motives of those who advocate for it in certain circumstances as morally bad. This is unfortunate and ethically problematic in its own right because it can disallow sterilization in situations where it indeed might be the best thing to do. Consider one of the cases described by Applebaum and La Puma.[75] Sonya is a 13-year-old severely retarded girl with the mental age of a 1 to 2-year-old child who is also blind and has marked neurological impairments. The child is unable to attend to any of her hygiene needs, experiences pain, and is irritable and confused during menstruation. Sonya lives with her grandmother who requested a hysterectomy, which would stop menstruation and also sterilize her. While medicine agreed that a hysterectomy would be in the best interests of the child, the court did not, ruling that the above factors were not sufficient to justify the procedure. Furthermore, the court ruled that the request for hysterectomy was primarily in the interest of the grandmother and such interests had no legal standing. Applebaum and La Puma suggested that the interests of families are legitimate and we concur with them in challenging the wisdom of the court's decision in this case. We would go further, however, in calling attention to the ethical implications of gendered work. Although a deeper discussion of this takes us beyond the scope of this chapter, we want to note that it is women who do the vast majority of caring labor in this society whether in the home or in institutions.[76-78] And there are several ethical issues embedded in these social arrangements including adequate resources and having a say in matters in which you are directly involved. In terms of sterilization, the ethical issues concern who makes the decisions, under what conditions, with what motivation, and to what end.

Another issue that illustrates the intersection of law, ethics, and social policy is confinement. In 1993, the U.S. Supreme Court upheld a Kentucky statute that makes it easier to involuntarily commit a mentally retarded person than it is a mentally ill person.[79] In other words, mentally retarded persons are held to lower standards. According to the majority opinion, the rationale for permitting these differences was claimed to lie in the ease of diagnosing mental retardation over mental illness, greater accuracy in predicting dangerous behavior among the mentally retarded, and less invasive treatment for mental retardation. Invasive treatment was considered to be psychotropic medication and psychotherapy that focuses on the inner life or psychological meanings for a person. The first of these assumptions is related to the use of intellectual tests that are supposedly objective and do not require an assessment of psychological phenomena such as motives and intentions. The second assumption rests on the long-term and irreversible nature of mental retardation. But as stated earlier, mental retardation is not a monolithic category; instead there is a range of functional capacity and individual differences within those ranges.

It is not clear, however, how the majority opinion reasoned regarding the third assumption. As dissenting author Justice Souter noted, psychotropic medication is used extensively with mentally retarded people. It has been estimated that 30 to 50 percent of mentally retarded adults in institutions and 25 to 35 percent of those in the community are receiving these medications.[80] Clearly, the majority opinion of Justice Kennedy recognizes psychotropic medication as a powerful means of social control. Yet in failing to recognize or acknowledge that mentally retarded people receive these drugs, they deny the extent to which the mentally retarded are subject to these controls and what this might mean in the day-to-day life of these people. One ethical issue concerns the degree of freedom of people to accept or refuse these drugs. Indeed, at least in some states, the involuntarily committed mentally ill cannot be forced to take medication except in an emergency. For example, in California, there is a special medication hearing called a Reese hearing that the patient must lose before he or she can be forced to take medication. Most times, therapists and the mentally ill person work together around medication while this is far less likely to be the case with the mentally retarded. Moreover, these drugs cause many uncomfortable, even toxic and irreversible side effects. A person who is cognitively impaired and, in addition, likely to experience speech difficulties may not be able to communicate that, or indeed, connect what is happening to them with the drugs.

More disturbing is the majority opinion's failure to appreciate, as invasive, the behavior modification and punishment to which the mentally retarded are subjected. As indicated in the previous section, there is literature addressing some of the issues related to these techniques. Here we specifically want to call attention to an extreme form of punishment documented in the literature. Although the case is recognized as extreme even by those in the field and is more than 20 years old, we relate it because it demonstrates severely invasive treatment. In our minds, it raises questions as to the ethics of treatment, even for very difficult and serious management problems such as self-injurious behavior (SIB). The following is taken from the section on punishment in Kiernan.[81] The presentation of the case is given in the context of a discussion of the effects of punishment that include "anger, aggression, withdrawal, general suppression of behavior, and ritualistic or inflexible behavior." The author reports that there is evidence for the same reactions among the mentally retarded. The case that Kiernan discusses was reported in the literature by Jones in 1974. The case is that of a 9-year-old girl who was treated with contingent electroshock in 1974 for self-hitting.

> During treatment, which was very prolonged, the child's repertoire of self-destructive behavior expanded to include 'pinching and jabbing with her fingers of sufficient intensity to open lesions in her sides, stomach, thighs and the back of her neck' (p 243). When this behavior was also punished with shock, jabbing increased, hitting reappeared and increased, and she refused food. Eventually the child was being tube-fed and was restrained with a neck collar and arm tubes.

It is distressing to read this but it speaks for itself—who could claim that this was not invasive treatment? We do not deny that the day-to-day care of some mentally retarded people pose marked challenges to our ingenuity, resources, and moral make-up. Although many, many ethical questions clamor to be answered about the above practice, our purpose is to inform nurses that such practices, although extreme, do exist. In this case, the practices are called treatment and treatment in whatever form it takes is not neutral—there are consequences and sometimes they can be extreme.

Values are embedded in all of our social practices, including the laws and social policies we adopt.[82] What are the values underlying the Americans with Disabilities Act (ADA) and how will they be enacted in day-to-day life for the disabled individual and the worlds of which they are a part? Kopelman provides a thorough discussion of the ethical assumptions underlying this legislation.[83] While the general values are fairness, equality of opportunity, and beneficence, there are significant ambiguities that arise because these values can conflict. For example, equality of opportunity can be understood in two ways. One school of thought holds that the standards used to evaluate someone must apply equally to everyone, independent of such things as "race, religion, gender, age, poverty, or physical or mental disability." [84] In this view, these factors cannot be used against anyone but neither can they be used to help. Another view holds that precisely because some people are more disadvantaged than others, it is unfair to treat everyone in the same way. These two perspectives illustrate the tension in the relationship between the individual and the group. When the individual is disabled, conflicts in values can be heightened. The example of the child who can attend a regular school but requires an educational aide in constant attendance illustrates this point. If the school board provides this service, will cuts need to be made elsewhere, cuts that might include services to all children? How the ideal of equal opportunity is understood has critical implications for the allocation of resources. In Kopelman's words: "The central moral and social question raised by the application of the ADA is: How can we remain committed to the rights and welfare of those with severe disabilities while placing limits on their claims?". The answer to this will continue to unfold as the ambiguities come to light and society makes choices.

GENETICS

Governments have special concerns for the health of citizens. For example, many nations have statutory programs to provide for the control of contagious diseases. There have also been times when the state legally forced a person to have treatment even when no discernible risk to society from the illness could be demonstrated. The boundaries of permissible government activities to regulate more generally the health of society as a whole have been delineated, in part, by such constitutional constraints as the guarantee of the freedom to religious convictions; the guarantee that no person will be deprived of life, liberty, or property without due process of the law; and the guarantee that no state shall deny to any person within its jurisdiction the equal protection of the law. The doctrine of Fundamental Interests holds that certain human activities not mentioned in the Bill of Rights deserve special judicial protection. One of these activities, privacy or the right to be left alone, has slowly expanded to include rights of personal decision-making.[85] No absolute and clear delineation of the outer limits of government action pursuant to the public health power can be made. The state's power to order an individual to undergo a medical procedure—such as immunization, sterilization, blood tests, and x-ray—has far-reaching implications. The potential of this power for both evil and good is obvious and any proposal for the extension of the power deserves very careful scrutiny.[86] Genetic screening legislation represents one such extension of this power.

Genetic screening is defined as the identification of those suffering from a genetically based disease or those possessing a certain genotype that may be inherited. Genetic screening may be done for several reasons: for the purpose of detecting disease; to gain reproductive information; to conduct epidemiological research.[87]

In screening for disease, the object is to discover persons with a specific disease or those who have genes that might lead to disease. Once such persons are identified, they are offered treatment, if available, to manage their disease or to reverse or prevent the adverse effects of a genetic disorder. In screening for reproductive information, the purpose is to discover persons within the population who have genes that, when joined with other genes, may lead to adverse genetic effects in offspring. The implicit assumption in this kind of screening is that persons may wish to include knowledge of their genotype and the possible risks of producing adversely affected children in their reproductive decisions. In screening for epidemiological purposes, public health authorities are monitoring the incidence of genetic disorders as a means to learning about their causes. This kind of screening may also be done for health purposes or to study the natural history of a genetic disorder for which there is currently no treatment.

While many believe in the benefits of screening for communicable disorders in this country, the questioning of the value of genetic screening extends back at least twenty years.[88] This has been due in part to the lack of specific criteria for screening programs and the lack of reliable testing materials to detect genetic disorders. These two problems are quite evident in the history of phenylketonuria (PKU) testing in the United States during the 1960s.

PKU is an inborn error of metabolism, which is an inherited disease of metabolism resulting from reduced or missing enzymes.[89] Undetected, PKU results in mental retardation but if discovered early enough, the mental retardation can be prevented by dietary restriction of phenylalanine. A diagnostic test for PKU was known in 1934 when it was discovered that the fresh urine from some mentally retarded children changed color in the presence of ferric chloride. Screening of all infants for PKU did not occur, however, until the bacterial inhibition assay for PKU was developed by Robert Guthrie in 1962.[90] PKU thus emerged as the first genetically determined condition for which there was both means of easy identification and treatment. In 1963, Massachusetts became the first state to mandate screening and within four years, forty states had legal requirements to screen for PKU.[91]

The phenomenal growth of PKU laws over a short period of time is rather interesting. Some analysts of health policy suggest that the small budget outlay required for a state PKU-testing program, combined with the unquestionable benefit of a plan to reduce mental retardation, provided special interest groups (such as the National Association for Retarded Children) with a powerful lobbying weapon that easily won support.[92] Others have suggested that it was the threat of mental retardation, not PKU *per se*, that impressed the state legislators to act so quickly.[93] Whatever the reasons, the growth of PKU screening and its surrounding controversies have provided important lessons that may apply to genetic screening in general. For example, the lack of counseling and follow-up in most early state-mandated PKU testing programs demonstrates that the planning for screening and intervention for all gene-related metabolic disease must be subjected to careful analysis before being instituted. The initial testing methodology for PKU was not of uniform quality from state to state. As a result, treatment for false positive reactions produced mental retardation in otherwise normal children who were wrongly placed on the PKU diet. In addition, few states required that affected children be placed on a low phenylalanine diet or gave statutory consideration to genetic counseling for families of affected children.[94]

Despite numerous problems in the PKU-testing experience, state genetic screening programs grew in number through the 1960s and 1970s. Screening for genetic disease was believed to be a desirable goal of society and was even emphasized in President Richard Nixon's 1971 health message to the nation. President Nixon noted the incidence of sickle cell anemia among the African-American population and asked the National Institutes of Health (NIH) to increase its funding for sickle cell anemia research.[95] Within a few months, reports of sickle cell anemia appeared in the national news media and there was an increase in federal funding for sickle cell anemia research. As sickle cell anemia moved to center stage in the genetic disease theater, state legislatures acted on hastily constructed sickle cell anemia screening proposals in much the same manner that they did on PKU screening proposals a few years before. By the end of 1976, other legislation had been passed related to Cooley's anemia, Tay–Sachs' disease, and other genetic disorders.[96]

Genetic disorder legislation, designed to influence childbearing decisions by heterozygous couples and to reduce the number of genetically defective children born, tended to overlook the dangers implicit in such laws. Because of the association of sickle cell anemia with only one race, screening laws confronted an unusual equal protection problem. This situation became further compounded by the fact that these laws failed to provide for confidentiality of test information—availability of competent, free genetic-counseling services, and programs to educate the general public about genetic disease. Similar problems encountered in other disease-specific legislation, such as laws regarding Tay-Sachs' disease and Cooley's anemia, raise larger questions as to the appropriateness and effectiveness of this multiplication of disease-specific laws.[97]

These ethical concerns, raised twenty years ago have not been addressed satisfactorily. In fact, they are greatly exacerbated with the Human Genome Project. The Human Genome Project is the ambitious undertaking to determine the molecular structure and location of all the genetic material of the human species. Although work in genetics has been conducted since the last century, it is only recent technical advances that have allowed for a large scale exploration. The reader is referred to *A Brief History of the Human Genome Project* for an excellent overview.[98] The Human Genome Project will have an extraordinary impact on social life. It will (and in fact, is) changing medicine, health care, insurance coverage, and conceptions of what it will mean to be a "normal" person. While there is undoubtedly some good that will come of this work, there is a potential for very great harm. We mention only a few harms. Before genetic screening and medicine, "patients" were people who were sick in the sense of not feeling well, not being able to carry out the routines of daily living. With the new genetics, however, patients will be those at risk for developing some disease. This is not without its dark side as patienthood submits the individual to the surveillance and control of others, medical, nursing, employers, and insurance. In many instances, those at risk will be the fetus. This will result in a shift of patienthood from the pregnant woman to the fetus. This may seem benign enough but it has the capacity to reduce women to being fetal containers.

Another significant issue is that the capacity for genetic diagnosis does now, and is likely to continue, to far exceed the capacity for treatment.[99] Most genetic diseases, unlike PKU, will not be so readily treated. Children are being tested for genetic diseases that do not present until adulthood and for which there is no treatment. What is being accomplished by this? What good can this do the child? People have already been denied both life and health insurance on the basis of genetic testing. If a woman is pregnant and the fetus is found to have some genetic abnormality, will she be forced to choose between an abortion and a denial of coverage. There is an extraordinary amount of money to be made in the genetic industry and there will be powerful interests at stake. Who will say what is "normal" and what must be done?

The creation of medical need will be endless. And of course, the powerful answers that medicine can provide will be a "wedge," in the words of sociologist Troy Duster, that will enable more and more control of human life to be directed on the basis of genetic information alone.[100] Who will get to say what is normal and what must be done about it? It will not be ordinary people, but is likely to be the wedding of powerful scientific elites and economic interests cloaked in the wrap of what is best for society. But the question, *who is society*? is a critical one. Even though attempts to legislate the use of genetic information are being made, they will not keep pace with the thrust of scientific and monetary interests.

It has been argued that we shift to the ancient concept of malady which refers to those evils for which we are at risk. The term would include disease, illness, and injury, as well as such things as short stature and low intelligence.[101] One geneticist has argued that it is those people with "genetic ailments of the mind" that will be most likely to suffer discrimination or worse.[102] All of these issues raise questions about the allocation of resources. We do not have limitless resources; if one area of health care is receiving a large portion, others are receiving less. Should our financial resources as a society be funneled into gene therapy when we pay people minimal wages to care for the retarded, the mentally ill, and the elderly? Take for instance, the little girl mentioned above who was 'treated' with electric shock. What if we paid enough people a sufficient living wage to care for her. Could she be restrained from injuring herself by the embrace of human workers who were skilled and wanted to be there, for whom this work was important? Of course, the argument could be made that with enough research money, we can find the genes for all of mental retardation or mental illness and therefore, these people won't have to be (implying a choice) or won't be (implying a prohibition) born. Is this how we want to address this type of medical need?

Another issue is that for all its complexity, the human genetics project is far easier to deal with than many of the social and environmental conditions such as poverty, homophobia or outright hatred, violence, and sexism.

Finally, we raise one last issue although there are others. Let us assume that in one way or another, we can eliminate all disease. What will we die from? Would we have to die? Should we die? If we don't die, how will we make room for the next generation? Will there be a next generation? In Shirley Jackson's chilling short story, *The Lottery*, we are never told why the lottery, the "winner" of which is stoned to death by her neighbors, takes place annually. Could it be a society where people do not die of disease? If there were such a place, would we invent some means? In the science fiction film, *Zardoz*, there is immortality but it is far from a happy society because everything is meaningless in a universe that is essentially static. In this imagined world, the violation of group norms are punished by aging, but dying remains an impossibility. Prisons are essentially wards of extremely old, incapacitated, demented, and suffering people. We have painted a rather dramatic picture, some might even call it extreme, but we live in a culture and historical period that assumes that technological advances are an unquestioned good.[103] A significant part of ethics concerns the kind of world we want to have.

Reflection on the social, political, and ethical aspects of the Human Genome Project is critical to the ethical practice of nursing, particularly as genetics becomes more "routine." Nurses are increasingly knowledgeable about genetics and involved in genetic counseling. This role originated with nurses working with the mentally retarded and[104] although nurses have been working in the area and publishing since the 1960s,[105,106] the last decade has seen a dramatic increase in nursing knowledge about genetics. A computer search for nursing and genetics revealed 245 citations. These ranged from specific disease entities such as inborn errors of metabolism[107,108] and cancer[109,110] to the Human Genome Project,[111] gene therapy,[112] the collaboration between nurses and genetic counselors,[113] infertility and reproductive technologies,[114–116] education,[117–119] psychiatry,[120,121] and ethics.[122–126] Recently formed is the International Society of Nurses in Genetics which, as of 1996, has 135 members in 36 states and nine members from four other countries. There are 26 specialty areas within this organization. The American Nurses Association has recently published ethical guidelines for dealing with genetic information.[127] There is no doubt that genetic knowledge will form the foundation of medical science for the 21st century and that nurses will have a significant role once that knowledge becomes routine.[128] Asking social, political, and ethical questions from a critical perspective is an essential aspect of an ethical practice in genetics.

ETHICAL IMPLICATIONS FOR NURSING PRACTICE

One of the major criticisms of our society's current enchantment with genetics is that it is seen as holding out an ideal of human perfectibility. The idea is that by appropriate counselling we will make wise choices so that our children will be close to "perfection." That we, as a society, believe in this idea of perfection has been documented by the sense of guilt and failure that parents feel when their children are born less than perfect.[129] Genetic counselors have described their work as "mopping up" the grief following parents' experience with one of *God's Mistakes*.[130] Encountering a less than perfect being confronts us with the knowledge that human life is fragile and such awareness can fill us with profound emotions. Why is it that so many of us avert our eyes from the physically different or the retarded or the mentally ill? When we encounter a disabled person, we can experience the encounter as an affront to our own personal integrity in that we realize the fragility of the world that we take for granted. The old adage, "There, but for the grace of God, go I," implies a universal vulnerability in a world over which we do not have absolute control. Even if genetics could give us absolute control, would we want it? Should we have it? An encounter with the mentally retarded can be experienced as an affront to the most fundamental core of our own personhood. We react to this affront with a variety of feelings, including thankfulness that we are as we are and guilt that we live in a world of "have" and "have nots." This latter world is not simply one of physical and cognitive intactness, however, it is also a political, social, and, above all, economic world. We live in a society that espouses economic individualism at a time when a significant portion of people believe that government cannot or should not be about helping people. Perhaps another aspect of the profound emotions that can be experienced with the loss of the perfect child is the fear of providing for the child in a society that is not structured to include the less than perfect.

In attempting to cope with such an encounter, commonly experienced feelings of repulsion and disgust not only can prevent us from examining the roots of our reaction, they can also have wide-ranging effects on our definition of the situation and on how or if we deal with the moral claims that the mentally retarded have on us as an individual, as nurses, and as citizens. Our attitudes also will determine how we think the resources of society should be allocated and how much and what we think the mentally retarded should receive. The concept of *distributive justice* provides us with a moral framework within which to make these decisions.

Obviously, the nurse must first sort out his or her own feelings about and attitudes toward the mentally retarded. Such a sorting out will need to take into account the concept of personhood and where one draws the line, if at all, with regard to the extent of the retardation and the consequences of such action. Questions raised will be:

- What attitudes do I have toward the mentally retarded?
- What attitudes should I have and why?
- Do I tend to stereotype all the mentally retarded and view them as a category rather than as individuals with differences?
- What moral principles have I used to think through my ethical position vis-a-vis the retarded?
- What moral claims do the retarded have on me as a professional?
- What moral claims do they have on society? How do we articulate these claims within the concept of distributive justice?

Parents have reported less than helpful reactions from others, ranging from too much sympathy, to denial of any sort of problem, to rejection.[131] These and other reactions grounded in negative attitudes toward the mentally retarded can hinder the nurse in performing the basic functions of his or her role, to say nothing of the quality of caring. It can only be assumed that the nurses working directly with the retarded and their families over a period of time have developed a moral position that enables them to provide all of the care required in the situation, while at the same time protecting the rights of these patients. Medicine has been accused of paternalism, but nursing also needs to examine its activities, especially with such patients as the mentally retarded and the mentally ill, to ascertain the extent of the paternalism that we inflict on others. In the sense in which any of us can ever be said to be at home in the world, we are at home not through dominating but through caring for others in ways that permit both to grow.

More problems may occur for those nurses in most other settings where encounters with the mentally retarded have been less frequent and of less intensity. In dealing with the ethical dilemmas of mental retardation, focusing on the rights of the retarded person may be helpful. The official statement of the American Association on Mental Deficiency makes the point that in all activities—designing facilities and organizing services, allocating funds and other resources, participating in the legislative or judicial process, teaching, conducting research, and "most of all, when participating directly in the treatment, training, and habilitation of retarded persons"— the rights of these individuals should serve as the foundation of all else.

For the nurse in the neonatal intensive care unit, the dilemma that he or she may face over the issue of letting a mentally retarded infant die will call for moral reasoning with regard to the part the nurse can or cannot play in this drama. It can only be hoped that the environment in such a unit will encourage open discussion of these ethical dilemmas in all their complex points.

As the field of genetics further advances, nurses—clinicians, educators, and researchers, both individually and collectively—along with other health professionals and concerned citizens must become more knowledgeable about the implications of this research. Decisions and research findings in this field affect all of us living now as well as future generations. The need to weigh the potential risks and possible benefits on the future course of human evolution is not of mere academic interest. Our deep-rooted concepts of ourselves and our relationship to the universe will be reappraised in this process. This has enormous consequences, not only for the mentally retarded but for all of us. Value judgments inevitably will play an important part in determining the direction society takes on this scientific and ethical issue. One can only wonder if the insights and humility gained from encounters with the mentally retarded will help in this awesome task before us.[132,133] As the largest segment of the health industry, nurses should have some valuable input for this debate. In all of these ethical dilemmas, the moral virtue of compassion and the moral principles of justice and utility, or the greatest possible balance of good over evil, have a part in our concept of obligations to the mentally retarded, as well as to the rest of us, now and in the future.[134]*

*The authors wish to thank Kathleen Schmidt Yule, RN, MS for her help with this chapter.

■ CASE STUDY I.

Cindy is a 26-year-old, low functioning, developmentally disabled woman living in a county-certified group home with other developmentally disabled clients. She tells the home operator that she was raped by a man also living in the home.

The police are contacted but refuse to make a police report because she would not be a competent witness and the case would never go to trial. Additionally, the accused man would never be deemed competent to stand trial and denies her claim. The local emergency department refuses to send out a rape kit and counselor since no police report has been filed. You are the nurse who case manages the home.*

Suggested Questions for Discussion

1. What are Cindy's rights in this situation? Are her rights lessened because she is developmentally disabled?

2. What are the obligations of the nurse? Are these reduced once the police are contacted? Should this be pursued as a criminal matter?

3. What is the best way to see that Cindy's needs are met in this situation?

4. What about the man involved in the rape, what are his needs and rights? How should these be addressed?

*Special thanks to Maurie Ange, MS, MFCC for this case.

■ CASE STUDY II.

Sheila is a 30-year-old woman living independently. She works in a workshop making hand crafted gifts. She was born with congenital heart and lung abnormalities that are progressively worsening. She was recently referred to a transplant center to be evaluated for a possible heart–lung transplant.

The referral center rejected her as a candidate saying that she would not be able to adequately manage her post-transplant care because of her mental retardation. Sheila has Down syndrome but is very high functioning. She appealed to a second center which accepted her. She received the transplant and is now doing very well.

Suggested Questions for Discussion

1. What is the responsibility of the transplant center in seeing that such a scarce resource as organs for transplantation are distributed fairly and equitably? Should such things as cognitive function, self-care capability, potential for social contribution be considered?

2. Is Sheila less worthy of a transplant than someone with a higher IQ?

3. As a result of Sheila's experience, state legislation barring discrimination in the allocation of organs for transplantation based on pre-existing mental or physical disability as defined by the American Disability Act was introduced. How would you respond to this type of legislative initiative?

REFERENCES

1. Downie RS, Telfer E: *Respect for Persons.* New York: Schocken Books; 1970.
2. Fletcher JF: Four indicators of humanhood—the enquiry matures. *Hastings Cent Rep* 4(6):4–7, 1974.
3. Teichmann J: The definition of person. *Philosophy* 60:175–185, 1985.
4. Trendelenberg A. A contribution to the history of the word person. *The Monist,* 20, 336–363, 1910.
5. Kant I: *The Fundamental Principles of the Metaphysics of Morals,* Paton HJ (trans). London: Hutchinson's University Library; 1948.
6. Downie RS, Telfer E: *Respect for Persons.* New York: Schoken Books; 1979.
7. Rorty AO: *The Identities of Persons.* Berkeley: University of California Press; 1976.
8. Goodman MF: *What is a Person?* Clifton, NJ: Humana Press; 1988.

9. Sapontzis S: A critique of personhood. *Ethics* 91:607–618, 1981.

10. Sapontzis S: *Morals, Reason, and Animals.* Philadelphia: Temple University Press; 1987.

11. Allmark P: An argument against the use of the concept of 'persons' in health care ethics. *J Adv Nur* 19:29–35, 1994.

12. Kleinig J: *Valuing Life.* Princeton: Princeton University Press; 1991.

13. Kopelman L: Respect and the retarded: Issues of valuing and labeling. In Kopelman L, Moskop J (eds): *Ethics and Mental Retardation.* Dordrecht: Kluwer; 1984, pp 65–86.

14. *Ibid.,* p 79.

15. Agich G: Reassessing autonomy in long-term care. *Hastings Cent Rep* 20(6):12–17, 1990.

16. *In the Matter of M.R.,* 638 A.2d 127, 1994 WL 117099 (N.J. 1994).

17. Hayes LJ, Adams M, Rydeen K: Ethics, choice, and value. In Hayes LJ, Hayes GJ, Moore S, Ghezzi P (eds): *Ethical Issues in Developmental Disabilities.* Reno: Context Press; 1994, pp 11–39.

18. Crocker AC, Cushna B: Ethical considerations and attitudes in the field of developmental disorders. In Johnston RB, Magrab PR (eds): *Developmental Disorders: Assessment, Treatment, Education.* Baltimore: University Park Press; 1976, p 496.

19. Friedman PR: *The Rights of Mentally Retarded Persons.* New York: Avon; 1976.

20. *Ibid.,* pp 97–135.

21. Scheerenberger RC: *A History of Mental Retardation: A Quarter Century of Promises.* Baltimore: Brookes Publishing; 1987.

22. Scheerenberger RC: *A History of Mental Retardation.* Baltimore: Brookes Publishing; 1983.

23. Bourguignon H: Mental retardation: The reality behind the label. *Cambridge Quart of Healthcare Ethics* 3(2):179–194, 1994.

24. Clarke AM, Clarke AD, Berg JM: *Mental Deficiency: The Changing Outlook.* 4th ed. New York: The Free Press; 1985.

25. Clarke AM, Clarke AD, Berg JM: *Ibid.,* p 47.

26. Stein Z, Susser M: Public health and mental retardation. In Begab MJ, Richardson SA (eds): *The Mentally Retarded and Society.* Baltimore: University Park Press; 1974.

27. Clarke AM, Clarke AD, Berg JM: *op. cit.,* p 27.

28. Rubin L: Diagnosis and disabilities. *J of Intellectual Disability Research* 36:465–472; 1992.

29. Milunsky A: *The Prevention of Genetic Diseases and Mental Retardation.* Philadelphia: Saunders; 1975.

30. *Americans with Disabilities Act,* 1990.

31. Clarke AM, Clarke AD, Berg JM: *op. cit.,* p 28.

32. Grossman H: *Manual on Terminology and Classification in Mental Retardation.* Washington, DC: American Association for Mental Deficiency; 1973.

33. Goffman I: *Stigma: Notes on the Management of Spoiled Identity.* Englewood Cliffs, NJ: Prentice-Hall; 1963.

34. Edgerton RB: *The Cloak of Competence: Stigma in the Lives of the Mentally Retarded.* Berkeley: University of California Press; 1967.

35. McCullough LB: The world gained and the world lost: Labeling the mentally retarded. In Kopelman L, Moskop J (eds): *op. cit.,* pp 99–118.

36. Rothman DJ: *The Discovery of the Asylum: Social Order and Disorder in the New Republic.* Boston: Little, Brown; 1971.

37. Dain N: *Concepts of Insanity in the United States, 1789–1865.* New Brunswick, NJ: Rutgers University Press; 1964.

38. Lazerson M: Educational institutions and mental subnormality: Notes on writing a history. In Begab MJ, Richardson SA (eds): *op. cit.,* p 37.

39. Wolfensberger W: The origin and nature of our institutional models. In Kugel RB, Wolfensberger W (eds): *Changing Patterns in Residential Services for the Mentally Retarded.* Washington, DC: President's Committee on Mental Retardation; 1969, pp 59–171.

40. Cremin LA: *The Transformation of the School.* New York: Knopf; 1962.

41. Spring J: *Education and the Rise of the Corporate State.* Boston: Beacon Press; 1972.

42. Lazerson M, Grubb WN: *American Education and Vocationalism, 1870–1970.* New York: Teachers College Press; 1974.

43. Haller M: *Eugenics: Hereditarian Attitudes in American Thought.* New Brunswick, NJ: Rutgers University Press; 1963.

44. Lazerson M, Grubb WN: *op. cit.,* p 49.

45. White House Conference on Child Health and Protection: Special Education. New York: Century; 1931.

46. Scheerenberger RC: *op. cit.,* 1987, p 116.

47. *Ibid.,* p 150.

48. Thomas JR: Quality care for individuals with dual diagnosis: The legal and ethical imperative to provide qualified staff. *Mental Retardation* 32(5):356–361, 1994.

49. Healey WC: Inclusion in childhood services: Ethics and endocratic oughtness. In Hayes LJ, Hayes GJ, Moore S, Ghezzi P (eds): *op. cit.,* pp 93–99.

50. Rock SL: Holding inclusion to a higher standard. In Hayes LJ, Hayes GJ, Moore S, Ghezzi P (eds): *Ibid.,* pp 100–102.

51. Brown D, Rosen D, Elkins TE: Sedating women with mental retardation for routine gynecologic examination: An ethical analysis. *J Clinical Ethics* 3(1):68–77, 1992.

52. Loewy EH: Limiting but not abandoning treatment in severely mentally impaired patients: A troubling issue for ethics consultants and ethics committees. *Cambridge Quart of Healthcare Ethics* 3(2):216–225, 1994.

53. Martyn SR: Substituted judgment, best interests, and the need for best respect. *Cambridge Quart of Healthcare Ethics* 3(2):195–208, 1994.

54. Is dying better than dialysis for a woman with Down syndrome? *Cambridge Quart of Healthcare Ethics* 3(2):270–276, 1994.

55. Longmore PK: Medical decision making and people with disabilities: A clash of cultures. *J Law Med Ethics* 23:82–87, 1995.

56. Bijou SW: Ethical issues concerning persons with developmental disabilities: A developmental perspective. In Hayes LJ, Hayes GJ, Moore S, Ghezzi P (eds): *op. cit.*, pp 69–75.

57. Swain MA: Developmental disabilities, change, and culture: Improving circumstances for children. In Hayes LJ, Hayes GJ, Moore S, Ghezzi P (eds): *Ibid.*, pp 76–79.

58. Kermani EJ, Kantor JE: Psychiatry and the death penalty: The landmark Supreme Court cases and their ethical implications for the profession. *Bull Am Academy Psych Law* 22(1):95–108, 1994.

59. Brown H, Hunt N, Stein J: 'Alarming but very necessary': Working with staff groups around the sexual abuse of adults with learning disabilities. *J Intellectual Disability Research* 38:393–412, 1994.

60. Kiernan C: Behavior modification. In Clarke AM, Clarke AD, Berg JM: *op. cit.*, pp 465–511.

61. Cuvo AJ: Gentle teaching: on the one hand . . . but on the other hand. *J Applied Behavior Analysis* 25(4):873–877, 1992.

62. Murphy G: The use of aversive stimuli in treatment: The issue of consent. *J Intellectual Disability Res* 37:211–219, 1993.

63. Van Houten R: The right to effective behavioral treatment. In Hayes LJ, Hayes GJ, Moore S, Ghezzi P (eds): *op. cit.*, pp 103–118.

64. Houmanfar R: How far is too far? In Hayes LJ, Hayes GJ, Moore S, Ghezzi P (eds): *Ibid.*, pp 119–120.

65. Mooney RP, Mooney DR, Cohernour KL: Applied humanism: A model for managing inappropriate behavior among mentally retarded elders. *J Gerontological Nurs* 21(8):45–50, 1995.

66. Mittler P, Serpell R: Services: An international perspective. In Clarke AM, Clarke AD, Berg JM: *op. cit.*, p 717.

67. Bourguignon H, *op. cit.*, p 182.

68. Duster T: *Backdoor to Eugenics.* New York: Routledge; 1990.

69. *Ibid.*

70. Scheerenberger, RC: *op. cit.*, 1987, pp 188–189.

71. Reilly PR: *The Surgical Solution–A History of Involuntary Sterilization in the United States.* Baltimore: Johns Hopkins University Press; 1991.

72. Bourguignon H: *op. cit.*, p 183.

73. *Ibid.*, p 195.

74. *Ibid.*, p 194.

75. Applebaum G, La Puma J: Sterilization and a mentally handicapped minor: Providing consent for one who cannot. *Cambridge Quart of Healthcare Ethics* 3(2):209–215, 1994.

76. Ruddick S: *Maternal Thinking: Towards a Politics of Peace.* New York: Ballantine Books; 1989.

77. Abel E, Nelson M: *Circles of Care: Work and Identity in Women's Lives.* New York: SUNY; 1990.

78. De Vault M: *Feeding the Family: The Social Organization of Caring as Gendered Work.* Chicago: University of Chicago Press; 1991.

79. *Heller v Doe*, 113 SCT 2637 (509 US 312).
80. Poling A: Pharmacological treatment of behavioral problems in people with mental retardation: Some ethical considerations. In Hayes LJ, Hayes GJ, Moore S, Ghezzi P (eds): *op. cit.*, pp 149–177.
81. Kiernan C: *op. cit.*, p 487.
82. Wallace J: *Moral relevance and moral conflict*. Ithaca: Cornell University Press; 1988.
83. Kopelman L: Ethical assumptions and ambiguities in the Americans with Disabilities Act. *J Med and Phil* 21:187–208, 1996.
84. *Ibid.*, p 191.
85. *Roe v Wade*, 410 US 113 (1973).
86. President's Commission for the Study of Ethical Problems in Medicine and Biomedical and Behavioral Research: *Genetic Screening*. Washington, DC: Government Printing Office; 1983.
87. Childs B: Genetic screening. In Roman HL (ed): *Annual Review of Genetics*. Palo Alto, CA: Annual Reviews; 9:67–89, 1975.
88. Lappe M: *Genetic Politics: The Limits of Biological Control*. New York: Simon & Schuster; 1979.
89. Schmidt K: A primer to the inborn errors of metabolism for perinatal and neonatal nurses. *J Perinat Neonatal Nur* 2(4):60–71, 1989.
90. *Ibid.*
91. Duster: *op. cit.*, p 39.
92. Bessman SP, Swazey JP: Phenylketonuria: A study of biomedical legislation. In Mendelsohn E, Swazey JP, Jarvis L (eds): *Human Aspects of Biomedical Innovation*. Cambridge, MA: Harvard University Press; 1971, pp 49–76.
93. Reilly P: State supported mass genetic screening programs. In Milunsky A, Annas GJ (eds): *Genetics and the Law*. New York: Plenum Press; 1976, p 160.
94. *Ibid.*, p 161.
95. *Ibid.*, p 65.
96. The National Sickle Cell Anemia, Cooley's Anemia, Tay–Sachs and Genetic Diseases Act, Pub L No. 92–278, 90 Stat, tit IV, ñ 401; 1976.
97. Reilly PR: The role of law in the prevention of genetic disease. In Milunsky A (ed): *The Prevention of Genetic Diseases and Mental Retardation*. Philadelphia: Saunders; 1975: pp 428–429.
98. Cahill GF: A brief history of the human genome project. In Gert B et al: *Morality and the New Genetics: A Guide for Students and Health Care Providers*. Sudbury, MA: Jones & Bartlett; 1996, p 5.
99. Muller-Hill B: The shadow of genetic injustice. *Nature* 362:491–2, Apr 8, 1993.
100. Duster: *op. cit.*
101. Culver CM: The concept of malady. In Gert B, et al: *op. cit.*, pp 147–166.
102. Muller-Hill B: *op. cit.*, p 492.
103. Drought T, Liaschenko J: Ethical practice in a technological age. *Crit Care Nur Clin N Am* 7:297–304, 1995.
104. Forsman I: Evolution of the nursing role in genetics. *J Obstet Gyn Neonat Nurs* 23:481–486, 1994.

105. Forbes NP: The nurse and genetic counselling. *Nurs Clin North Am* 1:12–26, 1966.

106. Hillsman GM: Genetics and the nurse. *Nurs Outlook* 14:34–39, 1966.

107. Schmidt K: *op. cit.*

108. Davidson A: Management and counseling of children with inherited metabolic disorders. *J Ped Health Care* 6:146–152, 1992.

109. Fitzsimmons ML, Conway TA, Madsen N, Lappe JM, Coody D: Hereditary cancer syndromes: Nursing's role in identification and education. *Onc Nur Forum* 16:87–94, 1989.

110. Kelly PT: Informational needs of individuals and families with hereditary cancer. *Onc Nurs* 8:288–92, 1992.

111. Lessick M, Williams J: The human genome project: Implications for nursing. *Medsurg Nur* 3:49–58, 1994.

112. Greener M: Gene therapy: The dawn of a revolution. *Prof Nurse* 8:784–787, 1993.

113. Lea DH, Williams JK, Tinley ST: Nursing and genetic health care. *J Genet Counsel* 3(2):113–24, 1994.

114. Gennaro S, Klein A, Miranda L: Health policy dilemmas related to high technology infertility services. *Image J Nurs Sch* 24:191–94, 1992.

115. Jones SL: Genetic based and assisted reproductive technology of the 21st century. *J Obstet Gyn Neonat Nurs* 23:160–165, 1994.

116. Jones SL: Assisted reproductive technologies: Genetic and nursing implications. *J Obstet Gyn Neonat Nurs* 23:492–497, 1994.

117. Forsman I: Education of nurses in genetics. *Am J Hum Gen* 43:552–558, 1988.

118. George JB: Genetics: Challenges for nursing education. *J Ped Nur* 7:5–8, Feb 1992.

119. Anderson GW: The evolution and status of genetics education in nursing in the United States 1983–1995. *Image J Nurs Sch* 28:101–106, 1996.

120. Simmons Alling S: Genetic implications for major affective disorders. *Arch Psych Nur* 4:67–71, 1990.

121. Scahill L, Ort S, Hardin M: Genetic epidemiology in child psychiatric nursing: Tourette's syndrome as a model. *J Child Adol Psych Men Health Nur* 4:154–161, 1991.

122. Jones SL: Decision making in clinical genetics: Ethical implications for perinatal practice. *J Peri Neonat Nur* 1:11–23, 1988.

123. White GD: Gene maps and ethical issues. *Nurs Connections* 1:18–24, 1988.

124. Doolittle ND: Presidential address: Advances in the neurosciences and implications for nursing care. *J Neurosci Nur* 23:207–210, 1991.

125. Bassford TL, Hauck L: Human Genome Project and cancer: The ethical implications for clinial practice. *Sem Onc Nur* 9:134–138, 1993.

126. Penticuff J: Ethical issues in genetic therapy. *J Obstet Gyn Neonat Nurs* 23: 498–501, 1994.

127. Scanlon C, Fibison W: *Managing genetic information: Implications for nursing practice.* Washington, DC: American Nurses Association, 1995.

128. Koenig B. The technological imperative in medical practice: The social creation of a "routine" treatment. In Lock M, Gordon D (eds): *Biomedicine Examined.* Dordrecht: Kluwer Academic Publishers; 1988, pp 465–496.

129. Duster: *op. cit.,* pp 137–159.

130. Bosk CL: *All God's Mistakes: Genetic Counseling in a Pediatric Hospital.* Chicago: University of Chicago Press; 1992.

131. Horoshak I: Where hope for mental retardees grows brighter: Eunice Kennedy Shriver Center for Mental Retardation. *RN* 39:39–43, 1976.

132. Hannam C: *Parents and Mentally Handicapped Children.* Baltimore: Penguin Books; 1975.

133. Mayeroff M: *On Caring.* New York: Harper & Row; 1971.

12

Policy, Ethics, and Health Care

Nurses, individually and collectively, are involved in development and implementation of policy in health care organizations and in the public sector. Examples range from policies that determine allocation of nursing care and expertise in hospitals, long-term care facilities, and home care to legislative actions related to advance treatment directives and the allocation of health care resources to and within health care delivery systems such as health maintenance organizations. Generally, policy refers to a course of action or inaction selected from among alternatives in a given context to guide present and future decisions and the implementation of those decisions. *Nursing's Agenda for Health Care Reform* (1992) is a document that was developed to influence health policy at the federal level.[1] Nursing's history and early leaders such as Florence Nightingale and Lillian Wald illustrate a long tradition of nursing involvement in efforts to influence health care policy of the past century.

Health policy issues involve ethical value dimensions that are often not considered explicitly in public debate that usually focuses on economic, legal, and political factors. Yet, ethical values such as fairness in the distribution of the benefits of health care and respect for persons should be considered in policy decisions. While more individualistic values such as professional autonomy, especially for physicians, were emphasized to a great degree during the last three decades, other values such as universal access to health care and more community-oriented values have not been realized. Values of social advocacy as enhancement of the public's health and advocacy for the most vulnerable and social solidarity as fostering a commitment to community inclusive of the different segments of our society are two examples of more community-oriented values.[2] Values may be viewed as a set of beliefs and attitudes for which logical reasons can be given. Values influence our perceptions of situations, guide our actions and behavior, are interrelated, and have consequences for individuals and society. Not all values are ethical or moral values. Political, economic, and even esthetic values are other types of values that enter into policy decisions in organizations and the wider society.

Arguments and decisions about health policy are ultimately based on underlying assumptions about what is valued in society and where health is placed on the list of societal priorities. This is significant to nurses as health care providers and to consumers of health care and nursing care, for it means that finite resources must be allocated among such competing societal interests as education, housing, defense, and welfare as well as health care. Curative and preventive care, education of health workers, and research represent competing interests and claims on health dollars.

Fuchs, an economist, points out in his now classic book *Who Should Live?* that resources are scarce, resources have alternative uses, and individuals have different wants and attach different levels of importance to satisfying these wants.[3] Notice that Fuchs talks about wants, not needs. Needs can be used as one basis for distribution of benefits and burdens in a just fashion in health care delivery as in the language of medical necessity used in managed care organizations to determine health plan benefit packages. The three factors mentioned by Fuchs indicate that choices must be made at personal and social levels in order to resolve issues such as the fairest distribution of resources to health care: who is to choose for communities and nations, how priorities will be set, and how needs and interests of individuals and society will be reconciled in policy development. These and numerous other challenges reflect value conflicts in our pluralistic society, such as individual freedom of choice in conflict with avoiding harm to others. These conflicts are also illustrated in the several goals of health care including containment of costs, quality of care, and access to health care for all.

Public policy consists of a course of action chosen by government.[4] The principles guiding the choice of such actions are or should be the concern of everyone in society. Two of the overall purposes of government, as found in the Preamble to the United States Constitution, are promoting the general welfare and establishing justice. Public policy is developed within this constitutional framework to meet these general goals. According to Strickland, the policy making process consists of deciding on goals for the public good and delineating and activating strategies for achieving these goals. This process requires agreement on both means and ends among those who have effective control over resources, such as money, personnel, and facilities.[5] A national health policy *per se* does not exist when one considers the following four aspects essential to policy: clear statement of purpose, working consensus to achieve the purpose, agreement on both means and ends, and continuing fiscal support of composite programs.[6] Much American medical care is still focused primarily on cure of disease and the use of increasingly sophisticated high tech procedures. Preventive activities are encouraged, yet most insurance still provides coverage only for hospital care and physicians' services in the hospital with Medicare as one example.

Relatively few people have insurance coverage for preventive, ambulatory, or long-term care and increasing numbers of individuals are uninsured or incompletely insured for medical care and mental health services. Trends to move more population groups into managed health care organizations do not automatically alleviate these problems. We also know that medical care does not automatically equal health care and that it is only one of several factors that affect health status. Other factors include socioeconomic circumstances, race, and age. Additionally, environmental health considerations involving the safety of homes, workplaces, and schools and the quality of air, food, and water must also be taken into account in order to realize comprehensive and ethically supportable health policies.

Even if the United States does not have a national health policy, the federal budget and health legislation for authorizing or withholding particular appropriations for grants and programs reflect implicit values about societal obligations in and to health care. They provide a foundation for policy making as they reflect the place of health and health care politically and economically in the overall societal picture. They impact the allocation of resources to medical care services, to education of health personnel, and to the provision of personal, community, and environmental health services. In other words, they have profound consequences for the lives and well-being of all people. Currently, resources for health care services are declining even as needs for health and health-related care are increasing. Consider AIDS, violence, and the increasing population of individuals over 85 as just three examples in the United States.

HISTORICAL, LEGISLATIVE, AND POLITICAL BACKGROUND

Historical and legislative aspects discussed here demonstrate the ways that values and value conflicts related to health have been part of our history as a country from its early beginnings. Health care has moved into an increasingly prominent place on the national public policy agenda as costs have escalated and various interventions, voluntary and mandated, have been used unsuccessfully in attempts to contain these costs over the past two decades. The increasing numbers of people who are uninsured or underinsured and lack adequate access to health care have also focused public concern on health and health care. Government's commitment to health care on the public policy agenda has changed over time and can be traced historically in legislation and funds actually appropriated to implement the legislation. These commitments have affected nursing education, nursing research, and the delivery of nursing care directly and indirectly.

Hints of a national health policy can be identified from the time of establishment of the Colonies. Early health measures passed by the Colonies in the 17th century had to do with quarantine for control of communicable diseases such as yellow fever. In the late 18th and early 19th centuries, debate focused primarily on state versus federal authority rather than health matters *per se*. Still, Congress went further in committing the federal government to more involvement with preservation of the health of citizens; a vaccination law was passed to make effective cowpox vaccine available to anyone requesting it free of charge. This law was repealed after the wrong vaccine was sent to the state of North Carolina, with disastrous results. But a precedent was set for involvement of the federal government in the health of individual citizens.[7]

In the late 1800s, the American Medical Association (AMA) made a definite distinction between public health and private, individual health. "State medicine" was to benefit communities by dealing with such communicable diseases as smallpox, which could only be controlled through public efforts. Even at that time in our history, there were problems in this public-or-private distinction that rapidly became blurred. Conflict began to develop between private groups, such as the AMA, and the government over governmental involvement in health. Another yellow fever epidemic in the 1870s influenced the authorization of a National Board by the federal government. The Board's duties were rather vague. But in the 4 years of its existence, it did authorize funds for biomedical research.[8]

Problems continued with the quarantine law and the authority to enforce it. Eventually, authority was given to the Marine Hospital Service, which became the United States Public Health Service in 1912. The Public Health Service was also authorized to do epidemiological research in order to control and prevent disease. Preventive medicine and the health of the public were still the bases of the general philosophy for government to be involved in health matters. Curative medicine and the health of individuals were considered to be primarily private concerns.[9]

European social and health insurance schemes began to receive attention in the United States in the early 1900s. The climate of economic reform in the United States, demands for better working conditions, emergence of labor unions, and passage of the National Health Insurance Act in Britain (1911) stimulated this interest. In the United States, the American Section of the International Association for Labor Legislation promoted the health insurance cause by calling for insurance against accidents, sickness, old age, and unemployment, further indication that health concerns require personal *and* collective action. Government recognition of social and health needs was also reflected in presidential messages, beginning early in the 20th century. Federally sponsored health insurance was at least mentioned in many of the presidential messages but was not activated through legislation. Early in the 20th century, the AMA was *not* opposed to some form of federal health insurance. This soon ended and AMA opposition continues almost a century later.[10] The failure of national health reform efforts during the Clinton administration of the early 1990s reflects this ongoing opposition.

The Great Depression and the passage of the Social Security Act in 1935 saw further federal concern over health, even though the Social Security

Board had no charge directly related to health insurance when the Act was passed in its final form. In 1939, Senator Robert F. Wagner introduced an amendment to the social security law called the National Health Act of 1939. This was followed in the early 1940s by several attempts to pass the Murray–Wagner–Dingell Bill, which would have created a system of federal compulsory health insurance and federal support of medical education. This proposal was strongly opposed by the private side of medical care, the AMA, and never came to a vote. However, the AMA did support the Hill–Burton Bill (1946) that provided grants-in-aid through the states for hospital construction. This program was steadily extended in the form of grants for such projects as research on hospital utilization, construction of nursing homes and other facilities, and hospital modernization projects.[11] This was part of an overall effort to improve services to citizens and demonstrates the philosophy of "sick care" in public policy making, rather than health care.

Legislative forerunners to Medicare and Medicaid appeared in the late 1950s and early 1960s. The Forand Bill provided hospital and medical care for the elderly through Social Security. The Kerr–Mills Bill did not use the social security mechanism for financing but provided federal aid to the states for payments for medical care of the "medically indigent" elderly.[12] When Medicare (an entitlement program) and Medicaid (a medical assistance program) were finally passed, they made no provisions for change in the actual structure of health care delivery. Under Medicaid provisions, matching federal grants are made available to the states for medical assistance to groups such as recipients of federally aided public assistance, recipients of supplemental security income benefits, the medically indigent in comparable groups (families with dependent children as defined for public assistance purposes, the aged, the blind, and the disabled), and other indigent children. Medicaid is usually administered through the Department of Public Welfare, Social Services, or Human Services at the discretion of the individual states.[13]

Various Social Security Act Titles passed during the past five decades demonstrate increasing involvement of the federal government in efforts to make health and medical care benefits available to an ever-increasing number of groups, such as the elderly, the disabled, and children. The Public Health Service Act of 1944, which legislated federally supported research including investigation of both physical and mental health problems and federal–state cooperation in prevention and control of communicable diseases, illustrates this trend.[14]

Federal Comprehensive Health Planning Amendments were legislated in the late 1960s to encourage state- and area-wide comprehensive health planning that included providers and consumers. These amendments still did not attempt to change the delivery of health care in any major way. The Health Maintenance Organization Act of 1973 provided financial assistance for the development of health maintenance organizations, which include prepaid group medical practice. This is the first deliberate legislative effort at the federal level to reorganize the delivery of health care.[15]

The 1972 Social Security Amendments are of particular note, as they made important changes in the Social Security Act, including Medicare and Medicaid. These Amendments also established Performance Standards Review Organizations (PSROs) directed to problems of control of cost, quality, and medical necessity of services. PSROs were established in states for review of professional activities of physicians and other providers. Another provision was for treatment of chronic renal disease under Medicare with reimbursement provided for hemodialysis and renal transplantation.[16]

The National Health Planning and Resource Development Act of 1974 combined many of the activities of the Hill–Burton Bill, Regional Medical Programs, and Comprehensive Health Planning into one single network of authority with Health Systems Agencies (HSAs) in designated health service areas. Federal funding, coming into a geographic area for planning and development of health services, went through agencies composed of providers and a majority of consumers on the HSA board or executive committee.[17]

Appropriation of increasing amounts of funding for medical research and development of the National Institutes of Health in the past few decades represented a significant level of governmental support for these activities. The amount of funding is now being cut drastically, reflecting a national change in support for health care and related activities. At the same time, states are being required to deal with decreased federal funding levels and the change from categorical grants to block grants, raising further issues of access and equity for millions of people. Even Medicaid and Medicare are under increasing attack as containment of health care costs and cutting the federal deficit are significant activities on the federal political agenda after failure of the Clinton administration health reform efforts.

This bird's-eye view of legislative activities related to health matters reflects value judgments and critical choices made over the years in allocation of finite societal resources, from control of communicable disease to development of medical research and health manpower, financing mechanisms for medical and health care, and efforts to alter health care delivery structures. Federal concerns about the health of citizens is also reflected in other kinds of legislation not discussed here, such as legislation for regulation of the pharmaceutical industry and health and safety in the work place.

HEALTH CARE POLICY—THE PAST TWO DECADES

Radical changes surrounding and influencing health care policy occurred in the 1970s and 1980s. Rapidly rising health care costs and unsuccessful attempts to deal with them in the context of the increasingly worrisome federal deficit have had the greatest role in shaping today's health care system. Managed care plans combining insurance and provider functions, horizontal integration of health care facilities into large multi-institutional organizations, expansion of hospitals into areas such as ambulatory surgery, home care, substance abuse clinics, restructuring of the hospital workforce, implementation of Medicare's Diagnostic Related Groups (DRG) system, and adoption of a resource-based relative-value scale (RBVS) for Medicare payments to physicians represent extraordinary changes in financing and delivery of health care in the United States. All of these efforts demonstrate a policy priority of trying to deal with escalating costs " . . . almost to the exclusion of any other policy objectives." [18] This priority and the efforts to put it into operation have obscured the impact that these changes have had on ethical values in medicine and health care such as professional autonomy, patient autonomy, advocacy for patients, and the fullest possible access to health care.[19] Such profound changes in the financing and delivery of health care point more clearly than ever to the interface of ethics and politics as society deals with issues such as the allocation and rationing of societal resources in and to health care. They also point to the ongoing need for nursing's involvement, in the role of patient advocate, in organizational and public policy development. What are some of the dimensions of ethically sensitive health and public policy?

ETHICAL DIMENSIONS OF HEALTH POLICY

Social scientists Kelman and Warwick, writing on the ethics of social intervention in the 1970s, presented elements for an ethical framework that is still significant to policy development and implementation. Social intervention is regarded by these authors as any planned or unplanned action that changes characteristics of an individual or the pattern of relationships among individuals, often a characteristic of nursing policies in health care organizations and public policy.[20] In this discussion, the focus is on changing patterns of relationships as we consider issues in social and political arenas related to health care policy and nursing's participation. This framework is also appropriate for identifying and evaluating ethical aspects of existing and developing policies in health care organizations, an issue in the domain of organizational ethics.

Warwick and Kelman discuss four areas of intervention that raise ethical concerns that should be addressed *before* policies are developed and implemented in order to develop more ethically responsible and responsive policy. The four areas are:[21]

1. The choice of policy goals that maximize or minimize specific values, as in capitated reimbursement systems that have cost containment as a major purpose, a goal that maximizes economic values

and minimizes human values such as respect for all persons in need of health care and those who provide that care.

2. The definition of the target of change, that is, who or what is supposed to change—clients, providers, organizations—and identification of how they are involved in the process of policy development or revision.

3. Identification of the means and methods chosen to develop and implement policy, ranging from those that are most coercive to those that are facilitative of what significant stakeholders have chosen to do and provide the necessary financial means to do so.

4. Assessment, to the extent possible, of direct and indirect consequences of a proposed policy such as attention to the economic, emotional, and psychological costs (a distributive justice concern) to all affected by a proposed policy, such as individual clients, families, caregivers, and communities.

One example might be a major effort by government to focus policies on preventive health activities in the areas of personal and environmental health. Such policy efforts would maximize the value of the greatest good for the greatest number, a more utilitarian or consequentialist view. At the same time, this might have negative effects on the values of equity and justice for the chronically ill elderly. In this example, the choice for targets of change might be individual life styles of the elderly and modifying carcinogenic elements in the environment. Methods of inducing change might impinge on values of individual freedom and autonomy or on the freedom of industry to maximize profits in our society. Conflict might occur between groups educating for life style changes, those working for healthier air and water, and those providing care for the acutely ill as they compete for finite resources. Finally, one has to assess the risks and benefits of various consequences of proposed policy changes on traditional values such as advocacy for individual patients and the emphasis in managed care on population-based interventions. If decision makers opt for expenditure of public funds on educating for life style changes emphasizing individual responsibility for health, there is the potential for developing a "victim blaming" focus in policy development. What, if any, values such as personal freedom are we willing or unwilling to give up or have modified in the interests of a healthier society, containment of health care costs, and preventing harm to the most vulnerable?

A key issue in examining goals for health policy development and the means chosen for implementing change is the extent to which affected population groups have their values and interests represented in the process—such as various socioeconomic groups, men, women, children, the employed, the unemployed, the healthy, the sick, providers, and payers. How much control should the affected groups and individuals have in the process of change? Whose interests are being served by proposed interventions, the providers of a community health program or the target population? Is the power of one group of patients or providers strengthened at the expense of another by some health interventions or policies? Such concerns should be considered in any process of social intervention with health policy development as one example. They often are not taken into consideration because of the difficulty in discerning which values should predominate and the difficulty of predicting consequences of particular actions on any selected value, such as the individual's freedom of choice or the overall welfare of society.[22]

Albert Jonsen, a prominent bioethicist, and Lewis Butler, a lawyer and public policy participant, suggest other ways in which ethical concerns might be an explicit part of policy debate. In doing so, they also acknowledge several problems that make such dialogue difficult:[23]

1. Exploring the ethics of a policy proposal does not provide ready-made answers for a single right action in any given situation.
2. Ethics has its own special language.
3. There is a common conception that ethics has to do primarily with personal behavior.
4. Policy makers have constituencies with loyalties and interests, which ethicists do not.
5. Policy makers use the technical expertise of others in making decisions but feel that in ethics and moral judgments individuals are their own experts.

Yet both ethicists and policy makers are concerned implicitly or explicitly about what is "good" for society and for individual members of that society. Concepts of politics include the idea that politics is a branch of ethics concerned with ethical relations and duties of governments and other social organizations with a focus on the interests of groups rather than individuals. Politics may also be defined as doing public ethics. These ideas negate ethics as *solely* a personal matter. Furthermore, politics deals with conflicting needs, interests, and values as does applied ethics.

Jonsen and Butler see "public ethics" as a subset of social ethics, that is, governmental decisions about matters of public concern such as equitable access to benefits of health care and dealing with pressing issues such as allocation and rationing of public funds. Three tasks of "public ethics" for public policy makers are:

1. To articulate the moral principles most relevant to the policy problem under consideration, such as justice, equity, and respect for persons
2. To examine proposed policy choices in view of identified relevant moral principles
3. To rank in order the moral options for a particular policy choice

This is rather like a "moral balance sheet" in terms of which social or economic arrangements enhance one moral principle and not another.[24]

In looking at the development of a national health insurance system, Jonsen and Butler considered two moral principles: distributive justice (fair distribution of harms and benefits in society according to standards of equity, desert, need, or contract) and respect for individuals (implies equal treatment for each person who has sets of liberties, rights, and obligations). What follows is one example of how a discussion might evolve between a member of Congress and an ethicist. In bringing the concept of distributive justice into a debate about national health insurance, many ethical concerns would be raised. They would include quesitons about the distribution of burdens and benefits to particular groups in society, whether or not equality is a criterion for distribution, the justification of unequal distribution according to merit or ability, and whether there is an "objective" way to determine a "fair" distribution in terms of the most medically needy.[25]

In clarifying policy options, one must, for example, consider the impact of deductibles and coinsurance on the poor, who may be particularly discouraged by them from seeking medical care. If relatively small deductibles are paid by patients, the money "saved" by government could be used for the seriously or chronically ill who must be institutionalized for care. However, wouldn't it be more just to still provide "free" care for the very poor? This might be considered unfair for those who do pay the deductible, because there would be less money "saved" to be used for the more expensive care. The ethicist might then show that the criterion of medical need takes preference over the criterion of equality, such as the need arising from poverty, which does influence negatively the distribution patterns of illness and disease. In the Rawlsian tradition, one might claim that it is not "unfair" to improve the position of the least advantaged in society. In view of fiscal constraints, some rationing of care is thought by some to be necessary. It might be more just to establish a health policy based on balancing the respective needs of the very sick, the very poor, and the uninsured. Deductibles would vary with income, so that the very poor would pay almost nothing. One can consider "equity" factors in various proposals in addition to economic evaluation of cost effectiveness, administrative implications, and changes in health care delivery patterns.[26] Such considerations would add an ethical dimension to health policy debate and decisions. This type of public debate did not occur in the most recent efforts to pass federal health reform legislation.

Further ethical considerations that should inform public policy debate about health care were developed in the report of the President's Commission for the Study of Ethical Problems in Medicine and Biomedical and Behavioral Research (1983) on access to health care and in the proposals made by philosopher Daniel Callahan in his book entitled *What Kind of Life: The Limits of Medical Progress* (1989). The President's Commission concluded that society has an ethical obligation to ensure equitable access to health care for all. This ethical obligation rests on the special importance of health care to relief of suffering, prevention of premature death, restoration of functioning, increasing opportunity, provision of information about individual health status, and showing evidence of mutual empathy and compassion.[27] Additional conclusions related to balancing societal and individual obligations to share fairly the costs of health care; ensuring that all citizens are able to secure an adequate level of care without excessive burdens; that the ultimate responsibility for ensuring that societal obligations are met rests with the federal government; and that while efforts to contain health care costs are important, they should not focus on limiting access to the most vulnerable population groups in our society.[28] Government, private organizations, and business continue to struggle with what constitutes an adequate level of health care benefits and how to fund them.

Callahan's proposals remind us that health is not an end in and of itself.[29] He asserts that health can only have meaning in the context of the overall welfare of our society, that is, the welfare of our social, educational, economic, and cultural institutions. He proposes a different vision of medical progress that gives the highest priority to caring for those who cannot be cured based on a variety of scientific, physiological, or economic realities. No one in need should be abandoned and individuals should always be treated with compassion as members of the human community. An additional priority would focus on the principles and practices of public health and primary care as they are most conducive to the common good at the least cost. Examples include good nutrition, disease prevention, immunizations, appropriate use of antibiotics, and emergency medicine. Callahan suggests that the last priority for society to pursue in health care is use of advanced forms of high technology medicine that tend to benefit fewer individuals at comparatively high costs and sometimes add a disproportionate burden to patient suffering. Organ transplants and advanced intensive care services for the very sick elderly are examples. These suggested priorities should guide policy development and implementation. They represent a radical shift from today's priorities of cure at almost any financial, emotional, or psychological costs and have profound implicatons for public and organizational health policy.

Allocation of societal resources to health care in relation to needs of other institutions such as education requires some degree of societal consensus about our health goals. Callahan raises the question of whether the search for unlimited medical progress may not lead to the impoverishment of the rest of our lives. He claims that we have drifted along for years " . . . creating a health care system that not only costs too much for what it delivers, but fails also to deliver what it could for millions of people . . . [and] has led us to spend too much on health in comparison with other social needs, too much on the old in comparison with the young, too much on the acutely ill in comparison with the chronically ill, too much on curing in comparison with caring . . . and too much on extending the length of life rather than enhancing the quality of life." [30]

In summary, any serious debates about health policy development and implementation must take account of ethical issues and aspects described above in order to develop ethically supportable policy recommendations that are more than simply attempts to deal with economic and cost considerations. More community-oriented ethical values such as community solidarity and personal security, as an obligation of the health care system to meet health needs without impoverishment, should inform policy decisions in public, private, and social arenas.[31]

FURTHER THOUGHTS FOR NURSING

The nurse collaborates with members of the health professions and other citizens in promoting community and national efforts to meet the health needs of the public. *ANA Code for Nurses, 1985*

Accountability to the patient or client and collaboration with other health professionals for purposes of assuring access to needed health and nursing care require a reasoned decision-making process and ethically supportable actions. Distributive justice is an ethical principle that nurses, individually and collectively, can use in looking at the interface of ethics and politics in policy development and implementation. The principle of distributive justice requires the fair distribution of burdens and benefits. Burdens in health care include economic costs and human energy costs of care. Provision of needed nursing and health care are benefits. Nurses and others must take issues of justice into account in attempting to meet the health and nursing needs of individuals, families, and communities through policy development and to ensure the survival of organizations to deliver health services. Nurses are becoming more knowledgeable and involved in public policy development and assessment.[32–36] Nursing values such as commitment to individual rights to health care and respect for human dignity provide a foundation for nursing involvement in health care policy development.[37] Medical and nursing needs may be used as a basis for distribution of benefits of health care and for a perspective on rights to and obligations in health care. If these needs are not met, people suffer and are not able to carry out their life plans. Needs might be considered on a spectrum extending from needs that arise in the individual such as those created by life-threatening illness, through needs for prevention of disease, to needs that arise from an unhealthy environment—the life support system of all of us. Health-related needs that arise in and from the environment include provision of safe water, safe food supplies, safe working conditions, and clean air. Meeting of these needs is required to carry out our life plans and for assuring the welfare of society. Meeting of health and health-related needs competes with other social needs and interests, such as public safety and education, for limited societal resources.

Nurses can and are taking leadership to articulate such needs in policy making in institutional and governmental arenas as demonstrated by the development of *Nursing's Agenda for Health Care Reform*.[38] This document issues a mandate for a restructured health care system and availability of essential health care services for everyone. While development of managed care organizations represents a major restructuring of health care services and their financing, such organizations generally consider their goals and obligations to be meeting needs of members and containing costs. The needs of the uninsured or incompletely insured go unmet.

There are several decisions that individual nurses, groups of nurses, and professional nursing organizations can make related to participation in policy development:

1. Decisions about the types of health and health-related organizations and at what level (local, state, national, or international) they will participate
2. Types of participation—ranging from financial support for groups working on goals that one supports to active participation in policy-making bodies
3. Whether or not the nursing profession will take an even stronger initiative in developing ethically responsible and responsive health policy in health care organizations and in society

Specific actions in the ethical domain related to policy development, implementation and assessment include:

1. Questioning the goals of proposed policies or changes in existing policies
2. Clearly identifying the persons or groups who are the targets of change and their participation in policy development, implementation, and assessment processes
3. Identifying the underlying ethical assumptions of policies
4. Discussing the means proposed to implement policy changes
5. Assessing the short- and long-term consequences of policy proposals or changes to the greatest degree possible
6. Identifying the moral principles and values that are at stake in policy changes

Taking such actions in health policy development and assessment processes can lead to different policy decisions from those that occur without such reflection and discussion.

Acting in the spirit of "preventive ethics" integrated with sensitivity to political power considerations will not lead automatically to one ethically acceptable decision or policy. Such analysis will rule out policy proposals that cannot be justified ethically, such as those that completely ignore the impact of a proposed policy on respect for individual autonomy or equity in access to health care for the most vulnerable.[39] It is a moral imperative that the impact of proposed and existing health policies on the sickest individuals, the dying, pregnant women, children, ethnic minorities, and the poverty stricken always be taken seriously as a consideration of justice, caring, and human rights. Nurses can and should become more knowledgeable about the interaction of social, ethical, legal, economic, and political aspects in institutional and public policy decisions. They can seek to influence these decisions individually and collectively through professional organizations or other community groups in both public and private sectors. Nursing expertise is one form of power. Choosing to do nothing about health policy development and implementation is a choice that has consequences for nursing and its clients. Making ethically responsible decisions for policy action requires a re-examination of values underlying the rhetoric of nursing and the behavior of nurses, individually and collectively, particularly in a time of radical change. A nursing focus on care of the individual patient is not adequate for the turbulent environments of patient care in the last decade of the 20th century. Yet, individual patients and their health care needs should not be abandoned in an era of managed care that focuses on population-based care decisions. The claim that nurses are patient advocates points to an obligation to participate and provide leadership in institutional policy making and development of adequate systems of nursing care for current and future patients.

The tasks involved in development of ethically responsible policy for all types of private and public health service arrangements are difficult and complex. They require the critical thinking and leadership of nurses and others in health care systems who affect and are affected by delivery of nursing care. A sense of powerlessness and moral distress in nursing often leads to inaction rather than the leadership necessary to meet patient and societal needs for nursing and health *care*. Such realities pose tremendous challenges to nursing's integrity as a profession, to nursing education, and to all organizations that provide nursing services in acute care, long-term care, psychiatric care, home care, prisons, schools, and the workplace.

Responses to these challenges must include an explicit focus on identification and clarification of ethical values in health care organizations such as service and compassion that might guide individual and organizational behaviors.[40,41] The Joint Commission Accreditation Manual for Hospitals (1996) requires attention to patient rights and responsibilities and the development of a code of ethics for organizational behavior as a requirement for accreditation.

Ethical obligations of the nursing profession in practice, education, research, and policy development are articulated in its ethical codes. As a society, we are more broadly challenged to develop health policies reflective of identified ethical principles and values that are individually and socially oriented. These are essential considerations in decisions about the allocation of finite resources at all levels of government and in health service organizations. While such deliberations are not easy in today's competitive and turbulent health care systems, such reflection and action are vital to meeting nursing's social mandate. Organizational and public policies related to health affect all of us as interconnected individuals in our pluralistic society and affect the environments in which we live, work, and play.

■ CASE STUDY I.

Mrs. D. is a 27-year-old woman pregnant for the first time. She and her husband are very excited about this pregnancy and faithfully follow all her physician's recommendations. When alpha-fetoprotein screening is offered—as mandated by state law—she willingly consents in the spirit of doing everything for her baby.

When the results come back, she is informed that the levels are elevated indicating a potential neural tube defect. Further tests are recommended and Mrs. D. agrees. The results of these tests confirm that the fetus does have spina bifida. The couple are told that given the size and location of the myelomeningocele the baby will have some disability affecting ambulation, bowel and bladder control, and possibly cognitive functioning, but the extent to which the baby will be affected is unknown. Mrs. D.'s obstetrician recommends they abort this child and try for a healthy baby.

Mr. and Mrs. D. are very distressed by the news and the recommendation. They say that if they had learned at birth that the baby was disabled, they would have been quite sad but able to deal with the situation. The knowledge gained through the testing has put them in the agonizing situation of having to make a choice. She now wishes she had never consented to the testing.*

Suggested Questions for Discussion

1. Is there an underlying presumption of abortion in the offering of prenatal screening of this type?

2. Do you think Mr. and Mrs. D. were adequately aware of the implications of pursuing prenatal testing?

2. What does it mean to give patients choices and is there an ethics of giving choices?

4. Should there be a public policy mandating the offering of such choices? What societal interest does it serve?

---

*Thanks to Barbara Loebel, MSW for assistance with this case.

■ CASE STUDY II.

California Proposition 187, a ballot initiative, denies the provision of education and other social services to undocumented immigrants. This includes health care except in the case of life-threatening emergencies or when the public health is threatened. The bill further requires that health care providers, including nurses, report suspected undocumented immigrants who present for care to the Immigration and Naturalization Service (INS). While this measure is undergoing judicial challenges, similar measures are being proposed in federal legislation.

Suggested Questions for Discussion

1. Is this an ethical issue for nurses as individuals, for organized nursing, or both? What is your reasoning?

2. What professional nursing values, if any, should be contemplated when considering this legislation?

3. What does it mean for nurses to be required to act as agents of the state? Should nurses consider engaging in acts of civil disobedience and if so, as a private citizen, as an individual nurse, or collectively as a profession?

4. What is the relationship between the values of the individual nurse as a person and those of the profession of nursing?

REFERENCES

1. American Nurses Association. *Nursing's Agenda for Health Care Reform.* Washington, DC: American Nurses Association Publishing; 1992.
2. Priester R: A values framework for health system reform. *Health Affairs* 11(1): 84–107, 1992.
3. Fuchs VR: *Who Shall Live?* New York: Basic Books; 1974.
4. Kalisch BJ, Kalisch PA: *Politics of Nursing.* Philadelphia: Lippincott; 1982.
5. Strickland SP: *Politics, Science, and Dread Disease,* Cambridge, MA: Harvard University; 1972.
6. *Ibid.,* p 255.
7. Chapman CB, Talmadge JM: The evolution of the right to health concept in United States. *Pharos* 34:31–33, 1971.
8. *Ibid.,* p 35.

9. *Ibid.*, pp 35–36.
10. *Ibid.*, pp 40–42.
11. Stevens R: *American Medicine and the Public Interest.* New Haven: Yale University Press; 1971.
12. Wilson FA, Neuhauser D: *Health Services in the United States.* 2nd ed. Cambridge, MA: Ballinger; 1982.
13. *Ibid.*, pp 172–179.
14. *Ibid.*, pp 187–189.
15. *Ibid.*, pp 208–210.
16. *Ibid.*, pp 176–180.
17. Novello DJ: The National Health Planning and Resources Development Act. *Nurs Outlook* 24:354–358, 1976.
18. Priester R: Health-care values buried by cost-control emphasis. *Minnesota J* 7:1, 1990.
19. The Center for Biomedical Ethics: *Rethinking Medical Morality: The Ethical Implications of Changes in Health Care Organization, Delivery, and Financing.* Minneapolis: University of Minnesota; 1989.
20. Warwick DP, Kelman HC: Ethical issues in social intervention. In Bennis WG, Benne KD, Chin R, et al (eds): *The Planning of Change.* 3rd ed. New York: Holt, Rinehart, & Winston; 1976, p 470.
21. *Ibid.*, p 471.
22. *Ibid.*, p 476.
23. Jonsen AR, Butler LH: Public ethics and policy making. *Hastings Cent Rep* 5(4): 19–31, 1975.
24. *Ibid.*, pp 23–24.
25. *Ibid.*, p 28.
26. *Ibid.*, pp 28–29.
27. President's Commission for the Study of Ethical problems in Medicine and Biomedical and Behavioral Research: *Securing Access to Health Care*, Report vol 1. Washington, DC: Government Printing Office; 1983, p 4.
28. *Ibid.*, pp 4–6.
29. Callahan D: *What Kind of Life? The Limits of Medical Progress.* New York: Simon & Schuster; 1989.
30. Callahan D: Modernizing mortality: Medical progress and the good society. *Hastings Cent Rep*, 20(1):28–32, 1990.
31. Priester R: A values framework for health system reform. *Health Affairs* 11(2): 84–107;1992.
32. Martin EJ, White JE, Hansen MM: Preparing students to shape health policy. *Nurs Outlook* 37(2):89–93, 1989.
33. Harrington C: Quality, access and costs: Public policy and home health care. *Nurs Outlook* 36(4):164–166, 1988.
34. Miramontes H: Needed: Effective national policy on AIDS/HIV infection. *Nurs Outlook* 36(6):262–263, 296, 1988.
35. Oda D: The imperative of a national strategy for children: Is there a political will? *Nurs Outlook* 37(5):206–208, 1989.

36. Mason DJ, Talbott SW, Leavitt JK: *Policy and Politics for Nurses.* 2nd ed. Philadelphia: W.B. Saunders; 1993.
37. Davis GC: Nursing values and health care policy. *Nurs Outlook* 36(6):289–292, 1988.
38. American Nurses Association: *op. cit.*
39. Aroskar MA: The interface of ethics and politics in nursing. *Nurs Outlook* 37(6): 268–272, 1987.
40. Norling RA, Pashley S: Identifying and strengthening core values. *Managed Care Quart* 3:11–28, 1995.
41. Reiser SJ: The ethical life of health care organizations. *Hastings Cent Rep* 24(6): 28–35, 1994.

Index

"A more comprehensive resource for comparable cost."*

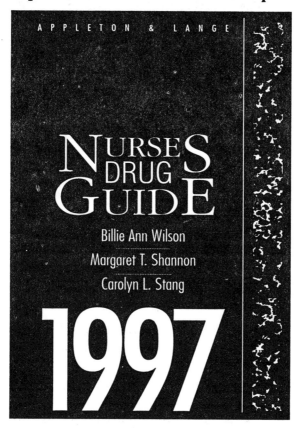

✔ Compact, comprehensive reference
✔ All the information for safe, accurate drug administration
✔ Updated annually
✔ Detailed information regarding IV dosages,
   preparation and administration, drug interactions, adverse reac-
   tions, and side effects
✔ Pertinent nursing implications including client
   assessment and client/family education
✔ Quick, logical access to practical, up-to-date
   drug information

1997, 1525 pp., Paperback, ISBN 0-8385-6985-4, A6985-4

Critical Care Nurse on previous edition

(More on Reverse)

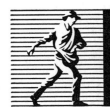